INFECTIOUS DISEASES
QUICK GLANCE

NOTICE

Medicine is an ever-changing science. As new research and clinical experience broaden our knowledge, changes in treatment and drug therapy are required. The authors and the publisher of this work have checked with sources believed to be reliable in their efforts to provide information that is complete and generally in accord with the standards accepted at the time of publication. However, in view of the possibility of human error or changes in medical sciences, neither the authors nor the publisher nor any other party who has been involved in the preparation or publication of this work warrants that the information contained herein is in every respect accurate or complete, and they disclaim all responsibility for any errors or omissions or for the results obtained from use of the information contained in this work. Readers are encouraged to confirm the information contained herein with other sources. For example and in particular, readers are advised to check the product information sheet included in the package of each drug they plan to administer to be certain that the information contained in this work is accurate and that changes have not been made in the recommended dose or in the contraindications for administration. This recommendation is of particular importance in connection with new or infrequently used drugs.

INFECTIOUS DISEASES QUICK GLANCE

FREDERICK S. SOUTHWICK, MD
Chief of Infectious Diseases
University of Florida College of Medicine
Gainesville, Florida

McGraw-Hill
MEDICAL PUBLISHING DIVISION

New York   Chicago   San Francisco   Lisbon
London   Madrid   Mexico City   Milan   New Delhi
San Juan   Seoul   Singapore   Sydney   Toronto

The McGraw·Hill Companies

INFECTIOUS DISEASES QUICK GLANCE

2 3 4 5 6 7 8 9 0   DOC/DOC   0 9 8 7 6 5

ISBN 0-07-143415-1

This book was set in Times Roman by Westchester Book Group.
The editor was Marc Strauss; the editorial assistant was Marsha Loeb.
The production supervisor was Rick Ruzycka.
The cover designer was Aimee Nordin.
Project management was provided by Westchester Book Services.
The index was prepared by Sandi Schroeder.
RR Donnelley was printer and binder.

This book is printed on acid-free paper.

Library of Congress Cataloging-in-Publication Data

Southwick, Frederick S.
    Infectious diseases quick glance / Frederick S. Southwick.
      p. ; cm.
    ISBN 0-07-143415-1
    1. Communicable diseases—Handbooks, manuals, etc. I. Title.
    [DNLM: 1. Communicable Diseases.   2. Bacterial Infections. WC 100
    S728ia 2005]
    RC112.S635   2005
    616.9—dc22   2004042111

To my parents, Ann and Wayne Southwick,
for all their love, encouragement, and generosity,

and

To my loving wife, Kathie Southwick,
whose gentle reminders and constant support
made this book possible.

CONTENTS

Preface   ix

Acknowledgments   xi

1. ANTI-INFECTIVE THERAPY   1

2. THE SEPSIS SYNDROME   71

3. THE FEBRILE PATIENT   79

4. PULMONARY INFECTIONS   97

5. EYE, EAR, NOSE, AND THROAT INFECTIONS   137

6. CENTRAL NERVOUS SYSTEM INFECTIONS   151

7. CARDIOVASCULAR INFECTIONS   169

8. GASTROINTESTINAL AND HEPATOBILIARY INFECTIONS   189

9. GENITOURINARY TRACT INFECTIONS AND SEXUALLY TRANSMITTED DISEASES (STDs)   217

10. SKIN AND SOFT TISSUE INFECTIONS   237

11. BONE AND JOINT INFECTIONS   247

12. PARASITIC INFECTIONS   261

13. ZOONOTIC INFECTIONS   287

14. BIOTERRORISM   303

15. SERIOUS ADULT VIRAL ILLNESSES OTHER THAN HIV   317

16. INFECTIONS IN THE IMMUNOCOMPROMISED
    HOST   331

17. HIV INFECTION   339

    Index   383

PREFACE

Anti-infective medications are widely prescribed. Unfortunately, all too often they are misused and as a consequence *Time* and *Newsweek* warn that we are nearing the "End of the Antibiotic Era." The majority of health care providers are unfamiliar with the principles of infectious diseases and the importance of a systematic approach to properly prescribing these agents. A large number of manuals are available that list the doses of various anti-infective agents; however, proper dosing represents only one small component for the proper management of infections. *Infectious Diseases Quick Glance* provides a full summary of the field of infectious diseases and includes all the key points discussed in the full-length textbook *Infectious Diseases in 30 Days*, also published by McGraw-Hill. In addition to providing proper dosage schedules for antibiotic, anti-fungal, and anti-viral agents, this pocket-sized manual includes all the key facts required to properly manage infectious diseases. Key facts about sepsis, fever of undetermined origin (FUO), emerging zoonotic infections, parasites, bioterrorist agents, the immunocompromised host, and serious viral infections are included. In addition, infections at various anatomic sites in the body are thoroughly covered, including the lungs, ears, nose, and throat (ENT), central nervous system, heart, gastrointestinal tract, genitourinary tract, soft tissues, joints, and bones. Tables summarize the antibiotic regimens recommended for infections at each anatomic site, and images illustrate important principles as well as useful physical and radiographic findings. *Infectious Diseases Quick Glance* is the first manual to provide all of the information required to help you prevent the "End of the Antibiotic Era."

ACKNOWLEDGMENTS

I wish to thank Dr. Paul Beeson, who first introduced me to the field of infectious diseases and instilled in me a lifelong love for scientific inquiry. I also want to thank Dr. Morton Swartz for teaching me infectious diseases, and for being such an inspiring role model. Finally, I wish to thank Dr. Jim McGuigan and Dr. Tom Stossel for their guidance and encouragement throughout my academic career.

INFECTIOUS DISEASES QUICK GLANCE

1

ANTI-INFECTIVE THERAPY

HIGHLIGHTS

- Too often antibiotics are prescribed to fulfill the patient's expectations, rather than to treat a true bacterial infection.
- The physician must differentiate infection from colonization.
- A single antibiotic cannot fulfill all infectious disease needs.
- Physicians ignore the remarkable adaptability of bacteria, fungi, and viruses at their patients' peril.
- Anti-infective therapy is dynamic and requires a basic understanding of microbiology.
- Narrow-spectrum antibiotics should be used whenever possible.
- Overuse of broad-spectrum antibiotics increases the risk of selecting for highly resistant pathogens such as vancomycin-resistant enterococcus (VRE) and methicillin-resistant *Staphylococcus aureus* (MRSA).
- The "shotgun" approach to infectious diseases must end, or we may truly experience the end of the antibiotic era.

MECHANISMS OF ANTIBIOTIC RESISTANCE

GENETIC MODIFICATIONS LEADING TO ANTIMICROBIAL RESISTANCE

Bacteria can quickly alter their genetic makeup by:

1. Point mutations—Develop as a consequence of inaccuracies in bacterial DNA polymerase.
2. Transfer of DNA by plasmid conjugation—A plasmid is a circular piece of DNA that can encode for antibiotic resistance. The donor bacteria containing the resistance plasmid forms a pilus on its outer surface. This pilus attaches to a second bacterium and serves as a bridge for the transfer of the plasmid DNA from the donor to the recipient bacterium (Fig. 1-1).
3. Transfer of DNA by bacteriophage transduction—Bacteriophages are protein-coated DNA segments that attach to the bacterial wall and inject DNA. These infective particles can readily transfer resistance genes to multiple bacteria (Fig. 1-1).
4. Transfer of naked DNA transposons by transformation—Linear segments of chromosomal DNA, called transposons, can be released by donor bacteria and taken up by other recipient bacteria where the new DNA is incorporated into the recipient's chromosome (Fig. 1-1).

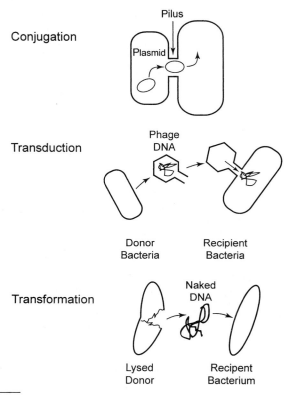

FIGURE 1-1
Mechanisms of bacterial transfer of antibiotic resistance genes.

The ability of bacteria to share their DNA provides a survival advantage, allowing them to quickly adapt to antibiotic exposure.

BIOCHEMICAL MECHANISMS FOR ANTIMICROBIAL RESISTANCE

1. β-Lactamases—These enzymes inactivate antibiotics by breaking the amide bond on the β-lactam ring. Plasmids and transposons primarily transfer β-lactamase activity. Extended-spectrum β-lactamases (**ESBLs**) readily destroy most cephalosporins including third-generation cephalosporins. Gram-negative bacilli produce a broader spectrum of β-lactamases than Gram-positive organisms, explaining why Gram-negative organisms more commonly arise in the patient who has been treated with prolonged broad-spectrum antibiotics. Enterobacter has an inducible β-lactamase that is expressed when the bacterium is exposed to cephalosporins. For this reason second- and third-generation cephalosporins are not recommended for serious Enterobacter infections.

2. Other enzyme modifications of antibiotics—Esterases can hydrolyze the lactone ring of erythromycin. Aminoglycosides can be inactivated by acetyltransferases. Phosphorylation and adenylation may also inactivate aminoglycosides. These resistance enzymes are found in many Gram-negative strains as well as enterococci, *S. aureus*, and *S. epidermidis*.
3. Alterations in bacterial membranes—The passage of hydrophobic antibiotics through the outer lipid coat of Gram-negative bacteria is facilitated by the presence of porins, or small channels. Mutations leading to the loss of porins decrease antibiotic penetration and lead to antibiotic resistance.
4. Production of efflux pumps—Transposons can encode for an energy-dependent pump that can actively pump antibiotics out of bacteria. Enteric Gram-negative bacteria use this mechanism to resist tetracycline, macrolide, and fluoroquinolone antibiotic treatment. *S. aureus*, *S. epidermidis*, *Strep. pyogenes*, group B streptococci, and *S. pneumoniae* also use efflux pumps.
5. Alterations of cell wall precursors—This mechanism is used by vancomycin-resistant enterococcus. Vancomycin and teicoplanin binding requires that D-alanine-D-alanine be at the end of the peptidoglycan cell wall precursors of Gram-positive bacteria. Resistant strains of *Enterococcus faecium* and *Enteroccus faecalis* contain the vanA plasmid that encodes a protein that synthesizes D-alanine-D-lactate. Loss of the terminal D-alanine markedly reduces vancomycin and teicoplanin binding.
6. Changes in target enzymes—Penicillins and cephalosporins bind to specific proteins in the bacterial cell wall called penicillin-binding proteins (PBPs). Penicillin-*resistant S. pneumoniae* demonstrate either decreased numbers of PBPs and/or PBPs that bind penicillin with lower affinity. Methicillin-resistant *S. aureus* (MRSA) produces a low-affinity PBP encoded by the mecA gene. Single amino acid mutations that alter DNA gyrase function cause fluoroquinolone resistance.
7. Alterations in ribosomal binding site—Resistance genes can encode for enzymes that demethylate adenine residues on bacterial ribosomal RNA and this activity inhibits tetracycline, macrolide, lincosamide, and aminoglycoside binding to and disruption of bacterial ribosome function.

Bacteria have multiple mechanisms to transfer DNA messages. This new DNA encodes proteins that destroy antibiotics, block their entry, pump them out, and interfere with their binding. Under the selective pressures of prolonged antibiotic treatment it is not a question of whether or not, but only a question of when resistant bacteria will take over.

FACTORS THAT DETERMINE ANTI-INFECTIVE AGENT DOSING

- Characteristics that need to be considered when dosing antibiotics include:
  1. Absorption (when dealing with oral antibiotics)
  2. Volume of distribution
  3. Metabolism and excretion
- Serum levels of the antibiotic should be maintained above the minimum inhibitory concentration > 50% of the time.
  1. The minimum inhibitor concentration (MIC)—determined by serially diluting the antibiotic into liquid media containing 10^4 bacteria per ml, and incubating overnight. The lowest concentration of antibiotic that prevents active bacterial growth (i.e., clear liquid media) constitutes the MIC (Fig. 1-2).
  2. The mean bactericidal concentration (MBC) is determined by taking each clear tube and inoculating the solution onto a solid media plate. The lowest

concentration of antibiotic that blocks all growth of bacteria (i.e., no colonies on solid media) represents the MBC (Fig. 1-2).

3. Serum antibiotic levels versus time can be plotted and the ratio of the area under the curve/MIC and time above the MIC can be determined (Fig. 1-3). Although it is recommended that antibiotic levels be maintained above the MIC for > 50% of the time, there are few human studies to support this recommendation.

4. Concentration-dependent killing is noted in vitro for aminoglycosides and fluoroquinolones; i.e., greater killing is observed the higher the antibiotic concentration exceeds the MIC.

5. Postantibiotic effect may be observed for aminoglycosides or fluoroquinolones in vitro studies; i.e., when the antibiotic is removed there is a delay the recovery of bacterial growth. The importance of concentration-dependent killing and postantibiotic effect have not been substantiated by controlled human clinical trials.

MIC & MBC

Inoculate all tubes with 10^4 bacteria incubate 38°C X 12 hrs

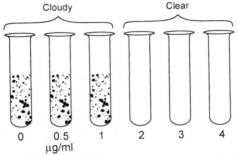

Minimal Inhibitory Concentration (MIC) = 2μg/ml

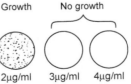

Then take a sample from each clear tube and inoculate a culture plate. Incubate 38° X 12 hrs.

Minimal Bactericidal concentration (MBC) = 3μg/ml

FIGURE 1-2

Determination of minimum inhibitory concentration (MIC) and mean bactericidal concentration (MBC).

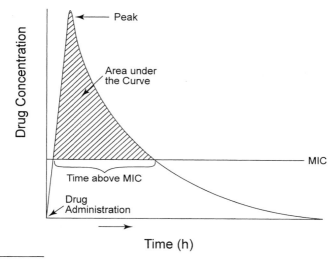

FIGURE 1-3
Pharmacokinetics of a typical antibiotic.

BASIC STRATEGIES FOR ANTIBIOTIC THERAPY
(FIG. 1-4)

1. *Decide whether or not the patient has a bacterial infection.* The peripheral white blood cell count (WBC) is low or normal in most viral infections and often elevated with an increased percentage of neutrophils and band forms in serious bacterial infection.
2. *Make a reasonable statistical guess as to the possible pathogens.* Determine the most likely anatomic site of infection and cover for the pathogens most likely to cause infection at this site (see subsequent chapters).
3. *Be aware of the susceptibility patterns in your hospital and community.* In certain areas of the country MRSA is found in the community. Many hospitals now have a high incidence of methicillin-*resistant S. aureus*. Other hospitals have a large percentage of Pseudomonas strains that are resistant to gentamicin, eliminating this antibiotic as a consideration for empiric treatment of possible Gram-negative sepsis.
4. *Take into account previous antibiotic treatment.* Prior antibiotic therapy selects for resistant pathogens. Therefore, a different antibiotic should be administered if infection develops within 2–3 weeks of prior antibiotic treatment.
5. *Take into consideration important host factors.*
   a. Penetration into the site of infection. Be aware of the blood-brain barrier, which blocks penetration by first-generation cephalosporins, gentamicin, and clindamycin.
   b. Peripheral white blood cell count. Patients with neutropenia have a high mortality rate from sepsis, and require immediate empiric broad-spectrum high-dose intravenous antibiotic treatment.

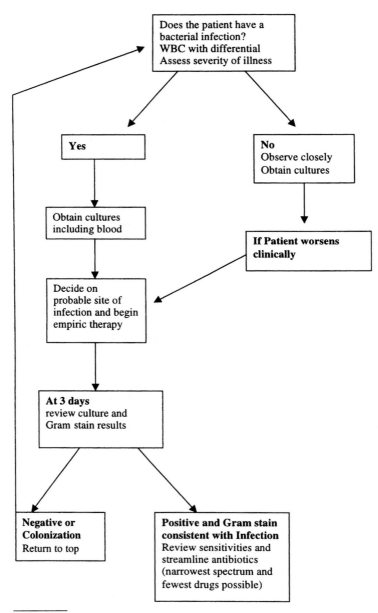

FIGURE 1-4
Algorithm for the initial use of anti-infective therapy.

   c. Age and underlying diseases. Elderly patients tend to more slowly metabolize and excrete antibiotics. Antibiotics primarily metabolized by the liver should generally be avoided or reduced in patients with significant cirrhosis. In patients with significant renal dysfunction, antibiotic doses need to be modified.

   d. Duration of hospitalization. Patients who have just arrived in the hospital tend to be colonized with community-acquired pathogens, while patients who have been in the hospital for prolonged periods and have received several courses of antibiotics are colonized with highly resistant bacteria as well as fungi.

   e. Severity of the patient's illness. The severely ill patient who is toxic and hypotensive requires empiric antibiotic therapy, while the patient who simply has a new fever without other serious systemic complaints or dysfunction can usually be observed off antibiotics.

6. *Use the fewest drugs possible.*

   a. Multiple drugs may lead to antagonism rather than synergy. The natural assumption that the more antibiotics, the more killing power often does not apply.

   b   Use of multiple antibiotics increases the risk of adverse reactions.

   c. Use of multiple antibiotics often increases the cost and increases the risk of administration errors.

   d. Use of multiple antibiotics increases the risk of infections with highly resistant organisms. Normal flora is killed and can no longer compete for nutrients, allowing resistant pathogens to overgrow.

7. *Switch to narrower-spectrum antibiotic coverage within 3 days.* Within 3 days of beginning a systemic antibiotic, the numbers and types of bacteria begin to significantly change. Resistant Gram-negative rods, Gram-positive cocci, and fungi begin to predominate. Generally by 3 days the pathogen or pathogens can be identified in the microbiology laboratory and a narrower-spectrum, specific antibiotic regimen initiated.

   Obey the 3-Day Rule—**Continuing broad-spectrum antibiotics beyond 3 days drastically alters the host's normal flora selecting for resistant organisms. After 3 days streamline your antibiotics. Use narrower-spectrum antibiotics to specifically treat the pathogens identified by culture and Gram stain** (see Table 1-1).

8. *When all things are equal, pick the least expensive drug.* Too often new, more expensive antibiotics are chosen over older generic antibiotics that are equally effective. In assessing cost, it is also important to factor in toxicity (see Tables 1-2 through 1-4).

TABLE 1-1
CLASSIFICATION OF ANTIBIOTICS BY SPECTRUM OF ACTIVITY

Narrow	Moderately Broad	Broad	Very Broad
Penicillin	Ampicillin	Ampicillin-sulbactam	Ticarcillin-clavulinate
		Amoxacillin-clavulinate	Piperacillin-tazobactam
Oxacillin/nafcillin	Ticarcillin	Ceftriaxone, cefotaxime	Imipenem
	Piperacillin	Ceftizoxime, ceftazidime	Meropenem
Cefazolin	Cefoxitin	Cefixime	Gatifloxacin
Cephalexin/cephradine	Cefotetan	Cefpodoxime proxetil	Moxifloxacin
Aztreonam	Cefuroxime-axitel	Cefepime	
	Cefaclor		
Aminoglycosides	Ciprofloxacin	Tetracycline	
		Doxycycline	
Vancomycin	Trimethorprim-sulfamethoxazole	Chlorampenicol	
Macrolides		Levofloxacin	
Clindamycin			
Linezolid			
Synercid™			
Metronidazole			

TABLE 1-2
COST RANGES FOR INTRAVENOUS AND ORAL ANTIBIOTICS

Intravenous Preparations (daily cost)

Low:	$20–60
Moderate:	$61–100
Moderately high:	$101–140
High:	$140–200
Very high:	> $200

Oral Preparations (cost for 10 days of treatment)

Low:	$10–40
Moderate:	$41–80
Moderately high:	$81–120
High:	$121–160
Very high:	> $160

TABLE 1-3
CLASSIFICATION OF PARENTERAL ANTI-INFECTIVES BY COST

Low	Moderate	Moderately High	High	Very High
Penicillin	Piperacillin-tazobactam	Ampicillin-sulbactam	Nafcillin	Synercid™
Ampicillin	Cefoxitin	Imipenam	Itraconazole	Amphotericin B lipid preparations
Oxacillin	Ceftizoxime	Meropenam	Acyclovir	Caspofungin
Ticarcillin-calvulinate	Fluconazole	Linezolid	Voriconazole	Cidofovir
Cefazolin	Ganciclovir	Daptomycin		Interferon-α
Cefotetan	Foscarnet			
Cefuroxime				
Ceftriaxone				
Cefotaxime				
Ceftazidime				
Cefepime				
Aztreonam				
Aminoglycosides				
Vancomycin				
Erythromycin				
Doxycycline				
Clindamycin				
Chloramphenicol				
Ciprofloxacin				
Levofloxacin				
Gatifloxacin				
Metronidazole				
Trimeth-sulfa				
Amphotericin B				

TABLE 1-4
CLASSIFICATION OF ORAL ANTIBIOTICS BY COST

Low	Moderate	Moderately High	High	Very High
Penicillin-VK	Cefadroxil	Cefuroxime-axetil	Amoxacillin-clavulinate	Vancomycin
Amoxacillin	Cefaclor	Cefpodoxime	Itraconazole	
Dicloxacillin	Clarithromycin	Clindamycin		Voriconazole*
Cephlexin	Azithromycin	Cycloserine		Ganciclovir
Cephradine	Ciprofloxacin	Fluconazole		Ribavirin
Cefixime	Levofloxacin			
Erythromycin	Gatifloxacin			
Tetracycline	Moxifloxacin			
Doxycycline	Rifabutiin			
Metronidazole	Terbinafine			
Trimeth-sulfa	Valacyclovir			
INH	Flucytosine			
Rifampin				
Pyrazinimide				
Ethambutol				
Ethionamide				
Griseofulvin				
Acyclovir				

* Potentially cost effective because it reduces the requirement for IV amphotericin B in Aspergillus infection.

DIFFERENTIATING COLONIZATION FROM INFECTION

- One of the most difficult and confusing issues for many physicians is the interpretation of culture results.
- Once a patient has been started on an antibiotic, the bacterial flora on the skin and in the mouth and sputum will change, and usually represent new flora that has colonized these anatomic sites. A change in antibiotics often is not required.
- Evidence for the onset of new infection include:
  1. A new fever or a change in fever pattern
  2. A rise in the peripheral white blood cell count with an increase in the percentage of PMNs and band forms (left shift)
  3. Increased inflammatory exhudate at the original site of infection
  4. Gram stain demonstrating increased number of PMN
  5. Correlation between Gram-stain bacterial morphology and culture
- Absence of these findings suggests colonization, and the current antibiotic regimen should be continued.

SPECIFIC ANTIBIOTICS

For each class of antibiotics it is important to know:

1. How the antibiotic kills or inhibits bacterial growth.
2. Each antibiotic's toxicities and how to monitor these side effects.
3. What bacteria the antibiotic kills or inhibits and its recommended uses. What is its overall spectrum of activity? (Narrow, intermediate, broad, or very broad.)
4. How the antibiotic is metabolized and cleared.
5. Dosing recommendations. Modifications with renal and hepatic dysfunction.
6. Cost.

- **The multiple potential toxicities of antibiotics, combined with the likelihood of selecting for resistant organisms, emphasize the dangers of overprescribing antibiotics.**

PENICILLINS

CHEMISTRY AND MECHANISMS OF ACTION

- Penicillins have a β-lactam ring (A) and thiazoladine ring (B). The side chain attached to the β-lactam ring (R) determines many of the antibacterial and pharmacologic characteristics of the specific penicillin (see Fig. 1-5).
- The β-lactam antibiotics bind to different penicillin-binding proteins (PBPs).
  - A family of enzymes important for bacterial cell wall synthesis.
  - Include carboxypeptidases, endopeptidases, transglycolases, and transpeptidases.
  - Binding to PBP-1, a cell wall transpeptidase, prevents the cross-linking of the cell wall peptidoglycans resulting in loss of the integrity of the bacterial cell wall and rapid bacterial death.
  - Binding PBP-3, a transpeptidase and transglycolase, acts at the septum of the dividing bacterium causes the formation of long filamentous chains of nondividing bacteria as well as bacterial death.
- Killing requires active bacterial growth and active cell wall synthesis.
- Bacteriostatic agents slow bacterial growth and antagonize β-lactam antibiotics.

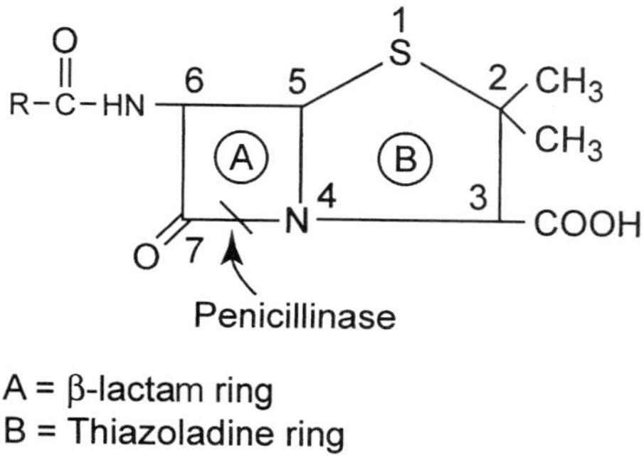

Penicillinase

A = β-lactam ring
B = Thiazoladine ring

FIGURE 1-5
Basic structure of penicillins.

TOXICITY

- Hypersensitivity reactions most common (0.7–10%).
  - Penicillin is the most common agent to cause drug allergies.
  - Breakdown products, particularly penicilloyl and penicillanic acid, form amide bonds with serum proteins and these antigens elicit allergic reactions.
  - Anaphylaxis and urticaria—Prior exposure can lead to immediate IgE-mediated hypersensitivity reaction. 400–800 fatalities occur per year in the United States. **Immediate hypersensitivity reactions = never give a β-lactam antibiotic**, including a cephalosporin or carbapenem.
  - Serum sickness—High levels of IgG antipenicillin antibodies can result in fever, arthritis and arthralgias, urticaria, and diffuse edema.
  - A macular pruritic rash involving the trunk and limbs is the most frequent allergic reaction. Immediately discontinue, because the rash can progress to exfoliative dermatitis.
  - Stevens-Johnson syndrome is rare, causing high fever, mucosal ulcerations, and erythema multiforme (target lesions on the trunk, palms, and soles followed by desquamation).
  - Other manifestations—Hemolytic anemia, agranulocytosis, thrombocytopenia, nephritis, pneumonitis, and vasculitis.
- Grand mal seizures—a less common side effect. High levels of penicillin lower the seizure threshold. Primarily observed in patients with renal failure.

NATURAL PENICILLINS

Bacterial Spectrum and Preferred Uses
- **Overall Spectrum of Activity: Narrow** (see Table 1-1)
  - Minimally disturbs the normal flora
- Indicated in place of broad-spectrum antibiotic for:
  - *Streptococcus pyogenes* (group A Streptococcus)
  - *Streptococcus viridans* group
  - *Streptococcus pneumoniae* sensitive to penicillin (MIC $< 0.1\,\mu g/ml$)
    Over 40% of strains are moderately resistant to penicillin (i.e., MIC 0.1–1 $\mu g/ml$). Use ceftriaxone, cefotaxime, or high-dose penicillin (≥ 12 million units/day). These strains possess a lower-affinity penicillin-binding protein that can be overcome by high serum levels of penicillin. Do not use for high-level penicillin-resistant *S. pneumoniae* (MIC $\geq 2\,\mu g/ml$); these require treatment with vancomycin.
  - Infections with mouth flora including *Actinomyces israelii*, *Capnocytophaga canimorsus*, and Fusobacterium.
  - *Clostridium perfringens, Clostridium tetani*
  - *Neisseria meningitidis*
  - *Erysipelothrix rhusiopathiae*
  - *Pasteurella multocida*
  - Spirochetes—syphilis and leptospira

Pharmacokinetics
- Serum half-life of < 30 minutes.
  - Intravenous penicillin G Q4H.
  - Intramuscular procaine penicillin Q12H.
  - Benzathine results in even more gradual release, every 15–20 days.

- Primarily excreted unmodified in the urine.
  - Probenecid slows renal excretion.
- Able to penetrate most inflamed body cavities.
  - In the absence of inflammation poor penetration of the blood-brain barrier.
  - With inflammation, therapeutic levels usually achievable in the cerebrospinal fluid.

Dose and Cost

Penicillin G in Sodium or Potassium salt
- 2 million to 4 million units IV Q4H
  - Creatinine Clearance (Cr Cl) < 10 cc/min the dose should be decreased by 1/2. Avoid potassium salt preparation in renal failure.
- **Cost: Low** (See Tables 1-2 through 1-4 for classifications)

Procaine Penicillin G
- 0.6 to 1.2 million units IM QD for moderate systemic infections

Benzathine Penicillin G
- 2.4 million units IM Q1 week × 3 weeks for late latent syphilis
- 1.2 million units IM × 1 dose for S. pyogenes pharyngitis
- **Cost of both IM preparations: Low**

Penicillin V-K
Oral absorption rates of 60%. Peak levels 1–2 hours after ingestion. Food delays absorption and lowers peak concentrations.

- 250–500 mg po Q6–8H × 10 days for S. pyogenes pharyngitis. Take 1 hour before or 2 hours after meals.
- 250 mg po BID for rheumatic fever prophylaxis.
- **Cost: Low**

AMINOPENICILLINS

Spectrum of Activity and Preferred Uses
- **Spectrum: Moderately broad**
- Ampicillin recommended for the treatment of:
  - *Listeria monocytogenes*
  - Penicillin-sensitive Enterococci, *E. faecium*, and *E. faecalis* (preferred over vancomycin); in endocarditis combine with gentamicin
  - *Proteus mirabilis*
  - Non-β-lactamase-producing *Haemophilus influenzae*
  - Sensitive strains of nontyphoidal Salmonella and *Shigella flexneri*
- Amoxacillin recommended for the treatment of:
  - Acute otitis media—Outpatient therapy
  - Acute bacterial sinusitis—Outpatient therapy
  - Fails to cover β-lactamase producing *H. influenzae* as well as *Moraxella catarrhalis*, common pathogens in otitis and sinusitis. If no improvement within 3 days switch to a broader-spectrum antibiotic such as amoxicillin-clavulanate (see below).

Pharmacokinetics
- Similar to penicillin, short half-life (1 hour)
- Primarily excreted unmodified in the urine
- Increases the resistance to stomach acid
- Can be given orally, intramuscularly, or intravenously
- Amoxacillin has excellent oral absorption that is not impaired by food (75% bioavailability as compared to 40% for ampicillin). The higher achievable peak levels allow a longer dosing interval for amoxacillin; it is a more convenient oral antibiotic than ampicillin.

Dose and Cost

Ampicillin
- 250–500 mg po Q6H given 1–2 hours before food
- Up to 14 grams IV per day given in Q6H doses. For meningitis 2 gm Q4H. Dosing is modified to Q8H for a Cr Cl of 30–50 cc/min and to Q12H for Cr Cl < 10 cc/min.
- **Cost: Low**

Amoxacillin
- 500–875 mg po Q12H P; when Cr Cl < 10 cc/min dose Q24H.
- **Cost: Low**

Amoxacillin-clavulanate (Augmentin)
- *Toxicity*: As compared to the other oral penicillins, more frequently associated with diarrhea.

Bacterial Spectrum of Activity and Preferred Uses
- **Spectrum: Broad**
- Amoxacillin combined with the β-lactamase inhibitor clavulanate kills many β-lactamase-producing bacteria.
- Effective against:
  ○ Methicillin-sensitive strains of *Staphylococcus aureus*
  ○ *Moraxella catarrhalis*
  ○ β-lactamase-producing *H. influenzae*
- Frequently used to treat:
  ○ Otitis media
  ○ Bacterial sinusitis
  ○ Higher cost and lack of proven superiority over amoxacillin
  ○ Preferred by pediatricians because it kills amoxacillin-resistant *H. influenzae*.

Pharmacokinetics
- Absorption and pharmacokinetics identical to those of amoxacillin.
- *Dose and Cost*
  ○ 500–875 mg po Q12H; when Cr Cl < 10 cc/min dose Q24H.
  ○ **Cost: High**

Ampicillin-sulbactam (Unasyn)
- Intravenous preparation with identical antibiotic spectrum to augmentin.
- Sulbactam, like clavulanate, inhibits β-lactamase activity.
- **Spectrum: Broad**
- *Dose and Cost*
  ○ 1.5–2 gm IV Q6H not to exceed 8 gm of ampicillin or 4 gm of sulbactam/day. Dosing adjustments for renal dysfunction are identical to those for ampicillin.
  ○ **Cost: High**

PENICILLINASE-RESISTANT PENICILLINS

Toxicity
- Methicillin is less potent and is associated with a higher incidence of interstitial nephritis, CNS toxicity, and bone marrow suppression than other penicillins. Not prescribed; used only for disk sensitivity testing.

Spectrum of Activity and Preferred Uses
- **Spectrum: Narrow**
- More resistant to the β-lactamases produced by *S. aureus*
- Reduced ability to kill anaerobic mouth flora as well as microaerophilic streptococci and Neisseria species
- Recommended for the treatment of:
  - Methicillin-sensitive *S. aureus*, drug of choice, should not use oral preparations for *S. aureus* bacteremia.
  - Cellulitis in which the most likely pathogens are *S. aureus* and *S. pyogenes*. Oral preparations only for mild soft-tissue infection or to complete therapy for resolving cellulitis.

Pharmacokinetics
- Same half-life as penicillin (30 min). Primarily hepatic clearance. Do not require adjustment for renal failure

Dose and Cost
- Nafcillin—500–2 gm IV. Q4H
  - **Cost: High**
- Oxacillin—1–2 gm IV. Q4H
  - **Cost: Low**
- Dicloxacillin and cloxacillin—250 mg–1 gm po Q6H taken 1 hour before or 2 hours after meals. (Dicloxacillin best absorbed. Food interferes with absorption.)
  - **Cost: Low**

CARBOXYPENICILLINS AND UREIDOPENICILLINS

Spectrum of Activity and Preferred Uses
- **Spectrum: Very broad**
- Ticarcillin and piperacillin resist Gram-negative β-lactamases allowing killing of:
  - Pseudomonas usually combined with an aminoglycoside.
  - Enterobacter
  - Morganella
  - Proteus-Providencia species
  - Anaerobes including *Bacteroides fragilis*; requires high doses.
- Available preparations also contain a β-lactamase inhibitor. Clavulinate is combined with ticarcillin (Timentin) and tazobactam is combined with piperacillin (Zosyn), allowing effective killing of methicillin-sensitive *S. aureus*.
- Recommended for the treatment of:
  - Mixed infections caused by methicillin-sensitive *S. aureus*, Gram-negative organisms, and anaerobes including:
    - In-hospital aspiration pneumonia
    - Moderately severe intra-abdominal infection
    - Mixed soft-tissue and bone infections
    - Ear, nose, and throat infections
    - Gynecologic infections

Pharmacokinetics
• Short half-life of approximately 1 hour. Renally cleared.

Dose and Cost
• *Ticarcillin-clavulinate*: 3.1 gm IV Q4–6H. The dose is modified for renal dysfunction: Cr Cl 10–50 cc/min dose Q6–8H, Cr Cl < 10 cc/min give 2 gm Q12H.
  ○ **Cost: Low**
• ***Piperacillin-tazobactam***: 3/0.25 or 4/0.5 gm IV Q6H. Adjustment for renal dysfunction: Cr Cl 10–50 cc/min, 3/0.25 gm Q6H. Cr Cl < 10 cc/min 3/0.25 gm Q8H. The higher dose recommended for *Pseudomonas aeruginosa* pneumonia.
  ○ **Cost: Moderate**

CEPHALOSPORINS

CHEMISTRY AND MECHANISMS OF ACTION

• Basic structure of cephalosporins is very similar to that of penicillin:
  ○ 4-member β-lactam ring connected to a 6-member dihydrothiazine ring.
  ○ Modified by substituting groups at positions 7 (R1 substitutions) and 3 (R2 substitutions) (Fig. 1-6).
    ▪ R1 substitutions change the antimicrobial spectrum:
      • Alter resistance to specific β-lactamases
      • Affect bacterial cell wall penetration
      • Change affinity for penicillin-binding proteins (PBPs).
    ▪ R2 substitutions affect the pharmacokinetics and metabolism of the antibiotic.
• Cephalosporins kill bacteria by the same mechanisms as penicillin (see above). Bind to bacterial penicillin-binding proteins and block cell wall synthesis causing lysis and death of bacteria.
• Require active bacterial growth to be bactericidal.

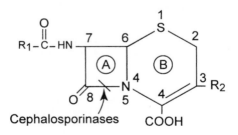

A = β-lactamase ring
B = Dihydrothiazine ring

FIGURE 1-6
Basic structure of cephalosporins.

TOXICITY

- Safest class of antibiotics.
- Hypersensitivity reactions are the predominant adverse reaction.
  - Incidence of serious immediate IgE-mediated hypersensitivity reactions much lower than with penicillin.
  - Delayed hypersensitivity reactions also less common.
    - Skin rash with or without eosinophilia in 1–3% of patients.
  - Cephalosporin allergic reactions occur in 1–7% of patients with a history of penicillin allergy, slightly higher incidence with first-generation cephalosporins.
    - In patients with a history of immediate IgE-mediated reactions to penicillin, cephalosporins should be avoided.
    - In patients with a history of delayed hypersensitivity reactions to penicillin, cephalosporins may be used if necessary, because allergic cross-reactions to cephalosporins are rarely severe.
  - Hematologic manifestations of cephalosporin allergy include eosinophilia (1–7%) and, following prolonged high-dose therapy, neutropenia (< 1%).
- Hypoprothrombinemia in cephalosporins with an R2 substitution containing a methyl group on the methylthiotetrazole (MTT) ring (cefamandole, cefoperazone, moxalactam, cefotetan). MTT ring also associated with an antibuse-like reaction.
- Nonspecific antibiotic-associated diarrhea develops in 2–5% of patients on cephalosporins.
- Ceftriaxone excretion through the biliary tract can form biliary sludge, usually asymptomatic, but can rarely develop symptoms of cholecystitis. Risk is higher in:
  1. Children
  2. Patients receiving high-dose ceftriaxone (> 2 gm/day)
  3. Patients receiving total parenteral nutrition
- Nephrotoxicity is rare. Potentiates the nephrotoxicity of aminoglycosides.

FIRST-GENERATION CEPHALOSPORINS

Spectrum of Activity and Treatment Recommendations
- **Spectrum: Narrow**
- Useful for treating:
  - Gram-positive cocci including methicillin-sensitive *S. aureus*
  - Community-acquired *Klebsiella pneumoniae*, *E. coli*, *Proteus mirabilis*, and *Moraxella catarrhalis*
  - Oral cavity anaerobes, not *Bacteroides fragilis*
- Recommended for:
  - Soft tissue infections caused by methicillin-sensitive *S. aureus* or *S. pyogenes*.
  - In surgical prophylaxis, cefazolin is the antibiotic of choice.
  - Do not cross the blood-brain barrier and should never be used to treat bacterial meningitis.
  - Oral first-generation cephalosporins commonly used to treat less severe soft tissue infections, including impetigo, early cellulitis, and mild diabetic foot ulcers.

Pharmacokinetics
- *Cephazolin*—Intravenously administered; half-life 1.8 hr, renally excreted.
- *Cephalexin and cephradine*—Very well orally absorbed, achieving excellent peak serum levels. The half-lives are short 0.9 hour for cephalexin and 0.7 hour for cephradine. Renally excreted.

Dose and Cost

- **Cefazolin**: 1–2 g IV or IM Q6–8H not to exceed 12 gm/day. Renal dosing: Cr Cl 10–50 cc/min 0.5–1 gm Q8–12H and for Cr Cl < 10 cc/min dose 0.25–0.75 gm Q18–24H.
    - **Cost: Low**
- **Cephalexin and cephradine**: 0.25–1 gm po Q6–8H for cephalexin and Q6H for cephradine.
    - **Cost: Low** for generic forms
- **Cefadroxil**: 0.5–1 gm Q12H. This antibiotic is 100% absorbed orally. The half-life is somewhat longer, 1.2 hour, than that of the above two agents allowing a longer dosing interval.
    - **Cost: Moderate**

SECOND-GENERATION CEPHALOSPORINS

Spectrum of Activity and Treatment Recommendations
- **Spectrum: Moderately broad**
- Use for treating:
    - *H. Influenzae*, *Neisseria meningitidis* and *gonorrheae*, and *Moraxella catarrhalis*.
    - Methicillin-sensitive *S. aureus* and nonenterococcal streptococci.
    - *E. coli*, *Klebsiella*, and some strains of Proteus: Cefoxitin and cefotetan have increased activity as compared to first-generation cephalosporins.
    - Anaerobic coverage including many strains of *B. fragilis* also provided by cefoxitin and cefotetan.
    - With the exception of cefoxitin and cefotetan, second-generation cephalosporins are rarely recommended as primary therapy.
- Cefoxitin and cefotetan recommended for:
    - Pelvic inflammatory disease in combination with doxycyline
    - Other gynecologic infections
    - Intra-abdominal infections
    - Mixed aerobic-anaerobic soft tissue infections including diabetic foot infections
- Cefuroxime
    - Used as an alternative treatment of *N. gonorrheae*, *H. influenzae*, or *S. pyogenes*.
    - Crosses the blood-brain barrier; however, randomized trial showed ceftriaxone to be superior to cefuroxime in the treatment of children with bacterial meningitis.
- Oral preparations recommended for:
    - Outpatient treatment of uncomplicated urinary tract infections.
    - Otitis media; however, β-lactamases produced by *H. influenzae* and *M. catarrhalis* are able to inactivate these agents.
    - Recommended only for mild to moderately severe infections.
    - Other less costly oral antibiotics effectively cover the same pathogens.

Pharmacokinetics
- Varies for each member of this class (see below under dose).

Dose

Intravenous
- **Cefoxitin**: Short half-life (0.8 hour) and requires frequent dosing; renally cleared.
    - Dose: 1–2 gm IV or IM Q4–6H not to exceed 12 gm/day. Renal dosing: Cr Cl 50–80 cc/min: 1–2 gm Q8–12H; Cr Cl 10–50 cc/min: 1–2 gm Q12–24H; Cr Cl < 10 cc/min: 0.5–1 gm Q12–48H.
    - **Cost: Moderate**

- **Cefotetan**: Cefotetan has an MTT group; however, treatment has not been clearly shown to increase the incidence of bleeding. Longer half-life than cefoxitin (3.5 hours vs. 0.8 hour).
  - Dose: 1–2 gm IV or IM Q12H. Renal dosing: Cr Cl 10–50 cc/min: 1–2 gm Q24H; Cr Cl < 10 cc/min: 1–2 gm Q48H.
  - **Cost: Low**
- **Cefuroxime**: Half-life of this drug is 1.3 hour; it is renally excreted.
  - Dose: 0.75–1.5 gm IV Q8H. Renal dosing: Cr Cl 10–50 cc/min: 0.75–1.5 gm Q12H, Cr Cl < 10 cc/min: 0.75 gm Q24H.
  - **Cost: Low**

Oral
- **Cefuroxime-axetil**: Esterification of cefuroxime increases its oral absorption to 30–50%. The peak levels achievable orally are approximately one-tenth that of intravenous administration. Food increases absorption.
  - Dose: 0.25–0.5 gm Q12H. Renal dosing: for Cr Cl < 10 cc/min: 0.25 gm Q24H.
  - **Cost: Moderately high**
- **Cefaclor**: Absorbed similarly to cephalexin, and has a similar half-life (0.8 hour). Its spectrum of coverage is somewhat broader. A slow-release tablet is available; however, peak serum levels are lower with this preparation. Food interferes with absorption, and cefaclor should be taken 1 hour before meals.
  - Dose: 0.25–0.5 gm Q8H; no requirement for adjustment in renal failure.
  - **Cost: Moderate**

THIRD-GENERATION CEPHALOSPORINS

Spectrum of Activity and Treatment Recommendations
- **Spectrum: Broad**
- Useful for treating:
  - Many aerobic Gram-negative bacilli, but do not cover *Serratia marcescens*, Acinetobacter, or *Enterobacter cloacae*.
  - *Pseudomonas aeruginosa* covered **only** by ceftazidime and cefoperazone.
  - *S. pneumonia* (including moderately penicillin-resistant strains), *S. pyogenes*, and other streptococci.
  - Methicillin-sensitive *S. aureus* except for ceftazidime.
  - *H. influenzae*, *M. catarrhalis*, *N. meningitidis*, *N. gonorrheae*.
  - Do not cover Enterococcus, methicillin-resistant *S. aureus*, highly penicillin-resistant Pneumococcus, or *Listeria monocytogenes*.
  - Problem of increasing bacterial strains with extended-spectrum β-lactamases (ESBLs) that promise to reduce the effectiveness of the third- and fourth-generation cephalosporins.
  - Specific recommendations for each antibiotic are outlined below.

Pharmacokinetics
- Varies for each member of this class (see below under dose).

Specific Antibiotics

- ***Ceftriaxone***
  - Recommended for:
    - Empiric treatment of community-acquired bacterial meningitis (see Chap. 5)
    - Empiric treatment of community-acquired pneumonia (see Chap. 4)
    - Empiric therapy of septic shock in combination with other antibiotics (see Chap. 2)
    - *N. gonorrhoeae*
    - Certain forms of bacterial endocarditis in combination with gentamicin (see Chap. 7)
    - Home intravenous therapy; once-a-day dosing schedule increases the feasibility and convenience
  - Pharmacokinetics, dose, and cost:
    - Prolonged half-life of 8 hours allows once-a-day administration for most infections; Q12H dosing recommended for meningitis. Achievable peak levels are very high (250 μg/ml following a 2-gm dose) enhancing delivery across the blood-brain barrier as well as in other, less penetrable body sites. Cleared by kidney and by the biliary tract. The potential for biliary sludging increases with higher doses and prolonged therapy, and is higher in children.
    - Dose: 1–2 gm Q12–24H; no adjustment required for renal failure.
    - **Cost: Low to moderate**
- ***Cefotaxime***
  - Recommended for the same indications as ceftriaxone. Requires Q8H dosing, making it less convenient. Preferred by some pediatricians concerned about biliary sludging associated with ceftriaxone.
  - Pharmacokinetics, dose, and cost
    - Half-life is 1 hour, necessitating Q8H dosing. At high doses (2 gm Q4H) cefotaxime reliably enters the cerebrospinal fluid. It is cleared renally and does not form sludge in the gallbladder.
    - Dose: 2 gm Q6–8H, for meningitis 2 gm Q4–6H, maximum dose 12 gm/day. Renal dosing: Cr Cl 10–30 cc/min Q8–12H, Cr Cl < 10 cc/min Q12–24H.
    - **Cost: Low to moderate**, depending on dose
- ***Ceftizoxime***
  - Treatment recommendations: Has a similar spectrum to ceftriaxone, but is somewhat less effective against *S. pneumoniae*. It covers a larger percentage of *B. fragilis* than cefotaxime or ceftriaxone. Primarily used to treat:
    - *Klebsiella pneumoniae*
    - Indole-positive Proteus (including *Providencia rettgeri*, *Morganella morganii*, and *Proteus vulgaris*)
  - Pharmacokinetics, dose, and cost
    - Half-life is 1.7 hours.
    - Crosses the blood-brain barrier, but not recommended as first-line therapy for meningitis.
    - Dose: 1–4 gm Q8–12H up to 12 gm/day. Renal dosing: Cr Cl 10–30 cc/min Q12H, Cr Cl < 10 cc/min Q24H.
    - **Cost: Moderate-high** depending on dose
- ***Ceftazidime***
  - Only third-generation cephalosporin with excellent activity against *Pseudomonas aeruginosa*. A weak inducer of β-lactamases and binds poorly to many β-lactamases. An effective agent for the treatment of Gram-negative bacilli. Has reduced activity against Gram-positive bacteria, particularly *S. aureus*. Also, has poor activity against *B. fragilis*.

- ○ Treatment recommendations:
  - Pyelonephritis
  - *Pseudomonas aeruginosa*, although ciprofloxacin is now considered first-line therapy.
  - *Klebsiella pneumoniae*
  - Indole-positive Proteus, and *E. coli*
  - *Pseudomonas aeruginosa* meningitis. Treatment of choice.
- ○ Pharmacokinetics, dose, and cost
  - Half-life 1.8 hours
  - Crosses the blood-brain barrier
  - Dose: 1–3 gm IV or IM Q8H up to 8 gm/day. Renal dosing: Cr Cl 10–50 cc/min 1 gm Q12–24H, Cr Cl < 10 cc/min 0.5 gm Q24–48H.
  - **Cost: Low to moderate;** spectrum: broad

Oral
- *Cefixime*
  - ○ Treatment recommendations:
    - Second-line therapy for community-acquired pneumonia.
    - An alternative to penicillin for the treatment of bacterial pharyngitis.
    - Covers:
      - *S. pneumoniae* (penicillin-sensitive)
      - *S. pyogenes*
      - *H. influenzae*
      - *M. catarrhalis*
      - Neisseria species
      - Many Gram-negative bacilli
      - Ineffective against *S. aureus*
  - ○ Pharmacokinetics, dose, and cost
    - Oral cephalosporin. Absorption is not affected by food.
    - Half-life of 3.7 hours allowing once-a-day dosing.
    - Dose: 400 mg QD or BID. Renal dosing: Cr Cl 10–30 cc/min 300 mg QD, Cr Cl < 10 cc/min 200 mg QD.
    - **Cost: Low**

- *Cefpodoxime proxetil*
  - ○ Treatment recommendations
    - Similar indications to cefixime, plus recommended as an alternative treatment for acute sinusitis.
    - Similar antimicrobial spectrum to cefixime but has moderate activity against *S. aureus*.
  - ○ Pharmacokinetics, dose, and cost
    - Half-life of 2.2 hours
    - Absorption is enhanced by food.
    - Dose: 200–400 gm BID. Renal dosing: Cr Cl 10–30 cc/min, 200–400 mg 3 ×/wk, Cr Cl < 10 cc/min 200–400 mg 1 ×/wk.
    - **Cost: moderately high**

FOURTH-GENERATION CEPHALOSPORINS

Cefepime is the only fourth-generation cephalosporin available in the United States. Cefipirome is available in other parts of the world.

Chemistry
• The R2 substitution contains both a positively and a negatively charged group that together have zwitterionic properties allowing penetration of the outer wall of Gram-negative bacteria and concentration in the periplasmic space.
• Resistant to most β-lactamases and only weakly induces β-lactamase activity.
• Bind Gram-positive penicillin-binding proteins with high affinity.

Spectrum of Activity and Treatment Recommendations
• **Spectrum: Very broad**
• Active against:
   ◦ Gram-negative bacilli including *Pseudomonas aeruginosa.* Comparable to ceftazidime for Pseudomonas. To maximize the likelihood of cure of Pseudomonas Q6H dosing recommended.
   ◦ Excellent coverage for *S. pneumoniae* including strains moderately resistant to penicillin.
   ◦ *S. pyogenes.*
   ◦ Methicillin-sensitive *S. aureus.*
   ◦ *H. influenzae* and *Neisseria* species.
   ◦ Not effective against *Listeria monocytogenes*, methicillin-resistant *S. aureus*, or *B. fragilis.*
   ◦ More resistant to β-lactamases, including the extended-spectrum β-lactamases (ESBLs), than third-generation cephalosporins.
• Recommended for:
   ◦ Febrile neutropenic patient as a single agent.
   ◦ Excellent agent for initial empiric coverage of nosocomial infections.
   ◦ Effectively used to treat Gram-negative meningitis.

Pharmacokinetics
• Half-life of cefepime 2.1 hours and cefpirome 2.0 hours.
• Cross the blood-brain barrier of inflamed meninges.

Dose and Cost
• Cefepime
   ◦ Dose: 0.5–2 gm Q8–12H. Renal dosing: Cr Cl 10–30 cc/min 0.5–1 gm Q24H, Cr Cl < 10 cc/min 250–500 mg Q24H.
   ◦ **Cost: Low moderate**
• Cefipirome: This drug not available in United States. Cefipirome has a similar antimicrobial spectrum to cefepime, although it is somewhat less active against *Pseudomonas aeruginosa.*
   ◦ Dose: 1–2 gm Q12H. Renal dosing: same as cefepime.

MONOBACTAMS

CHEMISTRY AND MECHANISMS OF ACTION

• Aztreonam is the only available member of this class of β-lactam antibiotic.
• Isolated from *Chromobacterium violaceum.*
• Has a single ring or monocyclic β-lactam structure making it distinctly different from the cephalosporins.
• Does not bind to the PBPs of Gram-positive organisms or anaerobes.
• Binds with high affinity to PBPs, particularly PBP-3 (responsible for septum formation during bacterial division), of Gram-negative bacilli including *Pseudomonas aeruginosa.*

SPECTRUM OF ACTIVITY AND TREATMENT RECOMMENDATIONS

- **Spectrum: Narrow**
- Effective against most Gram-negative bacilli including *Pseudomonas aeruginosa.* However, in some hospitals aztreonam-resistant Pseudomonas strains have developed.
- No activity against Gram-positive or anaerobic bacteria, and allows survival of the normal Gram-positive and anaerobic flora that can compete with more resistant pathogens.
- Has been marketed as a nonnephrotoxic replacement for aminoglycosides, but does not provide synergy with penicillins for Enterococcus.
- Recommended for treatment of:
  - Most infections due to Gram-negative bacilli
  - Pyelonephritis
  - Nosocomial Gram-negative pneumonia
  - Gram-negative bacteremia
  - Gram-negative intra-abdominal infections
  - When used for empiric treatment of the seriously ill patient, aztreonam should be combined with vancomycin, clindamycin, erythromycin, or a penicillin to treat for potential Gram-positive pathogens.
  - Useful in the penicillin-allergic patient. Aztreonam exhibits no cross-reactivity with other β-lactam antibiotics.

PHARMACOKINETICS

- Half-life 2 hours; primarily cleared by the kidneys.
- Penetrates tissues well and crosses the blood-brain barrier.

DOSE AND COST

- Dose: 1–2 gm IV or IM Q6H. Renal dosing: Cr Cl 10–30 cc/min 1–2 gm Q12–18H, Cr Cl < 10 cc/min 1–2 gm Q24H.
- **Cost: Low to moderate**

CARBAPENEMS

CHEMISTRY AND MECHANISMS OF ACTION

- Have a modified thiazoladine ring as well as a change in the configuration of the side chain that renders the β-lactam ring highly resistant to cleavage.
- Binds with high affinity to the high-molecular-weight PBPs of both Gram-positive and Gram-negative bacteria.
- Imipenem is combined in a 1:1 ratio with cilastatin to block rapid breakdown by renal dehydropeptidase-I. Meropenem is not significantly degraded by renal tubular dehydropeptidase and does not require coadministration with cilastatin.

TOXICITY

- Immediate hypersensitivity reactions the most frequent toxicity.
  - 3–7% of penicillin-allergic patients also experience allergic reactions.
  - Patients with a history of immediate hypersensitivity reactions to penicillin should not receive imipenem.

- Seizures are reported in 0.4–1.5% of patients. Less frequent with meropenem. Increased risk in patients with:
  ◦ Lesions in the central nervous system
  ◦ A prior history of seizures
  ◦ Renal insufficiency
  ◦ Old age
  ◦ Excessive doses
- Nausea and vomiting in 4% of patients, associated with rapid infusion or doses of > 2 gm/day.
- Diarrhea occurs in 3% of patients (only the minority are due to *C. difficile*).

SPECTRUM OF ACTIVITY AND TREATMENT RECOMMENDATIONS

- **Spectrum: Very broad**
  ◦ Kills nearly all normal flora, and the loss of normal flora increases the risk of nosocomial infections with resistant pathogens.
- Kills virtually all strains of Gram-positive and Gram-negative bacteria including anaerobes. Meropenem penetrates Gram-negative bacteria somewhat more efficiently than imipenem and is slightly more active against Gram-negative organisms, but slightly less active against Gram-positive organisms than imipenem. However, the two drugs are considered therapeutically equivalent.
- Effectively kills pathogens not covered by cephalosporins including:
  ◦ Listeria
  ◦ Nocardia
  ◦ Legionella
  ◦ *M. avium intracellulare*
  ◦ Enterococcus—has static activity against penicillin-sensitive enterococcus; does not cover penicillin-resistant strains.
- Resistance found with:
  ◦ Methicillin-resistant *S. aureus*
  ◦ Penicillin-resistant strains of *S. pneumonia*
  ◦ *C. difficile*
  ◦ *Stenotrophomonas maltophilia*
  ◦ *Burkholderia cepacia*
  ◦ Resistant in Gram-negative bacilli owing to:
    ▪ Loss of an outer membrane protein called D2 required for intracellular penetration of imipenem.
    ▪ Production of a β-lactamase that can hydrolyze carbapenem.
- *Treatment recommendations*
  ◦ Reserve for the seriously ill patient or the patient infected with a highly resistant bacterium that is sensitive only to carbapenems. Empiric therapy for sepsis, particularly if polymicrobial bacteremia is suspected.
  ◦ Severe intra-abdominal infections.
  ◦ Pyelonephritis if seriously ill.
  ◦ Infections due to Gram-negative bacilli resistant to cephalosporins and aminoglycosides may be sensitive to imipenem.
  ◦ Serratia.

PHARMACOKINETICS

- Half-life 1 hour.
- Readily penetrates tissues, has zwitterionic characteristics at physiologic pH, and is one of the smallest β-lactam antibiotics.

- Primarily cleared by the kidneys.
- Minimal concentrations are secreted into the bile.

DOSE AND COST

Imipenem
- Dose: 0.5–1 gm Q6H. Renal dosing: Cr Cl 50–80 cc/min, 0.5 gm Q6–8H; Cr Cl 10–50 cc/min, 0.5 gm Q8–12H; Cr Cl < 10 cc/min, 0.25–0.5 gm Q12H.
- **Cost: Moderately high to very high**

Meropenem
- Dose: 1 gm IV Q8H. Renal dosing: Cr Cl 10–50 cc/min 0.5 gm Q12H; Cr Cl < 10 cc/min 0.5 gm Q24H.
- **Cost: Moderately high**

AMINOGLYCOSIDES

CHEMISTRY AND MECHANISMS OF ACTION

- Originally derived from Streptomyces species.
- Have a 6-membered ring with amino group substitutions.
- Highly soluble in water.
- At neutral pH they are positively charged. Positive charge:
  - Causes them to interact with and precipitate DNA and other anionic components, contributing to their antibacterial activity.
  - Reduced by low pH, reducing antimicrobial activity.
  - Causes aminoglycosides to bind to and become inactivated by β-lactam antibiotics. Never store in the same solution with β-lactam antibiotics.
- Bind electrostatically to the bacterial outer membrane.
  - Competitively displace magnesium and calcium weakening lipopolysaccharide links.
  - Form temporary holes that allow the antibiotic to enter the bacterial cytoplasm.
  - Become trapped in the cytoplasm.
- Uptake is energy-dependent, requiring an electrochemical gradient of protons.
  - The greater the transmembrane potential, the greater the antibacterial effect of the aminoglycosides.
  - Acid pH, an anaerobic environment, and hyperosmolar conditions lower this potential.
- Also bind to the 30S subunit of bacterial ribosomal RNA and interfere with translation.
- The combined effects on the bacterial outer membrane and ribosome are bactericidal.

TOXICITY

- Aminoglycosides have a narrow therapeutic-to-toxic ratio and monitoring serum levels is generally required to prevent toxicity.
- Three major toxicities are observed:
  - Nephrotoxicity—Causes injury to the proximal convoluted tubules of the kidney decreasing creatinine clearance. Causes significant reductions of glomerular filtration in 5–25% of patients.

- Risk of nephrotoxicity includes:
    - Older age
    - Preexisting renal disease
    - Hepatic dysfunction
    - Volume depletion and hypotension
    - Reexposure to aminoglycosides, use of larger doses, more frequent dosing intervals, and treatment for more than 3 days
    - Coadministration of vancomycin, amphotericin B, clindamycin, piperacillin, cephalosporins, foscarnet, or furosemide
- Renal dysfunction usually reverses on discontinuation of the aminoglycoside.
- Aminoglycoside serum levels useful for detecting worsening renal function because these agents are excreted renally. Trough aminoglycoside serum levels often rise prior to the detection of a significant rise in serum creatinine.

○ Ototoxicity
- Enter the inner ear fluid and damage outer hair cells causing high-frequency hearing loss. Occurs in 3–14% of patients.
- Hearing loss is irreversible and can occur weeks after therapy has been discontinued.
- A genetic predisposition has been observed, certain families having a high incidence of deafness after aminoglycoside treatment.
- The risk of hearing loss is greater:
    - After prolonged treatment, most cases developing after 9 or more days of therapy.
    - With use of neomycin; associated with the highest risk of toxicity > gentamicin > tobramycin > amikacin > netilmicin.
    - With use of furosemide
    - With use of vancomycin
    - After exposure to loud noises
    - Once-daily dosing reduces the toxic risk.
- Also impair vestibular function by damaging type I hair cells in the semicircular canals.
    - Major problem for elderly patients, who often have visual deficits, as well a depressed proprioception and cerebellar function. Can result in a loss of the ability to walk without falling.
    - Incidence is estimated to be 4–6%.

○ Neuromuscular blockade
- Rare but potentially fatal complication.
- Block internalization of calcium into the presynaptic region of the axon, interfering with presynaptic release of acetylcholine.
- Also can interfere with postsynaptic receptors.
- Cause weakness of respiratory musculature, flaccid paralysis, and dilated pupils.
- Risk:
    - Higher in patients receiving curare-like agents, succinylcholine, or similar agents.
    - Potentiated by hypocalcemia or hypomagnesemia, and reversed by administration of calcium gluconate.
    - Can be prevented by slowly infusing the aminoglycoside over 20–30 minutes.
- **Given the high risk of toxicity, aminoglycosides should be utilized only when alternative antibiotics are unavailable**.

- When they are used, the duration of therapy should be as brief as possible.
- Monitor for toxicity. Pretreatment and periodic:
  - High-frequency hearing testing
  - Serum creatinine
  - Aminoglycoside serum levels

SPECTRUM OF ACTIVITY AND TREATMENT RECOMMENDATIONS

- **Spectrum: Narrow**
  - Cidal for most aerobic Gram-negative bacilli including Pseudomonas species.
  - Streptomycin most effective drug for treating *Yersinia pestis.*
  - Streptomycin or gentamicin effectively kills *Francisella tularensis.*
  - Spectinomycin can effectively kill many strains of *N. gonorrhoeae.*
  - Kill rapidly and killing is concentration-dependent; that is, the rate of killing increases as the concentration of the antibiotic increases.
  - Suppress bacterial growth for 1–3 hours after the antibiotic is no longer present. The higher the concentration of aminoglycoside, the longer the postantibiotic effect.
  - Once-a-day dosing takes advantage of concentration-dependent-killing and postantibiotic effect.
  - Demonstrate synergy with antibiotics that act on the cell wall (β-lactam antibiotics and glycopeptides).
    1. The effect of the drug combination is greater than the sum of each individual drug's antimicrobial effect.
    2. Synergy seen with:
       - Enterococci
       - *S. viridans*
       - *S. aureus*
       - Coagulase-negative Staphylococcus
       - *Pseudomonas aeruginosa*
       - *Listeria monocytogenes* in vitro
       - *Jeikeium Corynebacteria*
  - *Resistance*: Bacteria are able to resist aminoglycoside action by three mechanisms:
    1. Producing enzymes that modify and reduce the antimicrobicidal activity of aminoglycosides. Encoded by plasmids that can be transferred from one bacterial strain to another.
    2. Altering their ribosomal binding site reducing the ability of the antibiotic to impair translation.
    3. Altering their aminoglycoside transport pathways and preventing high concentrations of the antibiotic from entering the bacteria.
- *Treatment Recommendations*
  - Empiric therapy for the severely ill patients with the sepsis syndrome; used in combination with other antibiotics provides broad coverage for Gram-negative bacilli.
  - Empiric coverage of bacterial endocarditis in combination with penicillin.
  - Primary treatment of *Pseudomonas aeruginosa.* Tobramycin combined with an antipseudomonal penicillin or an antipseudomonal cephalosporin.
  - Tularemia as well as *Yersinia pestis.* Streptomycin or gentamicin is the treatment of choice.
  - *S. viridans* and *Enterococcus faecalis.* Gentamicin combined with penicillin is the treatment of choice.

PHARMACOKINETICS

- Half-life 1.5–3.5 hours.
- Following intravenous infusion takes 15–30 minutes to distribute throughout the body.
- Proper dosing of aminoglycosides is complicated and requires close monitoring.
  - Doses are calculated based on ideal body weight.
  - In the setting of renal dysfunction, dosing must be carefully adjusted and peak and trough serum levels monitored. As renal impairment worsens, the dosage interval should be extended.
- Once-daily aminoglycoside
  - Reduces the concentration of aminoglycoside that accumulates in the renal cortex and lowers the incidence of nephrotoxicity.
  - The high peak levels achieved with this regimen also increase the rate of bacterial killing and prolong the postantibiotic effect.
  - This regimen is simpler and less expensive to administer.
  - Not associated with a higher incidence of neuromuscular dysfunction.
- Monitoring of serum levels is recommended for both regimens.
  - With multidose therapy
    - A peak level should be drawn one-half hour after intravenous infusion is completed and a trough level drawn one-half hour before the next dose.
    - Peak and trough levels should be drawn after the third dose of antibiotic to assure full equilibration with the distribution volume. In the critically ill patient a peak level is recommended after the first dose.
  - For single-dose therapy
    - Trough levels need to be monitored to assure adequate clearance. Serum level at 18 hours should be < 1 μg/ml.
    - Alternatively, a level can be drawn between 6 and 14 hours and the value applied to a normogram to decide on subsequent doses.
    - In the serious ill patient a peak level one-half hour after completion of infusion.
    - Single-dose therapy is not recommended for the treatment of bacterial endocarditis and has not been sufficiently studied in osteomyelitis, pregnancy, or patients with cystic fibrosis.

DOSE AND COST

- *Multidose therapy*
  - Gentamicin and tobramycin: Loading dose: 2 mg/kg; maintenance dose: 1.7 mg/kg Q8H. Renal dosing: Cr Cl 80–90 cc/min, Q12H; Cr Cl 50–80 cc/min, Q12–24H; Cr Cl 10–50 cc/min, Q24–48H; Cr Cl < 10 cc/min, Q48–72H. Desired serum levels: peak: 4–10 μg/ml, trough: 1–2 μg/ml.
  - Netilmicin: Loading dose: 2 mg/kg; maintenance: 2 mg/kg Q8H. Renal dosing: dosing interval changes identical to those of gentamicin and tobramycin. Desired peak and trough levels identical to those of gentamicin and tobramycin.
  - Streptomycin: Loading dose: 7.5 mg/kg; maintenance: 7.5 mg/kg Q12H. Renal dosing intervals identical to those of gentamicin and tobramycin. Desired serum levels—peak: 15–30 μg/ml, trough: 5–10 μg/ml.
  - Amikacin: Loading dose: 7.5 mg/kg; maintenance 7.5 mg/kg Q12H. Renal dosing intervals identical to those of gentamicin and tobramycin. Desired serum levels: peak 15–30 μg/ml, trough: 5–10 μg/ml.

- *Once-a-day dosing*
  - Gentamicin and tobramycin: 5–6 mg/kg/day, adjust dose to achieve trough levels of < 0.5 μg/ml. Renal dose: Cr Cl 60–79 cc/min, 4 mg/kg/24H; Cr Cl 50 cc/min, 3.5 mg/kg/24H; Cr Cl 40 cc/min, 2.5 mg/kg/24H; Cr Cl < 30 cc/min; use multidose regimen.
  - Amikacin and streptomycin: 15–20 mg/kg/day. Renal dose: Cr Cl 60–79 cc/min, 12 mg/kg/24H; Cr Cl 50 cc/min, 7.5 mg/kg/24H; Cr Cl 40 cc/min, 4.0 mg/kg/24H; Cr Cl < 30 cc/min, use multidose regimen.
- **Cost:** Although the acquisition costs of aminoglycosides are low, when the monitoring costs and potential costs of nephrotoxicity are taken into account the cost of these agents is **high to very high**.
- Acquisition costs: Gentamicin: Low; Tobramycin: Low; Streptomycin: Low; Amikacin: Moderate

GLYCOPEPTIDE ANTIBIOTICS

CHEMISTRY AND MECHANISMS OF ACTION

- Complex glycopeptides of approximately 1,500 Da molecular weight.
- Primarily act at the cell wall of Gram-positive organisms.
  - Bind to the D-alanine-D-alanine precursor and prevent incorporation into the peptidoglycan.
  - Binding to this precursor blocks both transpeptidase and transglycolase enzymes and interferes with cell wall formation, increasing permeability.
  - Also interfere with RNA synthesis.
  - Bind rapidly and tightly to bacteria and rapidly kill actively growing organisms.
  - Have a 2-hour postantibiotic effect.

TOXICITY

Vancomycin
- Early preparations of vancomycin contained a high percentage of impurities, resulting in frequent adverse reactions.
- "Red man syndrome" is the most common side effect of vancomycin.
  - Occurs when vancomycin is infused rapidly, causing flushing of the face, neck, and upper thorax.
  - Caused by sudden histamine release secondary to local hyperosmolality.
  - Not a true hypersensitivity reaction.
  - Infusing vancomycin over 1 hour can usually prevent this reaction.
- Phlebitis is common. To prevent, infuse through an intravenous catheter that has been positioned in the right side of the heart.
- Deafness, the most serious side effect.
  - Loss of hearing is often preceded by tinnitus.
  - Infrequent when serum levels are kept below 30 μg/ml.
- Nephrotoxicity is uncommon.
  - Associated with excessively high serum levels.
  - Renal dysfunction generally reverses when the antibiotic is discontinued.
  - Incidence of aminoglycoside nephrotoxicity is increased by coadministration of vancomycin.

Teicoplanin
- Less experience with teicoplanin.
- Dose not cause significant thrombophlebitis.
- Skin flushing after rapid infusion is uncommon.
- Ototoxicity has been reported.

SPECTRUM OF ACTIVITY AND TREATMENT RECOMMENDATIONS

- **Spectrum: Narrow**
- Recommended for the treatment of:
    - Methicillin-resistant *S. aureus* (MRSA). Also treats methicillin-sensitive *S. aureus*; however, oxacillin, nafcillin, or cephazolin is preferred for MSSA. Vancomycin intermediately resistant strains of *S. aureus* (VIRSA) found in Japan, and also in Europe and the United States. Have MICs of 8–16 µg/ml and are cross-resistant to teichoplanin. The increasing use of vancomycin increases the risk of VIRSA, as well as vancomycin-resistant enterococcus (VRE).
    - Coagulase-negative Staphylococcus. Kills most strains. Used for coagulase-negative staphylococcal line sepsis and bacterial endocarditis. In endocarditis usually combined with an aminoglycoside and/or rifampin (see Chap. 7).
    - Penicillin-resistant and susceptible strains of *Streptococcus pneumoniae*. Recommended for empiric treatment of the seriously ill patient with pneumococcal meningitis to cover for highly penicillin-resistant strains.
    - *S. pyogenes*, GpB streptococci, *Viridans streptococci*, and *Streptococcus bovus* in the penicillin-allergic patient.
    - *Corynebacterium jeikeium* (previously called JK diptheroids).
    - *C. difficile* diarrhea. Oral vancomycin is used, IV administration does not achieve therpautic levels in the bowel. Because of the increased risk of developing VRE after oral vancomycin, it should be used only for cases that are refractory to metronidazole.
    - *Enterococcus faecalis* and *faecium*. Increasing number of strains have become resistant. Three gene complexes transfer resistance.
        - The Van A gene cluster directs peptidoglycan cell wall synthesis and coverts D-alanine-D-alanine (the site of action of vancomycin) to D-alanine-D-lactate, markedly reducing vancomycin and teichoplanin binding.
        - Van B and Van C result in vancomycin resistance, but do not impair teichoplanin activity.

PHARMACOKINETICS

- The half-life of vancomycin is 4–6 hours and that of teichoplanin is 40–70 hours. Both are primarily excreted by the kidneys.
- Unlike vancomycin, which is minimally bound to protein, teicoplanin is 90% protein-bound, accounting for its slow renal clearance.
- In the anuric patient the half-life of vancomycin is prolonged to 7–9 days.
- For vancomycin, peak levels should achieve concentrations of 20–50 µg/ml, and trough levels maintained at 10–12 µg/ml.
- Vancomycin penetrates most tissue spaces, but does not cross the blood-brain barrier in the absence of inflammation; however, therapeutic cerebrospinal levels are achieved in patients with meningitis.
- For teichoplanin, tissue penetration has not been extensively studied and there is little information on penetration of bone or peritoneal or cerebrospinal fluid.

DOSE AND COST

Vancomycin
* 1 g IV Q12H
    - Cr Cl 40–60 cc/min, give Q12–24H
    - Cr Cl 20–40, Q24–48H
    - Cr Cl 10–20, Q48–72H
    - Cr Cl < 10, Q3–7 days. Exact dosing is based on serum levels.
* **Cost: Low** (in patients requiring serum levels cost will be higher).
* Oral vancomycin:125–500 mg po Q6H (for *C. difficile* diarrhea)
* **Cost: High**

Teicoplanin
* 6 mg/kg loading dose followed by 3 mg/kg QD IV or IM (doses as high as 12 mg/kg have been given, but are associated with a higher incidence of toxicity).
    - Cr Cl 10–50 cc/min, 1/2 dose
    - Cr Cl < 10 cc/min, 1/3 dose
* **Cost: High**

MACROLIDES

CHEMISTRY AND MECHANISM OF ACTION

* Erythromycin a complex 14-member macrocylic lactone ring (giving rise to the class name macrolides) attached to two sugars.
* Azithromycin has a 15-membered lactone ring and a nitrogen substitution. Clarithromycin has a methoxy group modification at carbon 6 of the erythromycin molecule. These modifications enhance oral absorption and broaden the antimicrobial spectrum.
* Macrolides inhibit RNA-dependent protein synthesis by binding to the 50S ribosomal subunit. Binding prevents translocation of the peptide chain. Erythromycin is a weak base and its activity is greater at more alkaline pH.

TOXICITY

* One of the safest classes of antibiotics.
* Stimulate bowel motility and in young patients commonly cause abdominal cramps, nausea, vomiting, diarrhea, and gas. Symptoms are dose related and can occur with oral or intravenous administration of erythromycin. GI toxicity can be debilitating and force the drug to be discontinued. Primarily caused by erythromycin; the newer macrolides, azithromycin and clarithromycin, at standard doses less commonly cause this adverse reaction.
* Hypersensitivity reactions, including skin rash, fever, and eosinophilia, can occur with any of the macrolides.
* Reversible cholestatic jaundice in adults with estolate preparations of erythromycin.
* Transient reversible hearing loss, particularly in elderly patients associated with high doses of erythromycin.
* Prolong the QT interval and erythromycin administration has on rare occasions been associated with ventricular tachycardia.

Erythromycin

Spectrum of Activity and Recommended Uses
- **Spectrum: Narrow**
- Drug of choice for:
  - *Campylobacter jejuni* and *Bordatella pertussis*
  - *Legionella pneumophila*. Azithromycin and clarithromycin are more potent than erythromycin.
  - *Mycoplasma pneumoniae*, *Ureaplasma urealyticum*, *Chlamydia trachomatis*, and *Chlamydia pneumoniae*, all macrolides effective.
  - Bacillary angiomatosis, *Bartonella henselae*, and *B. quintani*
  - *Corynebacterium diphtheriae*
  - Community-acquired pneumonia: Primary therapy for outpatients combined with a third-generation cephalosporin for inpatients (see Chap. 4).
- In the penicillin-allergic patient can be used for:
  - *S. pneumoniae*, penicillin-sensitive stains; however, resistance is steadily increased, now ranging between 10 and 15%. Resistance more likely in intermediately penicillin-resistant strains (40% macrolide resistant) and highly penicillin-resistant strains (60% macrolide resistant).
  - *Streptococcus pyogenes* in penicillin-allergic patients. In most countries including the United States, 95% are sensitive to macrolides. However, in Japan, where macrolides are commonly used, 60% are resistant.
  - Not recommended for methicillin *S. aureus* (MSSA) despite being sensitive, because one step-resistant can develop to macrolides.
  - Mouth flora including anaerobes, but do not cover the bowel anaerobe *Bacteroides fragilis*.

Pharmacokinetics
- With oral forms, peak serum levels occur 3 hours after ingestion. Should be taken on an empty stomach. The base oral form is absorbed more erratically and peaks 4 hours after being taken.
- Intravenous preparations (lactobionate and gluceptate forms) peak within 1 hour.
- Penetrates most tissues including the prostate and middle ear.
- Clearance—concentrated in the liver and passed into the bowel via the biliary system. A small percentage is also excreted in the urine.

Dose and Cost
- Dose
  - Oral, 0.25–0.5 gm Q6H; IV, 0.5–1 gm Q6H. Renal dosing: No modifications required for renal dysfunction.
- **Cost: Low**

Clarithromycin

Spectrum of Activity and Recommended Uses
- **Spectrum: Narrow**
- Same recommendations as erythromycin
  - Equivalent activity against Legionella.
  - Somewhat greater activity against *H. influenzae*, *M. catarrhalis*, *C. trachomatis*, *U. urealyticum*, and *B. burgdorferi*.
  - Two to four times as active against *S. pneumoniae*, *S. pyogenes*, and methicillin-sensitive *S. aureus* compared to erythromycin.

- Preferred over erythromycin for:
  - *M. avium* complex; used in combination with other antibiotics for treatment and can be used alone as prophylaxis in HIV patients with CD4 count of $< 100/mm^3$.
  - *M. leprae*
  - *Toxoplasma gondii*

Pharmacokinetics
- Well absorbed orally. Improved absorption as well as the lower incidence of GI toxicity makes clarithromycin preferable to erythromycin in most instances.
- Half-life = 4 hours, the drug being primarily metabolized and cleared by the liver. A significant percentage is also excreted in the urine.
- Widely distributed in tissues achieving concentrations that are several times the peak concentrations achieved in the serum. Levels in the middle ear fluid are nearly 10 times higher than serum levels. Poorly penetrates the blood-brain barrier.

Dose and Cost
- Dose: 250–500 mg po Q12H
  - For Cr Cl < 10 cc/min give Q24H
- **Cost: Moderate to moderately high**

Azithromycin

Spectrum of Activity and Recommended Uses
- **Spectrum: Narrow**
- Same recommendations as erythromycin
  - Less active against *S. pyogenes*, *S. pneumoniae*, and *S. aureus* as compared to erythromycin.
  - Increased activity against Gram-negatives, particularly *M. catarrhalis* and *H. influenzae* as compared to erythromycin.
- Preferred over erythromycin for:
  - *Legionella pneumophila*. Has increased in vivo activity in animal studies and is the drug of choice.
  - *M. avium-intracelluare* (MAI), used in combination with other antibiotics. Used alone for MAI prophylaxis in HIV-infected patients with CD4 counts < 100 cells/mm^3.
  - Chancroid: a single high dose of azithromycin (1 gm) is effective.
  - *C. trachomatis* urethritis and cervicitis, single 1-gm dose.
  - *Ureaplasma urealyticum* urethritis, single 1-gm dose.
  - *H. pylori*. Azithromycin or clarithromycin combined with bismuth salts and either amoxicillin, metronidazole, or tetracycline and antacids are recommended for treatment (see Chap. 8).
  - Potential as prophylaxis against chloroquine-resistant *P. falciparum* and treatment of chronic *C. pneumoniae*, which may contribute to atherosclerotic coronary artery disease.

Pharmacokinetics
- Absorbed orally almost as well as clarithromycin; however, food interferes with absorption. Should be taken 1 hour before or 2 hours after meals. Aluminum- or magnesium-containing antacids slow absorption and should be avoided.
- Tissue concentrations exceed serum levels by 10–100-fold and the average half-life in tissues is 2–4 days.

- Therapeutic levels estimated to persist for 5 days after the completion of a 5-day treatment course.
- The majority of the drug is not metabolized, being excreted unchanged in the bile. A small percentage is also excreted in the urine.

Dose and Cost
- Dose: 500 mg loading dose, followed by either 250 or 500 mg × 4 days. Renal dosing: No data.
- **Cost: Low to moderate**

CLINDAMYCIN

CHEMISTRY AND MECHANISM OF ACTION
- Amino acid linked to an amino sugar.
- Binds to the same 50S ribosomal binding site as the macrolides blocking bacterial protein synthesis.

TOXICITY
- Diarrhea is a major problem:
  - Seen in 20% of patients taking clindamycin.
  - Highest with oral administration.
  - In up to half of these patients, the cause of diarrhea is pseudomembranous colitis, caused by the overgrowth of the anaerobic bacteria *Clostridium difficile* (see Chap. 8).
- Allergic reactions uncommon
- Hepatotoxicity rare
- Neutropenia and/or thrombocytopenia rare
- Hypotension very uncommon

ANTIMICROBIAL SPECTRUM AND TREATMENT RECOMMENDATIONS
- **Spectrum: Narrow**
- Recommended uses
  - No primary indications
  - In patients with pencillin allergies can be used for:
    - *S. pneumoniae.* Moderately penicillin-resistant *S. pneumoniae* are often sensitive to clindamycin.
    - *S. pyogenes*
    - Methicillin-sensitive *S. aureus*
    - Not recommended for otitis media because its activity against *H. influenzae* is limited.
  - Possesses excellent activity against *Bacteroides fragilis* as well as most other anaerobic bacteria.
    - May be used in combination with an aminoglycoside, aztreonam, or third-generation cephalosporin to treat fecal soilage of the peritoneum.
    - Other less toxic regimens are equally effective.
    - Effective for the treatment of anaerobic pulmonary and pleural infections.
  - For the sulfa-allergic patient an alternative for treatment of *Toxoplasma gondii.*

PHARMACOKINETICS

- Well absorbed orally.
- Intravenously can achieve higher peak serum levels.
- Penetrates most tissues, but does not enter the cerebrospinal fluid.
- Half-life 2.4 hours, being primarily metabolized by the liver and excreted in the bile. Small percentages of clindamycin metabolites are also excreted in the urine.
- Therapeutic concentrations of clindamycin persist in the stool for 5 or more days after discontinuation. The reduction of clindamycin-sensitive flora persists for up to 14 days.

DOSE AND COST

- Dose
  - Oral: 150–300 mg Q6H
  - Intravenous: 300–900 mg Q6–8H
  - Renal dosing: Usually no modification required
    - In anuric patient use 1/2 the dose.
- Cost
  - **Oral: Moderately high to high**
  - **Intravenous: Low to moderate**

TETRACYCLINES

CHEMISTRY AND MECHANISMS OF ACTION

- Four 6-member rings.
- Substitutions at the 4, 5, 6, and 7 positions alter the pharmacokinetics of the various preparations, but have no effect on the antimicrobial spectrum.
- Enter bacteria by passively diffusing through porins in Gram-negative bacteria.
- Bind to the 30S ribosomal subunit and block tRNA binding to the mRNA ribosome complex, inhibiting protein synthesis in bacteria.
- Inhibition of bacterial protein synthesis stops bacterial growth, but does not kill most bacteria. Therefore, tetracyclines are bacteriostatic agents.

TOXICITY

- Photosensitivity reactions consisting of a red rash over sun-exposed areas.
- Hypersensitivity reactions are less common than with the penicillins, but do occur.
- Enamel formation is impaired, and in children teeth often become permanently discolored. Not recommended for children aged 8 or younger or for pregnant women.
- Gastrointestinal side effects: esophageal ulcers, nausea, vomiting, and diarrhea.
- Hepatotoxicity is rare; high doses can cause fatty changes in the liver.
- Exacerbates azotemia in renal failure patients. Interferes with mammalian cell protein synthesis, particularly mitochondria, and this effect is thought to explain the increase in azotemia.
- Vertigo with minocycline, and this side effect has limited its use.
- Benign intracranial hypertension (pseudotumor cerebri), a rare neurological side effect.

ANTIMICROBIAL SPECTRUM AND TREATMENT RECOMMENDATIONS

- **Spectrum: Broad**
- Recommended uses
  - ○ Brucellosis: Doxycycline combined with gentamicin is the treatment of choice
  - ○ Vibrio infections
  - ○ *Mycobacterium marinum*
  - ○ Lyme disease (*Borrelia burgdorferi*) (see Chap. 13)
  - ○ Leptospirosis prophylaxis (see Chap. 13)
  - ○ Rickettsial infections (including Rocky Mountain spotted fever, Ehrlichiosis, Q fever, and typhus fever) (see Chap. 13)
  - ○ Chlamydia infections (including Chlamydia pneumonia, psittacosis, epididymitis, urethritis, and endocervical infections)
  - ○ Pelvic inflammatory disease in combination with other antibiotics (see Chap. 9)

PHARMACOKINETICS

- Well absorbed (70–80%) by the gastrointestinal tract.
  - ○ Food interferes with its absorption.
  - ○ Calcium- or magnesium-containing antacids, milk, or multivitamins markedly impair absorption of all preparations, and simultaneous ingestion of these products should be avoided.
  - ○ Doxycycline is nearly completely absorbed in the gastrointestinal tract.
- The half-life for clearance is 8 hours, the drug being primarily cleared by the kidneys. Doxycycline has a prolonged half-life of 18 hours and is primarily cleared by the liver.

DOSE AND COST

- Dose
  - ○ Tetracycline: 250–500 mg po BID–QID
    - ▪ Cr Cl 50–80 cc/min, Q8–12H
    - ▪ Cr Cl 10–50 cc/min, Q12–24H
    - ▪ Cr Cl < 10, Q24H
  - ○ Doxycycline 100 mg po BID
    - ▪ No renal adjustments required
- **Cost: Low for both drugs**

CHORAMPHENICOL

CHEMISTRY AND MECHANISMS OF ACTION

- Consists of a nitro group on a benzene ring and a side chain containing 5 carbons.
- Enters bacteria by an energy-dependent mechanism.
- Binds to the larger 50S subunit of the 70S ribosome, blocking attachment of transfer RNA, and inhibits bacterial protein synthesis.
- Bacteriostatic like the tetracyclines; although cidal for *H. influenzae*, *S. pneumoniae*, and *N. meningitidis*.

TOXICITY

- Significant bone marrow toxicity. Two forms:
  - Dose related
    - Commonly observed with doses of ≥ 4 gm/day.
    - Reticulocyte count decreases followed by anemia.
    - Elevated serum iron.
    - Leukopenia and thrombocytopenia are also common.
    - Reversed when the antibiotic is discontinued.
  - Irreversible aplastic anemia
    - Rare, but usually fatal.
    - Occurs weeks to months after the antibiotic is discontinued.
  - Required monitoring
    - Twice a week peripheral blood counts, WBC $<$ 2,500/mm^3 discontinue.
    - Increased serum iron often precedes neutropenia and anemia.
- Other side effects
  - Optic neuritis
  - Peripheral neuritis
  - Mental confusion
  - Hypersensitivity reactions
  - Nausea, vomiting, diarrhea
  - Bleeding secondary to vitamin K deficiency

SPECTRUM OF ACTIVITY AND TREATMENT RECOMMENDATIONS

- **Spectrum: Broad**
- Excellent activity against:
  - Gram-positive organisms except enterococci and *S. aureus*
  - *H. influenzae*, *N. meningitidis*, *N. gonorrhoeae*
  - Some strains of *E. coli*, Klebsiella, and Proteus
  - Salmonella strains including *S. typhi*
  - Shigella
  - Brucella
  - *Bordatella pertussis*
  - Anaerobes, including Peptostreptococcus, Clostridium species, *Bacteroides fragilis*, and Fusobacterium species
  - Spirochetes
  - Rickettsiae
  - Chlamydiae
  - Mycoplasmas
- Recommended Uses
  - Not considered the treatment of choice for any infection because of its bone marrow toxicity. Alternative less toxic agents are available for each indication.
  - Alternative therapy in the penicillin-allergic patient for:
    - Bacterial meningitis
    - Brain abscess
  - Alternative therapy for:
    - *Clostridium perfringens*
    - Psittacosis
    - Rickettsial infections including Rocky Mounted spotted fever
    - *Vibrio vulnificus*
    - Typhoid fever

PHARMACOKINETICS

- Oral preparations not available in the United States because oral administration is associated with a much higher incidence of idiosyncratic aplastic anemia as compared to intravenous administration. The drug is well absorbed and therapeutic serum levels can be achieved orally.
- Half-life is 4 hours.
- Metabolized by the liver.
- Diffuses well into tissues and crosses the blood-brain barrier of uninflamed as well as inflamed meninges.
- In patients with hepatic disease serum levels should be monitored and serum concentration maintained between 10 and 25 µg/ml.

DOSE AND COST

- Dose: 0.25–1 gm IV Q6H. Renal dose: No correction for renal insufficiency required. For liver failure monitor serum levels.
- **Cost: Low**

QUINOLONES

CHEMISTRY AND MECHANISMS OF ACTION

- Two six-membered rings with a nitrogen at position 1, a carbonyl group at position 4, and a carboxyl group attached to the carbon at position 3 (see Fig. 1-7).
- Potency greatly enhanced by adding fluorine at position 6.
- Gram-negative activity enhanced by addition of a nitrogen-containing piprazine ring at position 7.
- Inhibit two enzymes critical for DNA synthesis
  - DNA gyrase important for regulating the superhelical twists of bacterial DNA.
  - Topoisomerase IV responsible for segregating newly formed DNA into daughter cells.
  - Loss of these activities blocks DNA synthesis and results in rapid bacterial death.
- Resistance
  - Mutations in the DNA gyrase can reduce quinolone-binding affinity, described in *E. coli*.
  - Changes in outer membrane proteins that interfere with antibiotic penetration described in *E. coli* and Pseudomonas.
  - Efflux pumps expressed in both Gram-negative and Gram-positive bacteria can reduce the intracellular concentration of quinolones.

TOXICITY

- Serious adverse reactions are rare.
- Most common side effects are mild anorexia, nausea, vomiting, and abdominal discomfort.
- Diarrhea is less common and pseudomembranous colitis is rare.
- Mild headache, dizziness, insomnia, and seizures in association with theophylline.

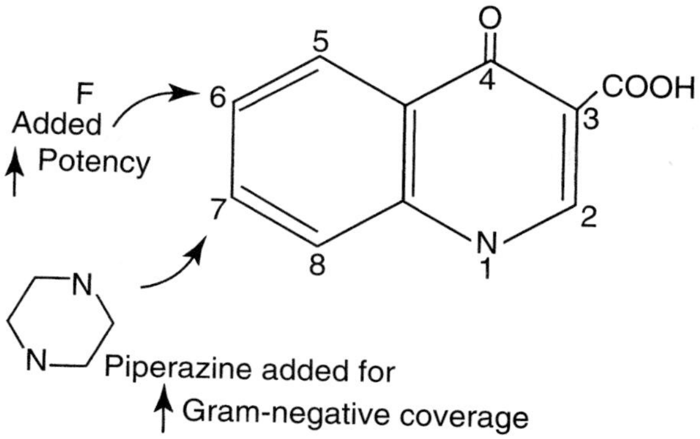

FIGURE 1-7
Basic structure of quinolones.

- Allergic reactions:
  - Skin rash most common, but less frequent than with penicillins or cephalosporins.
  - Fever, urticaria, serum sickness, interstitial nephritis, and anaphylactic reactions are rare.
  - Leukopenia and eosinophilia are also rare.
- Increased skin sensitivity to UV exposure can develop.
- Arthropathy and tendinitis due to cartilage damage.
  - A rare, but debilitating side effect that usually reverses weeks to months after the quinolone is discontinued.
  - Quinolones are not recommended for routine use in children because of concerns about cartilage damage.
- Hepatic toxicity:
  - Mild asymptomatic elevations of serum transaminase levels.
  - Serious hepatic toxicity was observed in several patients receiving trovofloxacin and as a result this antibiotic is no longer marketed.

Ciprofloxacin

Spectrum of Activity and Recommended Uses
- **Spectrum: Moderately broad**, does not kill anaerobes.
- Excellent activity against:
  - *Pseudomonas aeruginosa*, most potent quinolone
  - *E.coli*, Klebsiella, *Enterobacter cloacae*, Proteus, and Providencia
  - Salmonella, Shigella, Yersinia, and Campylobacter
  - *Neisseria meningitidis* and *gonorrhoeae*
  - *Moraxella catarrhalis* and *Haemophilus influenzae*
  - Legionella
  - *Mycoplasma pneumoniae* and *Ureaplasma urealyticum*
  - *Chlamydia pneumoniae* and *Chlamydia trachomatis*

- Variable activity against:
  - *Serratia marcescens*
  - *Morganella morganii*
  - *Burkholderia cepacia*
  - Aeromonas
  - Acinitobacter
  - Citrobacter species
- Recommended as primary antibiotic therapy for:
  - Urinary tract infections
  - Prostatitis, concentrates in the prostate
  - Traveler's diarrhea
  - *Salmonella typhi* (typhoid fever)
  - Salmonella gastroenteritis when antibiotic treatment is necessary
  - Cat scratch disease caused by *Bartonella henselae*
- Useful althernative therapy for:
  - Gonococcal urethritis in place of ceftriaxone

Pharmacokinetics
- Readily absorbed orally, achieving levels comparable to intravenous administration
- Half-life 4 hours
- Primarily cleared by the kidneys
- All quinolones demonstrate similar tissue penetration
  - Concentrate in prostate tissue, feces, bile, and lung tissue
  - Very highly concentrated in macrophages and neutrophils

Dose and Cost
- Dose: 250–750 mg Q12H orally, 200-400 mg Q12H IV. Renal dosing: Cr Cl 10–50 cc/min, Q18H dosing; Cr Cl < 10 cc/min, Q24H.
- **Cost: Moderately high po, low to moderate IV**

Levofloxacin

Spectrum of Activity and Recommended Uses
- **Spectrum: Broad**
- Similar Gram-negative coverage to ciprofloxin
- Greater Gram-positive acitivity than ciprofloxacin. Activity against:
  - *S. pneumoniae*
  - Other Streptococcus species including enterococcus
  - *S. aureus*
  - *S. pyogenes*
- Recommended as primary therapy
  - Community-acquired pneumonia in the otherwise healthy adult who does not require hospitalization. Cases of levofloxacin-resistant *S. pneumoniae* have been reported, raising concerns about overuse of this antibiotic. Some recommend reserving this antibiotic for elderly nursing home patients.
- Potential alternative therapy for:
  - Soft-tissue infections where a mixed infection including both Gram-positive and Gram-negative organisms is suspected.

Pharmacokinetics
- Well absorbed orally achieving equivalent levels to the intravenous preparation.
- Half-life of the drug is 6–8 hours.
- Cleared primarily by the kidneys.

Dose and Cost
- Dose: 500 mg 24H orally and intravenously. Renal dosing: Cr Cl 10–50 cc/min, 250 mg Q24H; Cr Cl< 10 cc/min, 250 mg Q48H.
- **Cost: oral, moderately high; intravenous, low**

Gatifloxacin and Moxifloxacin

Toxicity
Clinically significant prolongation of the QT interval has been reported with moxifloxacin, and less frequently with gatifloxacin. Potentially can cause life-threatening ventricular arrhythmias, particularly when combined with other drugs that prolong the QT interval.

Spectrum of Activity and Treatment Recommendations
- **Spectrum: Very broad**
- Activity against:
    - *S. pneumoniae*, including strains with high-level penicillin resistance. Gatifloxacin is 2–4 times and moxifloxaicin 4–8 times more active than levofloxacin.
    - Methicillin-sensitive *S. aureus*, but are not active against methicillin-resistant strains.
    - Anaerobes, both demonstrate moderate in vitro activity.
    - Spectrum of activity otherwise is similar to that of levofloxacin and ciprofloxacin. The exact indications for these agents are in evolution. Given their improved *S. pneumoniae* coverage, these new agents should be considered as a first-line regimen for community-acquired pneumonia not requiring hospitalization. Both agents are absorbed well orally. An intravenous preparation is available for gatifloxacin. Moxifloxacin is partly metabolized by the liver.

Dose and Cost
- Gatifloxacin: 400 mg Q24H po or IV. Renal dosing: Cr Cl 10–50 cc/min, 400 mg Q24–48H; Cr Cl < 10 cc/min, 400 mg Q48H.
- Moxifloxacin: 400 mg Q24H po. Renal dosing: No adjustments required.
- **Cost: po: both moderate; intravenous: low** (gatifloxacin)

OXAZOLIDONES

CHEMISTRY AND MECHANISMS OF ACTION
- Unique ring structure consisting of a five-membered ring containing an oxygen and nitrogen. The nitrogen connects to a six-membered ring and each specific compound has side chains added to both rings.
- Bind to the 50S ribosome preventing the nearby 30S subunit from forming the 70S initiation complex; block the initiation of protein synthesis.

Linezolid
The only oxalidone released to date.

Toxicity

- Reversible thrombocytopenia association with prolonged therapy. Monitor the platelet count for patients receiving 2 or more weeks of linezolid.
- Leukopenia
- Hepatic enzyme elevation
- Discoloration of the tongue
- Folliculitis
- Headache
- Diarrhea
- A weak inhibitor of monoamine oxidase; hypertension with ingestion of large amounts of tyramine. Avoid pseudoephedrine and selective serotonin reuptake inhibitors.

Antimicrobial Activity and Treatment Recommendations
- **Spectrum: Narrow**
- Active only against Gram-positive organisms. Bacteriostatic against:
    - Vancomycin-resistant *Enterococcus faecium* and *E. faecalis*
    - Methicillin-sensitive and -resistant *S. aureus*
    - Penicillin-resistant *S. pneumoniae*
- Recommended primarily for the treatment of vancomycin-resistant enterococcal infections.

Pharmacokinetics
- Well absorbed orally, peak serum levels being achieved in 1–2 hours. Food slows absorption, but does not lower peak levels.
- Half-life of 5 hours
- Partly metabolized by the liver and excreted in the urine

Dose and Cost
- Dose: 600 mg Q12H both po and IV. Renal dosing: No adjustment required.
- **Cost: Moderately high**

STREPTOGRAMINS

CHEMICAL STRUCTURE AND MECHANISMS OF ACTION

- Members of the macrolide family.
- Quinupristin derived from pristinamycin IA and dalfoprisitin derived from pristinamycin IIB.
- Syndercid is a combination of 30:70 quinupristin/dalfopristin that has synergistic activity.
- Inhibit bacterial protein synthesis by binding to the 50S bacterial ribosome.
    - Quinupristin inhibits peptide chain elongation.
    - Dalfopristin interferes with peptidyl transferase activity.

TOXICITY

- Myalgias and arthralgias
- Nausea and vomiting
- Diarrhea
- Experience with this drug remains limited.

ANTIMICROBIAL ACTIVITY AND TREATMENT INDICATIONS

- **Spectrum: Narrow**
- Primarily active against Gram-positive organisms. Effective against:
  - Vancomycin-resistant enterococci
  - Methicillin-resistant *S. aureus*
- Recommended for the treatment of vancomycin-resistant enterococcus.

PHARMACOKINETICS

- Administered intravenously
- Half-life 1.5 hours
- Primarily metabolized in the liver

DOSE AND COST

- Dose: 7.5 mg/kg Q8–12H IV. Renal dosing: No adjustment required.
- **Cost: Very high**

DAPTOMYCIN (CUBICIN)

CHEMICAL STRUCTURE AND MECHANISM OF ACTION

- A cyclic lipopeptide derived from *Streptomyces roseosporus.*
  - Chemical formula $C_{72}H_{101}N_{17}O_{26}$
  - 1,620 molecular weight
- Distinctly different mechanism of action than other antibiotics.
  - Binds to bacterial membranes.
  - Causes rapid depolarization of membrane potential.
    - Results in inhibition of protein, DNA, and RNA synthesis.
  - A cidal antibiotic that causes rapid concentration-dependent bacterial death.
- Synergy has been observed with aminoglycosides and β-lactam antibiotics for *S.aureus* and enterococci.

TOXICITY

- Muscle pain and weakness in 2.8% of patients as compared to 1.8% in patients treated with other antibiotics.
  - Associated with elevations of CPK.
  - CPK levels should be monitored weekly.
  - Drug should be discontinued if:
    - CPK > 1,000 U/L in association with symptoms of myopathy.
    - CPK ≥ 2,000 U/L in the absence of symptoms of myopathy.
  - Other drugs associated with rhabdomyolysis should not be coadministered with daptomycin, particularly HMG-CoA reductase inhibitors (statins).
- Neuropathy associated with decreases in nerve conduction velocity.
  - Can involve cranial or peripheral nerves (e.g., paresthesias, Bell's palsy).
  - A rare toxicity, but has also been observed in animal studies.

SPECTRUM OF ACTIVITY AND TREATMENT RECOMMENDATIONS

- **Spectrum: Narrow**
- Kills aerobic and facultative gram-positive microorganisms, including:
  - *Enterococcus faecalis* and f*aecium* (including vancomycin-resistant strains)
  - *Staphylcococcus aureus* (including MRSA)
  - *Staphylococcus epidermidis* (including methicillin-resistant strains)
  - *Streptococcus pyogenes*
  - *Corynebacterium jeikeium*
- At present approved only for the treatment of complicated skin and soft tissue infections by susceptible strains.
- Not approved for vancomycin-resistant enterococcus (insufficient clinical data).
- Should not be used for the treatment of pneumonia (poor entry into sputum).

PHARMACOKINETICS

- Intravenous administration of 4 mg/kg results in peak serum levels of 58 μg/ml.
- Half-life 8–9 hours
- 92% serum protein bound
- Primarily excreted by the kidneys.

DOSE AND COST

- Dose: 4 mg/kg IV Q24H. Renal dosing: Cr Cl< 30 cc/min, 4 mg/kg IV Q48H.
- **Cost: Moderately high**

METRONIDAZOLE

CHEMICAL STRUCTURE AND MECHANISMS OF ACTION

- A nitroimidizole
- Low molecular weight allows it to readily diffuse into tissues.
- Acts as an electron acceptor being quickly reduced in the bacterium. The resulting free radicals are toxic to the bacterium, producing DNA damage as well as damage to other macromolecules.

TOXICITY

- A disulfiram (antibuse-like) reaction with alcohol consumption.
- Seizures, encephalopathy, cerebellar dysfunction, and peripheral neuropathy are rare.
- Potential concern about induction of DNA mutations. However, multiple studies have failed to demonstrate significant DNA abnormalities. Not recommended in pregnancy.
- Impairs coumadin metabolism. Avoid in patients on coumadin.

SPECTRUM OF ACTIVITY AND TREATMENT RECOMMENDATIONS

- **Spectrum: Narrow**
- Trichomonas vaginitis effective both topically and orally.
- Amebiasis

- Giardiasis
- Anaerobic bacteria, cidal for most strains
- No significant activity against aerobes. Usually administered in combination with a cephalosporin for aerobic coverage.
- Recommended for:
  - Anaerobic bacteria, drug of choice
  - Pseudomembranous colitis due to overgrowth of *C. difficile*, first-line therapy, preferred over oral vancomycin
  - *Helicobacter pylori* gastric and duodenal infection in combination with other antibiotics (see Chap. 8)
  - Giardia
  - Amebiasis
  - Trichomonas vaginitis

PHARMACOKINETICS

- Rapidly and completely absorbed orally
- Therapeutic levels are achieved in all body fluids, including the cerebrospinal fluid and brain abscess contents.
- Half-life 8 hours
- Primarily metabolized by liver. Dose should be reduced to one half with severe hepatic failure.

DOSE AND COST

- Dose: Intravenous: 15 mg/kg loading dose followed by 7.5 mg Q6–8H not to exceed a maximum daily dose of 4 gm. Oral 500 mg Q6–8H. Renal dosing: no adjustment required.
- **Cost: Low**

SULFONAMIDES AND TRIMETHOPRIM

CHEMISTRY AND MECHANISMS OF ACTION

- Structure similar to para-aminobenzoic acid (PABA), a substrate required for bacterial folic acid synthesis (see Fig.1-8).
- A sulfonyl radical is attached to carbon 1 of the 6-membered ring and increases PABA inhibition.

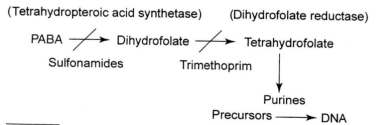

FIGURE 1-8
Effects of sulfonamides and trimethoprim on the bacterial folate pathway.

- Alterations in the sulfonyl radical determine many of the pharmacokinetic properties of the compounds.
- Inhibit bacterial folic acid synthesis by competitively inhibiting PABA incorporation into tetrahydropteroic acid.
- Bacteriostatic

TOXICITY

- Hypersensitivity reactions the most frequent and severe toxicity.
  - Macular papular drug rashes
  - Erythema multiforme and Stevens-Johnson syndrome
  - Vasculitis including drug-induced lupus, serum sickness-like syndrome
  - Anaphylaxis has been reported.
- Nausea, vomiting
- Diarrhea
- Headache
- Depression
- Jaundice and hepatic necrosis.
- Hemolytic anemia can be associated with glucose-6-phosphate dehydrogenase deficiency (G6PD-deficiency).
- Agranulocytosis, thrombocytopenia, and leukopenia rare.
- Avoid in the last month of pregnancy; displace bilirubin bound to plasma albumin and increase fetal blood levels of unconjugated bilirubin.

SPECTRUM OF ACTIVITY AND TREATMENT RECOMMENDATIONS

- **Spectrum: Moderately broad**
- Active against Gram-positive bacteria, but resistance is common.
  - Active against most strains of:
    - *Streptococcus pyogenes*
    - *Listeria monocytogenes*
    - *Bacillus anthracis*
  - Active against some strains of:
    - *Staphylococcus aureus*
    - *Streptococcus pneumoniae*
- Active against some Gram-negative strains, but resistance is widespread.
  - Active against many strains of:
    - *Escherichia coli*
    - Shigella species
    - *Haemophilus influenzae*
    - *Neisseria gonorrhoeae* and *Neisseria meningitidis*
  - Active against some strains of:
    - Klebsiella species
    - *Proteus mirabilis*
    - Salmonella
- Very active against *Chlamydia trachomatis*, *Nocardia asteroides*
- No anaerobic coverage
- Recommended for:
  - Empiric treatment of uncomplicated urinary tract infections. Ciprofloxacin is usually preferred, if cost is not an issue.
  - *Nocardia asteroides*
  - *Mycobacterium kansasii* in combination with other agents

PHARMACOKINETICS

- Classified as short-, medium-, and long-acting depending on their half-life.
- Sulfasoxazole is in the short-acting class, having half-life of 5–6 hours.
- Sulfamethoxazole and sulfadiazine are medium-acting, having half-life of 8–17 hours.
- Sulfadoxine is long acting, having half-life of 100–230 hours.
- Well absorbed orally.
- All metabolized by the liver, undergoing acetylation and glucuronidation. These metabolites are excreted in the urine.

DOSE AND COST

- Dose: Sulfasoxazole—1–2 gm po Q6H. Renal dosing: Cr Cl 10–50 cc/min, 1 gm Q8–12H; Cr Cl < 10 cc/min, 1 gm Q12–24H.
- Sulfadiazine—0.5–1.5 gm po Q4–6H. Renal dosing: Cr Cl 10–50 cc/min, 0.5–1.5 gm Q8–12H; Cr Cl < 10 cc/min, 0.5–1.5 gm Q12–24H.
- **Cost: Sulfasoazole: very low; sulfadiazine: low**

Trimethoprim

Chemistry and Mechanism of Action
- Two 6-membered rings, one with 2 nitrogens and 2 amino groups, and the other with 3 methoxybenzyl groups.
- Strongly inhibits dihyrofolate reductase and complements sulfonamides' inhibition of folate metabolism (see Fig. 1-8). Inhibition of bacterial dihydrofolate reductase is 100,000 × greater than its inhibition of the mammalian enzyme.

Spectrum of Activity and Treatment Recommendations
- Trimethoprim, usually administered in combination with sulfamethoxazole. This combination often results in significant activity against many Gram-positive bacteria:
  ○ *S. aureus*
  ○ *S. pneumoniae*
  ○ *S. pyogenes*
  ○ Enterococcus, only some strains
  ○ *Listeria monocytogenes*
- Trimethoprim-sulfamethoxazole (TMP-SMX) demonstrates excellent activity against many Gram-negative bacteria:
  ○ *E. coli*
  ○ *Proteus mirabilis*
  ○ Shigella species
  ○ Salmonella
  ○ *Burkholderia cepacia*
  ○ *Stenotrophomonas maltophilia*
  ○ *Yersinia enterocolitica*
  ○ *N. gonorrhoeae*
- Other pathogens
  ○ Chlamydia
  ○ *Pneumocystis carinii*

- Recommended for the treatment of:
  - Listeriosis in the penicillin-allergic patient.
  - Urinary tract infections, excellent for uncomplicated outpatient urinary tract infections. If cost not a concern, ciprofloxacin is preferred.
  - *Pneumocystis carinii* in immunocompromised hosts including AIDs patients. Also drug of choice to prevent Pneumocystis pneumonia in the immunocompromised host.
- Generally not recommended for:
  - Upper-respiratory-tract infections
  - Complicated urinary-tract infections
  - Plasmid-mediated resistance is common and treatment of Gram-negative pathogens should be initiated only after sensitivity is confirmed by microbiologic testing.

Pharmacokinetics
- Well absorbed orally
- Half-life of trimethoprim is 9–11 hours matching the half-life of sulfamethoxazole.
- Excreted primarily by the renal tubules and very high concentrations of active drug are found in the urine. Some trimethoprim is also excreted in the bile.

Dose and Cost
- Ratio of trimethoprim to sulfamethoxazole supplied is 1:5; single-strength tablet, 80 mg trimethoprim and 400 mg sulfamethoxazole, and double-strength tablet, 160 mg trimethoprim and 800 mg of sulfamethoxazole.
- Dose: Oral or parenteral: 1–5 mg/kg of the trimethoprim component Q6–12H. Renal dosing: Cr Cl 10–50 cc/min, half the oral dose, reduce the IV dose to 3–5 mg/kg Q12–24H; Cr Cl < 10, avoid administering.
- **Cost: Oral: low; intravenous: low to moderate**

ANTIMYCOBACTERIAL AGENTS

- Principles of antituberculous therapy
  - Therapy must be prolonged (months).
    - *M. tuberculosis* grow slowly and are intracellular.
    - Dormant bacteria are found in necrotic cavities, making them difficult to kill.
  - Two or more antimycobacterial agents should be administered.
    - 1×10^6 organisms are resistant to INH.
    - Cavitary lesions often contain 10^9–10^{10} organisms, assuring the survival and replicatation of resistant organisms.
    - Only 1×10^{12} organisms ($10^6 \times 10^6$) would be expected to be resistant to two antimicrobial agents.
  - The incidence of multidrug-resistant *M. tuberculosis* (MDR-TB) is increasing.
    - Resistant to isoniazid and rifampin.
    - Must be treated with three or more other antimycobacterial agents.
  - Agents classified as first-line and second-line drugs
    - First-line medications include isoniazide (INH), rifampin, pyrazinamide, streptomycin, and ethambutol.
      - More efficacious and less toxic than the second-line drugs.
      - Bactericidal with the exception of ethambutol.
      - Whenever possible first-line drugs should be employed for the treatment of *Mycobacterium tuberculosis*.
  - Standard therapy for drug-sensitive tuberculosis is a combination of three bactericidal agents—INH, rifampin, and pyrazinamide—for 6–9 months.

FIRST-LINE MEDICATIONS

Isoniazid (INH)

Chemistry and Mechanism of Action
- A hydrazide synthesized in 1952.
- Inhibits mycolic acid synthesis.
  - Mycolic acids are long-chain fatty acids found in the middle layer of the mycobacterial cell wall.
  - Damage to this layer results in bacterial death.

Toxicity
- Hepatocellular damage is the major toxicity.
  - 10–20% develop a transient rise in serum transaminase values on initiation of therapy. Discontinue if ≥ 3–5 × normal limit.
  - Levels usually return to normal.
  - Progressive hepatitis that can be fatal develops in a small percentage of cases when INH is continued.
  - The incidence of serious hepatitis is age-related, progressively increasing in patients over 35.
    - ≤ 0.3% in patients under 35 years
    - ≤ 1.2% age 35–49 years
    - ≤ 2.3% over age 50 years
  - The risk of hepatotoxicity increases in patients receiving rifampin, overusing alcohol, or taking acetaminophen.
  - Monitoring of hepatocellular enzymes remains controversial; however, monthly monitoring is recommended by some experts.
  - All patients should be warned to discontinue INH if they experience symptoms of early hepatitis: loss of appetite, nausea, malaise, and right-upper-quadrant or midabdominal pain.
- Peripheral neuropathy observed in malnourished patients.
  - Increases pyridoxine excretion.
  - Coadministering pyridoxine recommended as prevention.
- Hypersensitivity reactions.
- Arthritic disorders are less common.

Spectrum of Activity and Treatment Recommendations
- Active only against mycobacteria.
- At low concentrations INH is inhibitory and at higher concentrations is cidal to actively growing mycobacteria.
- INH should never be given alone in active infection.
  - INH resistance is observed in a significant percentage of primary isolates (7–8%).
  - Resistance more commonly observed in large cities.
  - Three or four drug regimens are commonly recommended until sensitivity to INH can be confirmed.

Pharmacokinetics
- Absorbed well orally or intramuscularly.
- Penetrates all body spaces including the blood-brain barrier.
- Metabolized by the liver.
  - The rate of metabolism depends on the capacity of the liver to acetylate INH.
    - Half-life is 3 hours in slow acetylators.
    - Half-life 1 hour in rapid acetylators.

- ○ Approximately half of American Caucasians are slow acetylators while only 5% of Eskimos fall into this category.
- ○ Both slow and rapid acetylators achieve therapeutic levels and cure rates with standard regimens.
- ○ Slow acetylators have a higher incidence of neurotoxicity.
- ○ Fast acetylators have a greater risk of developing hepatotoxicity.

Dose and Cost
- Dose: 300 mg or 5 mg/kg po QD. Renal dosing: Cr Cl $<$ 10 cc/min, slow acetylators 1/2 dose.
- **Cost: Low**

Rifamycins

Chemistry and Mechanism of Action
- Macrocyclic compounds that act as zwitterions capable of diffusing through lipids.
- Inhibit DNA-dependent RNA polymerase, preventing chain initiation. More active against bacterial RNA polymerase than mammalian mitochondrial polymerase.

Toxicity
- Hepatotoxicity
  - ○ Asymptomatic serum transaminase values observed in up to 14% of patients.
  - ○ Overt hepatitis develops in 1% in the absence of INH and in 2–3% when INH is coadministered with rifampin.
  - ○ The risk of hepatotoxicity increases with age, alcohol consumption, and malnutrition.
  - ○ Patients need to be instructed to discontinue if they experience the symptoms of early hepatitis (see INH above).
  - ○ A rise in serum bilirubin can occur in the absence of hepatitis in the first week of therapy owing to competitive inhibition of hepatic bilirubin metabolism.
- Skin rash
- Gastrointestinal complaints
- Renal dysfunction
- Orange discoloration of urine, sweat, and tears
- Organic brain syndrome
- Drug-drug interactions:
  - ○ A potent inducer of hepatic enzymes that shorten the half-life of a number of therapeutic agents, including:
    - Coumadin
    - Cyclosporin
    - Digoxin
    - Fluconazole
    - Anti-HIV protease inhibitors
    - Theophylline
    - Thyroxine
    - Zidovudine
  - ○ Trimethoprim-sulfamethoxazole increases rifampin levels.
  - ○ Before rifampin or rifabutin is administered, all other medications should be reviewed and potential interactions investigated.

Spectrum of Activity and Treatment Recommendations
- Excellent activity against *M. tuberculosis*, as well as some activity against *M. avium intracellulare*, *M. fortuitum*, *M. kansasii*, and *M. marinum*.
- Rifabutin, a semisynthetic derivative of rifampin, has better activity against *M. avium intracellulare* (MAI) than rifampin.
- Recommended in combination as first-line therapy for *M. tuberculosis*
  - Never use as monotherapy; rapid development of resistance is very frequent.
  - Always combined with other antimycobacterial agents.
- Rifabutin is the drug of choice for MAI.
  - Used alone for the prevention of MAI in HIV-infected patients.
  - More effective than rifampin in combination therapy for active MAI infections.
- Rifampin is active against a number of nontuberculous organisms, but cannot be used as monotherapy because of the high rate of rapid resistance. Excellent activity against:
  - *N. meningitidis*, one of the antibiotics recommended for meningococcal prophylaxis
  - *S. aureus*
  - *S. epidermidis*
  - *S. pyogenes*
  - Legionella
  - Chlamydia
- Recommended for therapy of:
  - Prosthetic valve endocarditis due to *S. epidermidis*; rifampin combined with vancomycin and gentamicin.
  - *S. aureus* bacteremia or endocarditis; use of rifampin remains controversial.
  - *Rhodococcus equi*. Can be used in combination with vancomycin.

Pharmacokinetics
- Oral preparations are almost completely absorbed. Peak serum levels are observed in 1–4 hours.
- Half-life 2–5 hours; half-life of rifabutin 16 hours.
- Both drugs taken up by the liver and deacetylated to an active metabolite and then excreted via the biliary tract.
- Penetrate all tissues and achieve excellent intracellular levels. They also cross the blood-brain barrier.

Dose and Cost
- Dose
  - Rifampin: 600 mg QD po, can increase to 600 mg BID for nontuberculous infections. Renal dosing: No adjustments required
  - Rifabutin: 300 mg QD po. Renal dosing: No adjustments required.
- **Cost: Rifampin: low; rifabutin: moderate**

Pyrazinamide

Chemistry and Mechanism of Action
- A pyrizine analogue of nicotinamide.
- Its mechanism of action is unknown.
- Most active in an acidic environment such as the low pH of the macrophage phagolysosome where tubercle bacilli are commonly found.

Spectrum of Activity and Recommended Uses
- Cidal against replicating *M. tuberculosis*.
- Should never be used as monotherapy because resistance rapidly develops.
- Recommended for the treatment of tuberculous meningitis.

Toxicity
- Most common side effects:
  - Nausea and vomiting
  - Hepatitis is dose related, and is uncommon with current dosing recommendations.
  - Interstitial nephritis
  - Polymyalgia, rhadomyolysis
  - Photosensitivity
  - Decreases tubular secretion of urate and asymptomatic hyperuricemia in approximately half of patients.

Pharmacokinetics
- Well absorbed
- Readily distributes throughout the body including the cerebrospinal fluid.
- Hepatic metabolized and the kidneys primarily excrete metabolites.
- Half-life is 10–16 hours.

Dose and Cost
- Dose: 15–30 mg/kg QD po. Renal dosing: Cr Cl < 10 cc/min, lower dose to 12–20 mg/kg QD.
- **Cost: Low**

Ethambutol

Chemical Structure and Mechanism of Action
- An 8-carbon noncyclic molecule that was specifically synthesized as an antituberculous agent.
- Inhibits arabinosyl transferases that are important for mycobacterial cell wall synthesis.
- Ethambutol is a static agent.

Toxicity
- Optic neuritis resulting in loss of visual acuity and defective red-green color vision.
  - Dose related being more common with doses of 25 mg/kg than 15 mg/kg.
  - On high-dose ethambutol, monitoring of visual acuity and color perception is recommended every 4–6 weeks.
  - Also monitor those with baseline visual dysfunction receiving 15 mg/kg.

Pharmacokinetics
- Well absorbed orally
- Broad tissue distribution, including the CSF
- Half-life of 3–4 hours
- Metabolized by the liver and the resulting metabolites excreted by the kidneys

Dose and Cost
- Dose: 15–25 mg/kg QD po. Renal dosing: Cr Cl 50–80 cc/min, 15 mg/kg Q24H; Cr Cl 10–50 cc/min, 15 mg/kg Q24–36H; Cr Cl < 10 cc/min, 15 mg/kg Q48H.
- **Cost: Low**

Streptomycin
- This aminoglycoside has the same mechanism of action as the other aminoglycosides.
- Similar toxicities:
  - Nephrotoxicity and hearing loss are less common.
  - Higher incidence of vestibular dysfunction.
    - If tinnitus, decreased hearing, or dizziness develops, the drug should be stopped.
- Cidal for extracellular *M. tuberculosis*, but fails to achieve therapeutic intracellular levels.
- This agent should never be given alone because resistance develops rapidly with monotherapy.
- Half-life of 2–5 hours
- Excreted by the kidneys
- The need for parenteral administration, usually intramuscularly, causes some inconvenience for outpatient therapy.
- Dose: 1–2 gm QD, IM or IV. Renal dosing: Cr Cl 50–80 cc/min, 15 mg/kg Q24–48 hr; Cr Cl 10–50 cc/min, 15 mg/kg Q72–96H; Cr Cl < 10 cc/min, 7.5 mg/kg Q72–96H.
- **Cost: Moderate**

SECOND-LINE MEDICATIONS

Quinolones
- Often cidal for mycobacteria.
- Ciprofloxacin and ofloxacin are frequently used for the treatment of multiresistant *M. tuberculosis*.
- The recommended doses are ciprofloxacin 750 mg BID or ofloxacin 400 mg BID.

Other Aminoglycosides
- Capreomycin, amikacin, kanamycin, and viomycin have all been used for the treatment of multidrug-resistant *M. tuberculosis*.
- Capreomycin is less toxic than other aminoglycosides and is the preferred drug in this category
  - Only given intramuscularly and is excreted unaltered by the kidneys.
  - Major side effects are nephrotoxicity and ototoxicity.
  - Multiresistant strains exhibiting resistance to streptomycin are generally sensitive to capreomycin.
- Amikacin is the most active aminoglycoside against *M. tuberculosis*.
  - High incidence of nephrotoxicity and ototoxicity associated with prolonged therapy limits its usefulness.
- Kanamycin and viomycin are less commonly used because they exhibit cross-resistance to capreomycin and amikacin, and are more toxic.

Dose and Cost
- Dose: Capreomycin: 1 g QD IV or IM. Renal dosing: Cr Cl 10–50 cc/min, 7.5 mg/kg Q24–48H; Cr Cl < 10 cc/min, 7.5 mg/kg twice per week.
- **Cost: Very high**
- Dose: Amikacin 7–10 mg/kg IV or IM (not to exceed 1 gm) 5 times per week. Renal dosing: Dose based on serum levels.
- **Cost: Low**

Cycloserine
- Bacteriostatic agent is usually not effective against multidrug-resistant strains.
- Has been used in primary drug-resistant *M. tuberculosis*.
- Severe central nervous system toxicity including seizures, somnolence, headache, and severe depression.
  - Should not be given to patients with a history of seizures or depression.
- Well absorbed orally and distributes to all tissues and readily crosses the blood-brain barrier
- Renally excreted
- Half-life of 8–12 hours
- Dose: 250–500 mg BID po. Renal dosing: Cr Cl 10–50 cc/min, 250–500 mg QD, Cr Cl< 10 cc/min, 250 mg QD.
- **Cost: Moderately high**

Para-aminosalicylic Acid (PAS)
- Inhibits folate metabolism of tuberculous organisms and is a static agent.
- Use limited by the frequent occurrence of nausea and vomiting.
- Other side effects include hypersensitivity reactions, e.g., a lupus-like syndrome, lymph node hypertrophy, and hepatitis.
- Incompletely absorbed orally.
- Excreted in the urine.
- The drug is available through the Centers of Disease Control.
- Usual dose is 10–12 gm/day in 3–4 divided doses.

Ethionamide
- Derived from isonicotinic acid and is tuberculostatic, interfering with mycolic acid synthesis.
- Toxicity frequent:
  - Often causes nausea and vomiting.
  - Neurologic side effects are common, including peripheral neuropathy and psychiatric disorders.
  - Reversible hepatotoxicity
- Well absorbed orally and penetrates all tissues including the blood-brain barrier.
- Metabolized by the liver and metabolites are excreted in the urine.
- Half-life 2–4 hours
- Dose: Initial dose 250 mg BID increasing 250 mg/day to reach a final dose of 500 mg BID. Renal dosing: Cr Cl < 10 cc/min, 5 mg/kg Q48H.
- Cost: Low

ANTIFUNGAL AGENTS

- A major difference between fungi and eukaryotes is the primary sterol building block used to form the plasma membrane.
  - Fungal plasma membrane consists of ergesterols.
  - The major sterol component of the human plasma membrane is cholesterol.
- Two classes of drugs exploit these differences.
  - Polyenes act by binding to ergesterol and disrupting the fungal membrane. They are fungicidal.
  - Azoles inhibit ergesterol synthesis and lower ergesterol levels, resulting in fungal membrane breakdown. These agents are usually fungistatic.

AGENTS FOR TREATMENT OF SYSTEMIC FUNGAL INFECTIONS

Amphotericin B

Chemical Structure, Mechanisms of Action, and Spectrum of Activity
- A long cyclic polyene compound forms a large rod-like structure.
- Bind to ergesterol in the fungal membrane, and form pores that result in leakage of intracellular potassium and fungal cell death.
- Fungicidal action is rapid and does not require active growth.
- Effective against most fungal infections and remains the most effective agent for systemic fungal infections.
- Resistance to amphotericin B has been demonstrated among:
  - *Candida lusitaniae*
  - Fusarium species
  - *Pseudallescheria boydii*
- Alterations in sterol structure required for amphotericin B resistance often reduce tissue invasiveness, such strains being capable of growing only on mucosal surfaces or in the urine.

Toxicity
- Nephrotoxicity is the major complication associated with the conventional deoxycholate form of the drug (amphotericin B deoxycholate [ABD]).
  - Causes vasoconstriction of renal arterioles resulting in a reduction in glomerular filtration rate.
  - Also impairs proximal and distal tubular reabsorption causing potassium, magnesium, and bicarbonate wasting.
  - These effects are often reversible.
  - Permanent loss of nephrons and permanent damage to tubular basement membranes are also observed; correlate with the total dose of ABD administered.
  - Renal dysfunction occurs in all patients; serum creatinine levels of 2–3 mg/dl are to be expected.
  - Hydration with normal saline prior to infusion reduces nephrotoxicity.
- Fever is commonly associated with administration. Often associated with chills, fever, and tachypnea, particularly if the drug is infused too rapidly.
  - Administered over a minimum of 2–3 hours. A more rapid infusion of lipid-complexed amphotericin B is required to prevent drug precipitation.
  - Fever and chills diminish with each ensuing dose.
  - If fever persists, can premedicate with acetaminophen or by the addition of 25–50 mg of hydrocortisone to the solution.
  - A febrile response does not represent an allergic reaction and should not be misinterpreted as anaphylaxis.
  - A 1-mg test dose prior to administration of the full dose is no longer recommended; this strategy delays achievement of therapeutic antifungal serum and tissue levels.
- Nausea, vomiting, and anorexia
- Phlebitis is common when the drug is administered by a peripheral vein. Therefore, a centrally placed intravenous line is recommended.

Pharmacokinetics
- Insoluble in water at physiologic pH and is stored as a powder that is dispersed as coloidal suspension in a 5% dextrose solution. The addition of electrolytes aggregates the colloids, making the solution cloudy.

- Binds to lipoproteins in the serum and then leaves the circulation.
- Stored in the liver and other organs and subsequently released into the circulation.
- Lipid-complex amphotericin B is ingested by macrophages, resulting in high intracellular levels in this cell type.
- Poorly penetrates the blood-brain barrier and brain.
- Therapeutic levels are detectable in inflamed pleural fluid, peritoneum, and joint fluid.
- Slowly degraded and degradation is not affected by hepatic or renal dysfunction.
- Initial half-life of the drug is 24 hours; over time extends to 15 days.

Efficacy of Different Amphotericin B Preparations
- Clinical trials of liposomal preparations of amphotericin B demonstrate comparable efficacy to amphotericin B deoxycholate.
- Lipid-complexed amphotericin B markedly reduces nephrotoxicity. Use in:
  ○ Patients with significant preexisting renal dysfunction.
  ○ Patients who develop progressive renal failure (serum creatinine above 2.5 mg/dl) while being treated with amphotericin B deoxycholate.

Dose and Cost
- Dose: Amphotericin B deoxycholate, 0.3–1.4 mg/kg QD. Renal dosing not required.
  Amphotericin B lipid complex, 3–5 mg/kg QD. Renal dosing not required.
- **Cost: Amphotericin B deoxycholate: Low. Amphotericin B lipid complex, all three preparations: Very high** (liposomal preparation > $1,000/day; Lipid complex preparation $270/day)

Azoles

Chemical Structure and Mechanism of Action
- Triazoles are the class of azoles preferred for systemic fungal infection.
- Inhibit a cytochrome P450–dependent demethylation system that results in decreased production of ergesterol and accumulation of intermediate sterols.
  ○ Alter fungal membrane permeability.
  ○ Disturb activity of membrane surface enzymes and retention of metabolites.
- Fungistatic rather than fungicidal activity.
- Itraconazole can antagonize amphotericin B activity by reducing its binding target, ergesterol.

Toxicity
- Ketoconazole the most toxic of the triazoles; as a consequence rarely used.
  ○ Higher doses also interfere with testosterone and cortisone production. Gynecomastia and loss of libido are common.
  ○ Nausea and vomiting
  ○ Hepatotoxicity
    ▪ Asymptomatic increases in serum transaminase levels.
    ▪ Severe hepatitis can develop; patient should be warned to discontinue if he experiences the symptoms of hepatitis (anorexia, malaise, nausea, and vomiting).
- Fluconazole minimal toxicity:
  ○ Headache
  ○ Anorexia
  ○ Reversible alopecia
  ○ Asymptomatic increases in serum transaminase levels

- Itraconazole also has an excellent toxicity profile:
  ○ Nausea and abdominal discomfort
  ○ Hypokalemia, mild hypertension, and edema in association with daily doses of 400 mg or higher.
- Voriconazole infusion is associated with transient loss of light perception.
  ○ This symptom resolves with subsequent doses.
  ○ Visual hallucinations less commonly occur.
  ○ Decreases metabolism of coumadin. Affects the metabolism of many drugs metabolized by the cytochrome P450 system.

Spectrum of Activity and Treatment Recommendations
- Fluconazole
  ○ Active against most strains of *Candida albicans*, but natural resistance observed with:
    ▪ *C. glabrata*
    ▪ *C. krusei*
    ▪ Any strain of Candida can develop resistance due to increased production of demethylase as well as increased drug efflux.
  ○ No activity against Aspergillus species.
  ○ Recommended for the treatment of:
    ▪ Oropharyngeal candidiasis
    ▪ Vulvovaginal candidiasis
    ▪ Uncomplicated candidemia in the nonimmunocompromised host can give intravenous fluconazole.
      • Therapeutically equivalent to amphotericin B in this group.
      • In immunocompromised (including neutropenia) host, and for seriously ill patients with deep-tissue Candida infection, amphotericin B is the treatment of choice.
    ▪ Cryptococcal meningitis in AIDs patients.
      • Used to complete therapy after initial therapy with amphotericin B with or without flucytosine for 2 weeks
      • Fluconazole (400 mg QD) treatment is recommended for 2 months followed by daily fluconazole maintenance therapy (200 mg QD).
      • The role of fluconazole in non-AIDs patients has not been defined.
    ▪ Prophylaxis in neutropenic allogeneic bone marrow transplant patients.
      • Reduces mortality and the incidence of invasive Candida infections.
      • No effect on the incidence of Aspergillus infections.
    ▪ Prophylaxis for leukemia patients.
      • Reduces the incidence of invasive Candida infections but does not affect mortality.
    ▪ Not proven to be efficacious for surgical intensive-care-unit patients.
      • Increases the prevalence of fluconazole-resistant fungi, including *C. krusei* and *C. glabrata*.
    ▪ Not recommended for prophylaxis in HIV-infected patients.
- Itraconazole
  ○ Increased activity against:
    ▪ Histoplasmosis
    ▪ Coccidiomycosis
    ▪ Blastomycosis
    ▪ Sporotrichosis
  ○ Recommended for:
    ▪ Acute and chronic vaginal candidiasis
    ▪ HIV-associated oral and esophageal candidiasis

- Consolidation and maintenance therapy for cryptococcal meningitis in AIDS patients, although fluconazole preferred
- Lymphocutaneous sporotrichosis
- Nonmeningeal, non-life-threatening histoplasmosis, blastomycosis, and coccidiomycosis
- Not recommended for deep-seated candidal infections or candidemia. Efficacy has not been proven.
- Amphotericin B recommended for disseminated histoplasmosis and coccidiomycosis.
- Primary prophylaxis and secondary prophylaxis to prevent relapse of histoplasmosis in AIDS patients.
- Voriconazole
  ○ Increased activity against Aspergillus.
  ○ Treatment of choice for:
    - Invasive Aspergillus
    - Empiric antifungal therapy for the neutropenic patient with persistent fever; a suitable alternative to amphotericin B

Pharmacokinetics

- Fluconazole
  ○ Well absorbed orally and serum levels after ingestion of the oral preparation are comparable to those after intravenous administration.
  ○ Penetration into tissues and body fluids including the cerebrospinal fluid is excellent.
  ○ Excreted primarily in the urine; smaller amounts are released into the feces.
  ○ The half-life of fluconazole is 27–34 hours.
- Itraconazole
  ○ Variable oral absorption
    - Requires stomach acidity for adequate absorption.
    - Capsule absorption is enhanced by food.
    - Reduced by agents that reduce stomach acidity.
  ○ Penetrates most tissues but does not cross the blood-brain barrier and minimally enters ocular fluids.
  ○ Primarily metabolized by the liver and metabolites excreted in the feces.
  ○ Half-life of this drug is 20–60 hours.
- Voriconazole
  ○ Well absorbed orally
  ○ Good tissue penetration
  ○ Metabolized by the cytochrome P450 system of the liver
  ○ Half-life of 6 hours

Dose and Cost

- Dose: Fluconazole oral: 100–400 mg QD; intravenous: 100–400 mg QD. Renal dosing: Cr Cl 10–50 cc/min, reduce dose by 50%; Cr Cl < 10 cc/min, 25–50 mg QD.
  Itraconazole oral: 200–400 mg QD; intravenous: 200 mg QD. Renal dosing not required.
  Voriconazole oral: 200–400 mg Q12H; intravenous: 200 mg QD. Renal dosing not required.
- **Cost: Fluconazole oral—Moderately high to very high** depending on dose
  Fluconazole IV—Moderate to moderately high
  Itraconazole oral—High to very high, depending on the dose
  Itraconazole IV—High to very high

Voriconazole oral—Very high (however, often cost effective, because it eliminates the requirement for IV amphotericin B in Aspergillus infection)
Voriconazole IV—High

Flucytosine (5-FC)

Chemical Structure and Mechanism of Action
- Fluorine analogue of cytosine
- Multistep conversion, including deamination and phosphorylation, forms 5-fluorouracil (5-FU).
  - ○ Inhibitor of thymidylate synthetase, impairing DNA and RNA synthesis.
  - ○ 5-FC is not as toxic to humans because they lack the deaminase required for conversion to 5-FU.

Toxicity
- Bone marrow suppression leading to neutropenia, anemia, and thrombocytopenia.
  - ○ Dose related and usually occurs when serum levels exceed 125 µg/ml.
  - ○ Higher risk in patients with diminished bone marrow reserve (AIDs patients and patients receiving cancer chemotherapy).
  - ○ Commonly 5-FC is administered in combination with amphotericin B. As amphotericin B impairs renal function, serum levels of 5-FC increase.
  - ○ Monitoring of peak (2 hours after oral administration) and trough levels (just prior to the next dose) with renal dysfunction maintaining serum levels between 20 and 100 µg/ml.
- Nausea and vomiting
- Diarrhea
- Abdominal pain
- Hepatitis.

Spectrum of Activity and Treatment Recommendations
- Effective against:
  - ○ *Candida albicans*
  - ○ *Cryptococcus neoformans*
  - ○ Chromomycosis
- 15% of *C. albicans* strains and 3–5% of *C. neoformans* resistance.
- 5-FC is usually fungistatic.
- Inferior activity compared to amphotericin B.
- Never use alone because resistance rapidly develops with monotherapy.
- Combination of 5-FC and amphotericin B demonstrates additive or synergistic activity for cryptococcal infections and is the recommended treatment.
  - ○ Combination therapy sterilizes the CSF faster than amphotericin B alone in cryptococcal meningitis.
  - ○ In vitro and animal testing also suggest that combination therapy for Candida may be of benefit; however, efficacy has not been proven in human patients.

Pharmacokinetics
- Well absorbed orally
- A small molecule that penetrates tissues well and crosses the blood-brain barrier achieving therpeutic levels in the cerebrospinal fluid, aqueous humor, joint fluid, and respiratory secretions
- Half-life of 3–5 hours
- Cleared by the kidneys

Dose and Cost
- Dose: 25 mg/kg Q6H po. Renal dosing: Cr Cl 10–50 cc/min, 25 mg/kg Q12–24H; Cr Cl < 10 cc/min, adjust dose using serum levels (see above).
- **Cost: Moderate**

Caspofungin

Chemical Structure and Mechanism of Action
- Derived from echinocandin B
- A semisynthetic lipopeptide that blocks synthesis of β-(1,3)-D-glucan, a critical component of the cell wall of many pathogenic fungi

Toxicity
- Fever, rash
- Nausea and vomiting
- Phlebitis has been reported.
- Flushing of the face has also been observed during infusion.
- One case of anaphylaxis has been reported.
- Drug-drug interactions
  - Plasma levels are increased by coadministration of cyclosporin.
  - Plasma levels decreased by efavirenz, nelfinavir, Dilantin, Tegretol, rifampin, and dexamethasone.
  - Reduces serum levels of tacrolimus, but does not interact with mycophenolate mofetil (Cell Cept), amphotericin B, or itraconazole.

Spectrum of Activity and Treatment Indications
- Active against:
  - Aspergillus sp.
  - Candida sp., including isolates that are resistant to other antifungal agents
  - Less effective versus *C. parapsolosis* in vitro
- Not active against Cryptococcus
- Approved for the treatment of:
  - Invasive aspergillosis in patients who fail or are unable to tolerate amphotericin B or itraconazole.
  - Oral candidiasis that is refractory to azole or amphotericin B therapy.

Pharmacokinetics
- Not absorbed by the gastrointestinal tract and must be administered intravenously
- Half-life of 9–11 hours
- Metabolized by the liver

Dose and Cost
- Dose: 70 mg first day, followed by 50 mg QD IV. Infused over 1 hour. Renal dosing not required. Moderate hepatic failure: reduce dose to 35 mg QD.
- **Cost: Very high**

ANTIVIRAL DRUGS
(OTHER THAN ANTIRETROVIRAL AGENTS)

- Most antiviral agents target viral nucleic acid synthesis.
- Resistance may develop during treatment because most antiviral agents act at a single target. Development of resistance is favored by:
    ○ A high viral load
    ○ A high intrinsic viral mutation rate (more common in RNA than DNA viruses)
    ○ A high degree of selective pressure (i.e., prolonged antiviral therapy or repeated courses of treatment)
- A second method for controlling viral infection is by modifying the host immune response.
    ○ Antibody infusion
    ○ Interferon administration

Acyclovir and Valacyclovir

Chemical Structure and Mechanisms of Action
- Synthetic analogues of guanine (a side chain has been substituted for a sugar moiety).
- Phosphorylated by viral thymidine kinase forming a monophosphate compound.
    ○ As a consequence, concentrations of acyclovir triphosphate are 40–100 times higher in infected than uninfected cells.
- Host cell kinases, then add two additional phosphates
    ○ Allows acyclovir triphosphate to add to replicating DNA.
    ○ The acyclic side chain prevents the addition of subsequent nucleic acids to DNA causing premature termination.
    ○ Acyclovir triphosphate also selectively inhibits viral DNA polymerase.
- Resistance
    ○ Most common cause: reduction in viral thymidine kinase
        ▪ Loss or reduction in viral thymidine kinase activity impairs acyclovir phosphorylation.
        ▪ Also renders the virus resistant to penciclovir and ganciclovir, which also require activation by viral thymidine kinase.
- Less common mechanisms of resistant
    ○ Alterations in viral thymidine kinase substrate specificity (phosphorylates thymidine, but not acyclovir)
    ○ Mutations in viral DNA polymerase

Toxicity
- Minimal toxicity
- Rarely causes rash, hematuria, headache, and nausea.
- Neurotoxicity in 1–4% of patients receiving intravenous acyclovir. Usually associated with renal dysfunction resulting in high drug serum levels. Can result in:
    ○ Lethargy, obtundation, coma
    ○ Hallucinations
    ○ Seizures
    ○ Autonomic instability
    ○ Coadministration of zidovudine and acyclovir increases the risk of developing lethargy.
- Crystalluria and crystalline nephropathy associated with IV administration, particularly if the patient is dehydrated.
- Cyclosporin increases the risk of nephrotoxicity.

Antiviral Activity and Therapeutic Indications
- Excellent activity against herpes simplex-1 and -2
- Significant activity against varicella; however, higher drug concentrations are required to kill this virus.
- Modest activity against cytomegalovirus
- Some activity against Epstein-Barr virus, but is generally not recommended for therapy.
- Topical acyclovir generally not effective and not recommended.
- Oral acyclovir recommended for:
  - Treatment and prevention of genital herpes
  - Treatment and prevention of recurrent ocular herpes simplex.
- Intravenous acyclovir recommended for:
  - Herpes simplex encephalitis; treatment of choice. Reduces morbidity and mortality.
  - Varicella and herpes zoster in the immunocompromised host.
  - Varicella pneumonia or encephalitis in the previously healthy adult.
  - Modest protection against cytomegalovirus; however, ganciclovir is more effective and is preferred.

Pharmacokinetics
- Oral absorption of acyclovir is limited, only 15–20% of the drug being bioavailable.
  - Poorer in transplant patients, necessitating higher oral dosing.
- Valcyclovir, an oral acyclovir prodrug, well absorbed.
  - Rapidly and completely converted to acyclovir by hepatic and intestinal valcyclovir hydrolase
  - Achieves acyclovir serum levels that are 3–5 times higher than those with oral acyclovir
- Widely distributed in tissues and fluids. Therapeutic levels can be achieved in:
  - Cerebrospinal fluid
  - Saliva
  - Vaginal secretions
  - Aqueous humor
- Primarily excreted unchanged in the urine
- Mean half-life of 2.5–3 hours
  - Probenecid reduces renal clearance and increases the half-life.

Dose and Cost
- Oral acyclovir: 200–800 mg 3–5 × per day (see specific infections for dosing). Renal dosing: Cr Cl 10–50 cc/min, 800 mg Q8H maximal dose; Cr Cl < 10 cc/min, 200 mg Q12H; for varicella infection, 800 mg Q12H.
- **Cost: Low–very high** depending on dose
- Oral valacyclovir: 500–1000 mg BID to TID. Renal dosing: Cr Cl 10–50 cc/min, 500–1,000 mg Q12–24H; Cr Cl < 10 cc/min, 500 mg QD.
- **Cost: Moderate to high** depending on dose
- Intravenous acyclovir: 5–10 mg/kg Q8H. Renal dosing: Cr Cl 10–50 cc/min, 5–12 mg/kg Q12–24H; Cr Cl < 10 cc/min, 2.5–6 mg/kg Q24H.
- **Cost: Very high**

Penciclovir and Famciclovir

Chemical Structure and Mechanism of Action
- Penciclovir is an acyclic guanosine analogue similar to acyclovir and has similar mechanisms of action.
  - Not a DNA chain terminator.
  - Acts primarily as a viral DNA polymerase inhibitor.
    - A less potent inhibitor than acyclovir
  - Concentrations in virally infected cells are much higher and persist longer than acyclovir. Explains its potent antiviral effect.
- Resistance
  - Requires viral thymidine kinase for activity.
  - Acyclovir-resistant strains due to deficient thymidine kinase demonstrate cross-resistance to penciclovir.
- Famciclovir is the diacetyl ester of penciclovir.
  - Quickly converted to penciclovir following oral absorption.

Toxicity
- Side effects are similar to those of oral acyclovir.
  - Headache, nausea, and vomiting
  - Hallucinations and confusion in the elderly
  - Neutropenia and elevated serum transaminase levels reported

Antiviral Spectrum and Treatment Recommendations
- Comparable antiviral activity to acyclovir.
- Excellent activity against herpes simplex-1 and -2
- Good activity against varicella-zoster virus
- Limited activity against cytomegalovirus
- Same indications as oral acyclovir. In addition, can be used for:
  - Hepatitis B virus
    - DNA levels and serum transaminase values reduced in patients with chronic hepatitis B
    - Additive when combined with interferon
    - Used to treat recurrent hepatitis B after liver transplantation
  - Topical treatment of recurrent orolabial herpes
    - Topical 1% penciclovir cream shortens healing by 0.5–1 day in healthy patients.

Pharmacokinetics
- Famciclovir well absorbed orally. The only systemic preparation.
  - Purine is quickly deactylated and oxidized by liver and intestine to form penciclovir.
- Excellent tissue penetration
- Half-life of 2–3 hours
- Primarily excreted by the kidneys

Dose and Cost
- Dose: 125 Q12H po for herpes simplex and 500 mg Q8H po for varicella-zoster Renal dosing: Cr Cl 10–50 cc/min, 125 mg Q24H for herpes simplex and 500 mg Q12–24H for varicella-zoster; Cr Cl < 10 cc/min, 125 mg Q48H for herpes simplex and 250 mg Q48 for varicella-zoster
- **Cost: Moderate to very high** depending on dose

Ganciclovir and Valganciclovir

Chemical Structure and Mechanisms of Action
- A guanine analogue-like acyclovir
  ◦ Has an additional hydroxymethyl group on the acyclic side chain.
  ◦ Converted to the monophosphate form by viral thymidine kinase followed by host cell kinase phosphorylation to produce the active triphosphate form.
  ◦ Valganciclovir is a more completely orally absorbed L-valyl ester of ganciclovir that is rapidly converted to ganciclovir.
- Triphosphate competitively inhibits viral DNA polymerase incorporation of guanosine triphosphate into elongating DNA.
  ◦ Does not act as a chain terminator.
  ◦ Intracellular concentrations of ganciclovir triphosphate are 10-fold higher in infected cells as compared to acyclovir triphosphate.
  ◦ Triphosphate persists, having a intracellular half-life of 16–24 hours.
  ◦ Higher intracellular concentrations may account for its greater activity against cytomegalovirus.
- Resistance
  ◦ Requires viral thymidine kinase activity for conversion to the active triphosphate form.
  ◦ Acyclovir-resistant viral strains with decreased thymidine kinase activity are also less sensitive to ganciclovir.
  ◦ Mutations that alter the structure of the viral DNA polymerase confer ganciclovir resistance as well as foscarnet and cidofovir resistance.

Toxicity
- Ganciclovir triphosphate concentrates in uninfected as well as virally infected cells.
  ◦ Bone marrow progenitor cells affected.
  ◦ Incorporates into cellular DNA and blocks host cell DNA replication.
  ◦ Neutropenia and thrombocytopenia are commonly observed in AIDs patients.
    ▪ Close monitoring of their white blood cell and platelet counts required during therapy.
    ▪ Coadministration of zidovudine increases the risk.
    ▪ Risk lower but significant in transplant patients.
    ▪ Discontinue if the absolute neutrophil count drops below 500 cells/mm^3.
- Central nervous system side effects also common and include:
  ◦ Headache
  ◦ Confusion, psychosis, coma
  ◦ Seizures
- Less common side effects: rash, fever, phlebitis, abnormal liver function tests.

Spectrum of Activity and Treatment Indications
- Highest activity against cytomegalovirus (CMV).
- Also active against:
  ◦ Herpes simplex-1 and -2
  ◦ Varicella zoster
  ◦ Epstein-Barr virus

- Recommended for:
  - CMV infections
    - Treatment of choice for retinitis, pneumonia, and colitis
    - Prophylaxis in transplant patients
    - Maintenance therapy in AIDs patients with persistently low CD4 lymphocyte counts
  - Not recommended for other viral infections because of problems of bone marrow toxicity.

Pharmacokinetics
- Oral ganciclovir absorption is poor (5–9% bioavailability).
  - Can achieve low therapeutic serum levels.
  - Absorption is improved by taking with food.
- Valganciclovir, a prodrug of ganciclovir, has better oral bioavailability (60%).
  - Rapidly hydrolyzed to ganciclovir by esterases in intestinal and hepatic cells.
  - When taken with food, 900-mg dose is equivalent to 5 mg/kg of IV ganciclovir.
  - High-fat food significantly increases bioavailability and increases serum levels.
- Intravenous administration is recommended for active CMV infection and oral administration for maintenance and prophylaxis. Oral valganciclovir achieved similar response rates to IV ganciclovir in CMV retinitis.
- Readily penetrates all tissues and fluids, including the brain and cerebrospinal fluid.
- Ganciclovir primarily excreted unmodified in the urine.
- Half-life of 2–5 hours

Dose and Cost
- Ganciclovir: Oral: 1,000 mg TID. Renal dosing: Cr Cl 50–80 cc/min, 500 mg TID; Cr Cl 10–50 cc/min, 500 mg QD; Cr Cl< 10 cc/min, 500 mg 3× per week.
- Intravenous: induction—5 mg/kg Q12H; maintenance—5 mg/kg QD. Renal dosing: Cr Cl 50–80 cc/min, induction—2.5 mg/kg Q12H; maintenance—2.5 mg/kg QD; Cr Cl 10–50 cc/min, induction—2.5 mg/kg QD; maintenance—1.2 mg/kg QD; Cr Cl < 10 cc/min, induction—1.25 mg 3× per week; maintenance—0.6 mg/kg 3× per week.
- Valganciclovir: induction—900 mg po BID; maintenance—900 mg QD. Renal dosing: Cr Cl 40–59 cc/min, induction—450 mg BID; maintenance—450 mg QD; Cr Cl 25–39 cc/min, induction—450 mg QD; maintenance—450 mg Q48H; Cr Cl 10–24 cc/min, induction—450 mg Q48H, maintenance—450 mg twice/week.
- **Cost: Ganciclovir oral: Very high; intravenous: moderate; Valganciclovir oral: Very high**

Cidofovir

Chemistry and Mechanism of Action
- Analogue of deoxycytidine monophosphate
- Inhibits viral DNA synthesis.
  - Acts as a competitive inhibitor of viral DNA polymerase.
  - Also adds to DNA, substituting for deoxycytidine triphosphate (dCTP), causing premature chain termination.
- Does not require viral kinase for activity.
  - Converted by cellular enzymes to its active diphosphate form.
  - Viral thymidine kinase mutants do not impair cidofovir activity.
- Resistance conferred through viral DNA polymerase mutations.
  - Results in cross-resistance to ganciclovir and less commonly to foscarnet.

Toxicity
- Highly nephrotoxic
  - Causes proteinuria in half of patients.
  - Azotemia and metabolic acidosis in a significant number.
  - Vigorous saline hydration and coadministration of probenecid reduces nephrotoxicity.
  - Discontinue if proteinuria of 3+ or higher develops or if the serum creatinine increases by > 0.4 mg/dl.
- Neutropenia less common.
- Other side effects include nausea, vomiting, diarrhea, rash, anterior uveitis, and headache.

Spectrum of Activity and Recommended Uses
- Activity against many DNA viruses:
  - CMV
  - Herpes simplex
  - Herpesvirus 6 and 8
  - Varicella-zoster virus
  - Pox viruses including smallpox, papilloma viruses, polyoma viruses, and adenoviruses
- Approved for the treatment of CMV retinitis in AIDs patients.
  - Parenteral use of this drug in other viral infections is likely to be limited because of its highly toxic profile.
  - Topical therapy may prove efficacious in acyclovir-resistant HSV infections in AIDs patients.
  - Being studied for the treatment of anogenital warts.

Pharmacokinetics
- Half-life of 17–65 hours
- Cidofovir is cleared by the kidneys

Dose and Cost
- Dose: 5 mg/kg IV Q 2 weeks; contraindicated in patients with Cr Cl < 50 cc/min.
- **Cost: Very high**

Foscarnet

Chemical Structure and Mechanism of Action
- An inorganic pyrophosphate analogue, trisodium phosphonoformate
- Reversibly blocks the pyrophosphate binding site of viral DNA polymerase, inhibiting the polymerase from binding deoxynucleotide triphosphates (dNTPs).
- Resistance is rare. Due to mutations to the viral DNA polymerase.

Toxicity
- Nephrotoxicity most common serious side effect
  - Azotemia, proteinuria
  - Rarely acute tubular necrosis
  - Usually develops during the second week of therapy and reverses when the drug is discontinued.
  - Dehydration increases the incidence and saline loading reduces this complication.

- Metabolic abnormalities are frequent.
  - Hypocalcemia due to chelation by foscarnet
    - Reduced ionized calcium can cause CNS disturbances, tetany, paresthesias, and seizures.
  - Hypophosphatemia
  - Hypomagnesemia
  - Hypokalemia
  - To minimize, intravenous infusion should not exceed 1 mg/kg/min.
  - Electrolytes, magnesium, phosphate, and calcium should be closely monitored.
- Other common side effects include: fever, headache, nausea, vomiting, and abnormal liver function tests.

Spectrum of Activity and Treatment Indications
- Active against:
  - Cytomegalovirus
  - Herpes simplex
  - Varicella-zoster virus
  - Epstein-Barr virus
  - Herpesvirus 8
- Approved for the treatment of:
  - Cytomegalovirus retinitis
  - Acyclovir-resistant mucocutaneous herpes simplex

Pharmacokinetics
- Poorly absorbed orally and is administered intravenously.
- Penetrates all tissues and fluids, achieving excellent levels in the CSF and vitreous humor.
- Half-life of 4–8 hours
- Renal excreted unmodified

Dose and Cost
- Dose: Induction—60 mg/kg Q8H IV (maintenance—90–120 mg/kg QD). Renal dosing: Cr Cl 50–80 cc/min: induction—40–50 mg/kg Q8H (maintenance—60–90 mg/kg QD); Cr Cl 10–50 cc/min: induction—20–30 mg/kg Q8H (maintenance—50–80 mg/kg QD); Cr Cl < 10 cc/min, contraindicated for both induction and maintenance.
- **Cost: High for induction, moderate for maintenance**

Ribavirin

Chemical Structure and Mechanism of Action
- A guanosine analogue that contains the D-ribose side chain.
- Inhibits both DNA and RNA viruses.
- Mechanisms of inhibition are complex and not completely understood.
  - Phosphorylated to the triphosphate form by host cell enzymes and the triphosphate form interferes with viral messenger RNA formation.
  - Monophosphate form interferes with guanosine triphosphate synthesis, lowering nucleic acid pools in the cell.

Toxicity
- Dose-related red blood cell hemolysis
- High doses suppress the bone marrow.
  - Anemia reverses when the drug is discontinued.

- Other side effects include: rash, pruritus, nausea, cough, and depression.
- Aerosolized ribavirin can cause:
  - Conjunctivitis
  - Bronchospasm can lead to deterioration of pulmonary function.
  - Teratogenic and embryotoxic effects noted in some animal studies. Pregnant health care workers should not administer.

Spectrum of Activity and Treatment Recommendations
- Active against a broad spectrum of DNA and RNA viruses including:
  - Respiratory syncytial virus
  - Influenza and parainfluenza virus
  - Herpes
  - Adenovirus
  - Poxviruses
  - Bunyavirus and arenaviruses
- Approved in the United States for:
- Aerosol treatment of RSV bronchiolitis and pneumonia in hospitalized patients
- Treatment of chronic hepatitis C. Oral ribavirin in combination with interferon.
- Intravenous administration is not approved in the United States, but available for patients with Lassa fever and some other forms of hemorrhagic fever.

Pharmacokinetics
- One third of orally administered ribavirin is absorbed.
- Penetrates all tissues and body fluids.
- The triphosphate becomes highly concentrated in erythrocytes ($40 \times$ plasma levels) and persists within them for prolonged periods.
- Prolonged half-life of 300 hours
- Cleared by both the kidneys and liver
- Aerosolized ribavirin results in high levels in the respiratory secretions that have a half-life of up to 2.5 hours.
  - A special aerosol generator is required for proper administration.

Dose and Cost
- Dose: Oral—1.0–1.2 gm QD. Renal dosing: Cr Cl < 10 cc/min, not recommended.
- **Cost: Very high**

Interferons

Chemical Structure and Mechanism of Action
- Interferons (IFN)
  - 16–27,000 Da molecular weight proteins synthesized by eukaryotic cells in response to viral infections.
  - Stimulate host antiviral responses.
  - INF receptors regulate approximately 100 genes and rapidly produce dozens of proteins.
  - A wide variety of RNA viruses are susceptible.
  - Most DNA viruses are only minimally affected.

Toxicity
- Mild side effects with doses below 5 million units
  - Influenza-like syndrome
    - 1–2 million units can cause an influenza-like syndrome, particularly severe during the first week
    - Reduced by premedication with antipyretics such as aspirin, ibuprofen, and acetaminophen
- Higher doses (> 5 million units) cause more serious toxicities:
  - Bone marrow suppression doses > 5 million units: granulocytopenia and thrombocytopenia
  - Neurotoxicity leading to confusion, somnolence, and behavior disturbances
  - Hepatoxicity
  - Retinopathy
- Local irritation at injection sites frequent after subcutaneous and intramuscular injection

Spectrum of Activity and Treatment Recommendations
- Effectiveness of INFs has been limited by the frequent side effects.
- Approved for the treatment of:
  - Chronic hepatitis C
  - Chronic hepatitis B
  - Kaposi's sarcoma
  - Condyloma acuminatum

Pharmacokinetics
- INF-α is well absorbed intramuscularly and subcutaneously.
  - Other interferons have more variable absorption.
- Activity that persists for 4 days after a single dose.
  - Pegelated forms result in slow release and result in more prolonged activity, allowing once-per-week administration.

Dose and Cost
- Dose: IFN-α 2A or 2B: 3 million units 3× per week (hepatitis C); 30–35 million units/week (hepatitis B); 30–36 million units 3–7× per week (Kaposi's sarcoma); 1 million units intralesional 3× per week (condyloma acuminata)
- Peginterferon-α 2B: Pegintron—1.5 µg/kg SC Q 1 week + ribovirin; Pegasys—180 mg SC Q 1 week + ribovirin (both for treatment of hepatitis C)
- **Cost: Very high**

ANTI-INFLUENZA VIRAL AGENTS

Amantadine and Rimantadine

Mechanism of Action
- Effective only against influenza A.
- Amantadine and rimantadine bind to and inhibit the M2 protein, a viral protein important for viral particle assembly expressed on the surface of infected cells.

Toxicity
- Amantadine causes moderate CNS side effects, especially in the elderly
  - Insomnia, inability to concentrate, and dizziness
  - Increases the risk of seizures in patients with a past history of epilepsy.
- Rimantadine causes CNS side effects less frequently.

Treatment Recommendations
- Must be given within 48 hours of the onset of symptoms to be effective.
- Efficacy has been proven in healthy adults.

Dose and Cost
- Dose: Amantadine: 200 mg po QD × 3–5 days. Renal dosing: 100 mg QD in patients with impaired renal function and in the elderly.
- **Cost: Low**
- Rimantadine: 200 mg po QD × 3–5 days. Renal dosing: 100 mg QD in patients with renal impairment and in the elderly.
- **Cost: Moderate**

Neuramidase Inhibitors

Mechanism of Action
- Block viral neuramidase activity of both influenza A and B.

Toxicity
- Zanamivir inhaler commonly causes bronchospasm, limiting its usefulness.

Treatment
- Must also be given within 48 hours of the onset of symptoms to be effective.

Dose and Cost
- Zanamivir: 10 mg QD intranasally for 5 days
  - **Cost: Moderate**
- Oseltamivir is well absorbed orally; oral dose is 75 mg OD for 5 days.
  - **Cost: Moderate**
- Amantadine, rimantadine, or oseltamivir can be given for longer duration as prophylaxis in patients at risk of serious complications from influenza.
- Influenza vaccine is preferred for prophylaxis.

FURTHER READING

Antibiotic Handbooks
Bartlett JG: *Pocket Book of Infectious Disease Therapy*. Philadelphia: Lippincott Williams and Wilkins, 2001.
Gilbert DN, Moellering RC Jr., Sande MA: *Sanford Guide to Antimicrobial Therapy*. Hyde Park, VT: Antimicrobial Therapy, Inc., 2001.

PDA Sources
EPocrates and ePocrates ID. Web address: www.epocrates.com.
Johns Hopkins Division of Infectious Diseases Antibiotic Guide. Web address: www.hopkins-abxguide.org.

Other
The choice of antibacterial drugs. *The Medical Letter* 1999; 41: 95–104.
Hardman JG, Limbird LE: *Goodman & Gilman's The Pharmacological Basis of Therapeutics*. New York: McGraw-Hill Medical Publishers, 2001.
Mandell GL, Bennett JE, Dolin R: *Principles and Practice of Infectious Diseases*. Philadelphia: Churchill Livingstone, 2000.

CHAPTER

2

THE SEPSIS SYNDROME

HIGHLIGHTS

- Associated with a high mortality.
- Toll-like receptors play a key role in the innate immune response to sepsis.
- Bacterial cell wall components and exotoxins produce a "cytokine storm."
- Early broad-spectrum antibiotics and volume replacement play critical roles in reducing mortality.
- Drotrecogin alpha–activated protein C should be used only in severely ill patients with Apache scores ≥ 25.

POTENTIAL SEVERITY

- Life-threatening syndrome.
- Must be recognized and treated quickly to prevent progression to irreversible shock.

PREVALENCE

- A problem of increasing magnitude in the United States
- 300,000–500,000 cases per year
- 15–60% mortality, the risk of death is related to:
  - Underlying diseases
  - Age
  - Infecting organism
  - Appropriateness of empiric anti-infective therapy
- The sepsis syndrome caused by:
  - Bacterial infections are most common
  - Viral infections, e.g., dengue fever
  - Fungal infections, e.g., candidemia
  - Noninfectious diseases, e.g., pancreatitis, can mimic the sepsis syndrome

Based on Chapter 2 by Dr. Reuben Ramphal in *Infectious Diseases in 30 Days*, F Southwick, ed.

DEFINITIONS OF SEPSIS

- Best defined as the "systemic inflammatory response syndrome" (SIRS) caused by:
  - ○ Microbial products from viable or dead organisms.
  - ○ Entities other than infection causing tissue necrosis and inflammation.
- Severe sepsis = sepsis with organ dysfunction.
- Septic shock = hypotension due to sepsis that is unresponsive to initial attempts at volume expansion.
- Bacteremia is often called sepsis; however, only some bacteremias result in the sepsis syndrome, and all sepsis syndromes are not caused by bacteremia.
- Approximately 40% of patients with the sepsis syndrome have a proven infection.

PATHOGENESIS

- Activation of cellular pathways that trigger innate immune responses and the coagulation cascade.
- Bacterial cell wall components bind to specific host cell receptors and activate the innate immune response.
  - ○ Gram-negative bacteria have lipopolysaccharide (LPS), also called endotoxin, linked to their outer membrane.
    - This product alone can produce the syndrome.
    - Endotoxin (LPS) is found in the bloodstream of patients with gram-negative bacteremia.
    - Endotoxin (LPS) blood levels correlate with the clinical severity of the sepsis syndrome.
  - ○ Gram-positive bacteria produce peptidoglycans and lipoteichoic acid that mimic endotoxins in their effects on the host.
  - ○ Gram-positive bacteria also secrete exotoxins.
    - *S. aureus* can secrete toxic shock syndrome toxin-1 (TSST-1).
    - *S. pyogenes* secretes streptococcal pyrogenic exotoxin A (SPEA).
  - ○ Fungal cell walls can also activate the innate immune response.
- Host cell receptors that respond to bacterial and fungal cell wall components.
  - ○ The monocyte-macrophage is the first cell to respond to endotoxin.
    - Endotoxin first binds to LPS-binding protein produced by the liver in response to inflammation and this protein complex binds to two surface receptors on mononuclear cells.
      - CD14
      - Toll-like receptors (TLR)
  - ○ TLR are able to recognize substances produced by multiple pathogens.
    - TLR2 recognizes peptidoglycans, mannans, and lipotechoic acids
    - TLR4 recognizes LPS
    - TLR5 recognizes bacterial flagellin
  - ○ TLR receptor binding results in signal transduction and cell activation, leading to cytokine release.

- Cytokines and other inflammatory mediator cascades
  - Stimulated monocytes-macrophages produce proinflammatory cytokines (i.e., stimulate inflammation).
    - Tumor necrosis factor-α (TNF)
    - IL-1, IL-6, IL-8
    - Followed by interferon-γ
  - Infection activates the complement and coagulation pathways.
  - Infection stimulates neutrophils and monocytes to produce reactive oxygen intermediates.
- How infection leads to septic shock (see Fig. 2-1)
  - Release of the inflammatory mediators described above leads to:
    - Endothelial damage resulting in fluid leakage
    - Loss of vascular resistance
    - Reduced cardiac inotropy
    - Extensive coagulation and disseminated coagulopathy
  - End result is end organ damage that eventually will lead to organ failure and death.
  - The larger the inoculum of the challenge molecule, the more rapid the progression of these events.
    - The potency of the various cell wall products to stimulate the innate immune system varies.
    - Endotoxin is a more powerful stimulant than the cell walls of enterococci or coagulase-negative staphylococci.

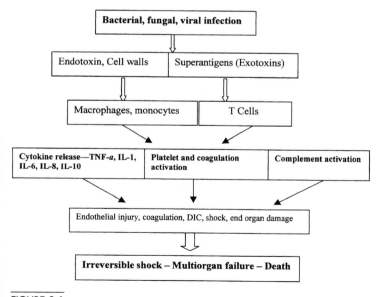

FIGURE 2-1
Pathophysiology of the sepsis syndrome.

CLINICAL MANIFESTATIONS OF THE
SEPSIS SYNDROME

- Fever
  - Usually the first and most common manifestation of sepsis.
  - The greater the height of the temperature, the more likely a patient is bacteremic.
  - Hypothermia and normal body temperature can be seen in patients who are bacteremic.
    - Hypothermia is a poor prognostic indicator in bacteremic patients.
- Hemodynamic changes
  - Tachycardia in association with fever is to be expected.
  - Bradycardia is unusual, being found in typhoid fever and brucellosis.
  - Hypotension the most important determinant of outcome.
  - Preshock the stage at which hypotension is reversible.
    - Characterized by warm skin, diminished mentation (often worse in the elderly), and oliguria.
    - Failure to reverse hypotension in its early stages results in serious end organ damage.
  - Persistent hypotension often not reversed by antibiotics and other measures.
    - Characterized by cool skin, acute renal failure, and, later, hepatic injury.
- Acid-base disturbances
  - Reduced tissue perfusion results in shift from aerobic to anaerobic metabolism causing lactic acid accumulation.
  - Respiratory alkalosis usually seen first as a consequence of tachypnea (see below). The first pronounced change, signaling impending shock.
    - Seen at the time when hemodynamic changes are reversible with fluid resuscitation.
    - Critical to recognize this early reversible stage of septic shock.
  - Metabolic acidosis develops just prior to or accompanies hypotension.
    - Signals the beginning of a fatal downward spiral.
    - Reflects severe organ hypoperfusion and failure.
- Respiratory changes
  - Tachypnea is a common feature of early sepsis.
    - Caused by stimulation of the CNS respiratory center by cytokines, elevated body temperature, and the accumulation of lactic acid.
  - Adult respiratory distress syndrome (ARDS) is common in severe cases.
    - Can be induced by endotoxin
      - Activates neutrophils that become trapped in the small vessels of the lung
      - Release of toxic neutrophil oxygen products and proteases causes vessel wall damage and leakage of fluid into the alveoli
    - Chest X-ray changes mimic cardiac pulmonary edema
    - Accompanied by severe hypoxemia
  - Pneumonia may be seen on chest X-ray, and infection of lungs can be accompanied by bacteremia and the sepsis syndrome (see Chap. 4).

- Toxic shock syndrome
  - Caused by the exotoxin toxic shock syndrome toxin-1 (TSST-1) produced by some strains of *S. aureus*.
  - Can be seen in association with menstruation in young women with vaginal *S. aureus* infection, usually associated with tampons.
  - Also seen with TSST-1 producing strains of *S. aureus* causing soft tissue infection.
    - Fever and profound shock are followed by:
      - Conjunctival hyperemia
      - Palmar hyperemia and desquamation
- Necrotizing fasciitis due to *Streptococcus pyogenes*
  - Streptococcal pyrogenic exotoxin A (SPEA). Causes:
    - Shock
    - Tissue necrosis, including the fascia, resulting in necrotizing fasciitis
  - TSST-1 and SPEA are superantigens.
    - Proteins capable of bypassing the macrophage are termed "superantigens."
    - Superantigens directly activate lymphocytes to release cytokines.
    - Unlike conventional antigens, they do not require processing by macrophages and dendritic cells, the cytokine cascade being triggered at the level of T cells.

DIAGNOSIS OF THE SEPSIS SYNDROME

- Early diagnosis is difficult.
- Laboratory studies recommended in patients with suspected sepsis syndrome:
  1. Two blood cultures, urine culture, and sputum culture if a patient has chest X-ray abnormalities
  2. Complete blood count with differential and platelet
  3. Coagulation studies to include INR, fibrinogen, and D-dimers or fibrin split products
  4. Blood gases and metabolic panel
- Common clinical and laboratory findings indicative of sepsis include:
  1. Temperature $< 36°C$ or $> 38°C$
  2. Pulse rate > 90/min
  3. Respiratory rate > 20/min
  4. $PaCO_2 < 32$ with pH > 7.45 (early sepsis)
  5. WBC $< 4,000$/mm^3 or $> 12,000$ with a band count $> 10\%$
  6. Chills, lethargy, hemorrhagic skin lesions
- Fever, tachycardia, and tachypnea with or without leukocytosis = SIRS
- SIRS combined with a positive blood culture, preferably two (excluding coagulase-negative staphylococci) = sepsis syndrome
- Exceptions made in patients in whom there is clear clinical evidence of an intra-abdominal infection such as peritonitis
- Other findings may include:
  - Hypotension not due to hypovolemia, or a recent cardiac event. In more severe cases accompanied by increased cardiac output and changes in peripheral vascular resistance.
  - Thrombocytopenia
  - Evidence of fibrinogen consumption and clot lysis

TABLE 2-1
EMPIRIC ANTIBIOTIC THERAPY FOR THE SEPSIS SYNDROME

Site of Infection	Pathogens to Be Covered	Antibiotics
Lung (hospital acquired)	*Pseudomonas aeruginosa* Enterobacter	Cefepime or ticarcillin/ clavulanate Piperacillin/ tazobactam + aminoglycoside
Abdomen Pelvis	Gram-negative rods Anaerobes	Ticarcillin/ clavulanate or piperacillin/ tazobactam + aminoglycoside Imipenem/ meropenem
Urinary tract	*E. coli* Klebsiella Proteus	Ciprofloxacin Ceftriaxone
Skin	*S. aureus* *S. pyogenes*	Oxacillin or vancomycin Ticarcillin/ clavulanate
	Mixed aerobic/anaerobic Necrotizing fasciitis	Piperacillin/ tazobactam Imipenem/ meropenem
Bacteremia of unknown source (hospital acquired)	*S. aureus* (MRSA) Gram-negative rods	Cefepime + vancomycin
Bacteremia of unknown source (community acquired)	*S. aureus* *S. pneumoniae* *E. coli* Klebsiella Proteus	Vancomycin + ceftriaxone or cefepime

TREATMENT OF THE SEPSIS SYNDROME

ANTIBIOTIC THERAPY

- Empiric antibiotics are critical.
- Therapy must treat the most probable site of the infection and cover the most likely pathogens from that site (see Table 2-1).
- Other findings may help direct empiric therapy:
  - Petechial skin rash must consider:
    - Meningococcemia or gonococcemia
    - *S. aureus* bacteremia or localized *S. aureus* infection
- Coverage for every possible pathogen is not possible, and certain pathogens in certain locations are unlikely to cause the sepsis syndrome and do not need to be covered:
  - Enterococci at most sites
  - *S. aureus* in the respiratory tract
- Empiric therapy must be adjusted to reflect antibiotic sensitivities of the hospital bacterial flora.
- In 24–48 hours after blood culture results are available, the antibiotic regimen needs to be adjusted and narrower-spectrum antibiotics utilized (see Chap. 1).

MANAGEMENT OF PATIENTS WITH SIGNS OF SEVERE SEPSIS

- In addition to prompt administration of antibiotics, volume expansion, initially with normal saline.
- Immediate surgical consultation must be sought if there is:
  - A possible undrained infected intra-abdominal site (see Chap. 8)
  - Gas present in soft tissues or clinical evidence of a necrotizing soft tissue infection (see Chap. 10)
- Intravascular catheters must be removed and cultured (see Chap. 7).
- If the patient is to be treated on conventional ward, the parameters to be followed include:
  - Hourly measurements of vital signs and urine output
  - Two-hourly measurements of arterial blood pH, $PaCO_2$, and PaO_2
  - Blood lactate and coagulation parameters initially, and every 4–6 hours until the patient is clinically stable
- Transfer to the intensive-care unit for closer monitoring if:
  - Persistent hypotension
  - Accumulation of lactate
  - Increasing hypoxemia
  - Laboratory signs suggesting a coagulopathy
- If BP fails to increase with volume replacement, vasopressors recommended.
  - Begin with dopamine.
  - Progress to norepinephrine.
  - Aggressive fluid resuscitation is continued with specific attention to central venous pressure and pulmonary vascular congestion.

ADJUNCTIVE THERAPIES

- Many adjunctive measures have failed to improve mortality in large studies:
  - Anti-inflammatory agents such as corticosteroids and ibuprophen
  - Narcotic antagonists
  - Monoclonal antibody against the core of the endotoxin molecule
  - Antibody against TNF and the TNF receptor
  - IL-1 receptor antagonists
  - Platelet-activating factor antagonists

DROTRECOGIN ALPHA

- Protein C levels are often low in septic patients.
  - Protein C plays a key role in inhibiting coagulation.
  - May be an important inhibitor of monocyte activation.
- Infusion of activated protein C reduces the mortality of lethal *E. coli* infections in animals.
- Infusion in humans is associated with a 6% reduction in mortality in severe septic shock (Apache score ≥ 25): 30.8% in placebo vs. 24.7% in treated patients.
- Infusion in patients with less severe sepsis (Apache score < 25) is not cost effective.
- Activated protein C (Drotrecogin alpha), is approved by the FDA for the treatment of severe sepsis as an adjunct to standard therapy.
- Should be ordered only by intensive-care and infectious disease specialist because:
  - Inclusion criteria are complex.
  - Cost is very high.
  - Bleeding complications can develop.
- Contraindication for this agent is recent surgery; the risk of bleeding complications is prohibitively high.

REFERENCES

Abraham E, Reinhart K, Opal S, Demeyer I, Doig C, et al: Efficacy and safety of tifacogin (recombinant tissue factor pathway inhibitor) in severe sepsis: A randomized controlled trial. *JAMA* 2003; 290:238–47.

Balk RA: Sepsis and septic shock: Definitions, epidemiology and clinical manifestations. *Crit Care Clin* 2000; 16:179–92.

Bernard GR, Vincent JL, Laterre PF, LaRosa SP, Dhainaut JF, Lopez-Rodriguez A, Steingrub JS, Garber GE, Helterbrand JD, Ely EW, Fisher CJ Jr.: Efficacy and safety of recombinant human activated protein C for severe sepsis. *N Engl J Med* 2001; 344:699–709.

Kreger BE, Craven DE, McCabe WR: Gram-negative bacteremia IV. Reevaluation of clinical features and treatment in 612 patients. *Am J Med* 1980; 68:344–55.

Manns BJ, Lee H, Doig CJ, Johnson D, Donaldson C: An economic evaluation of activated protein C treatment for severe sepsis. *N Engl J Med* 2002; 347:993–1000.

Pittet D, Li N, Woolson RF, Wentzel RP: Microbiological factors influencing the outcome of nosocomial bloodstream infections: A 6 year validated, population based model. *Clin Infect Dis* 1997; 24:1068–78.

Wheeler AP, Bernard GR: Treating patients with severe sepsis. *N Engl J Med* 1999; 340:207–14.

THE FEBRILE PATIENT

HIGHLIGHTS

- Fever is probably protective and is an indicator of ongoing inflammation.
- Fever may be reduced in the elderly and young children, patients with cardiac or pulmonary diseases.
- When fever is reduced, aspirin, acetaminophen, or NSIDS should be given as a standing dose rather than PRN.

TEMPERATURE REGULATION

- Regulated by the anterior hypothalamus near the optic chiasm in combination with:
  - ◦ Brain stem
  - ◦ Spinal cord
  - ◦ Sympathetic ganglia
- The anterior hypothalamus has a distinct temperature set point.
  - ◦ Below this set point body metabolism increases, shivering and chills develop.
  - ◦ Above this set point peripheral blood flow increases, and sweating develops.
- "Normal" body temperature is 98.6 °F or 37 °C.
  - ◦ The set point follows a normal distribution.
    - ▪ Some individuals have a lower set point.
    - ▪ Others have a higher set point than the mean "normal" temperature.
  - ◦ Core temperature varies during the day, lower in the morning and higher in the evening.
- Diagnosis of fever must take into account the individual patient's normal set point and diurnal variation in core temperature.

MECHANISMS UNDERLYING THE FEBRILE RESPONSE

- The set point of the anterior hypothalamus is increased by inflammatory mediators:
  - ◦ Interleukin-1 (IL-1)
  - ◦ Tumor necrosis factor-α (TNF-α)
  - ◦ Interleukin-6 (IL-6)
  - ◦ Interferon-γ (IFN-γ)
- Cytokines are released by monocytes and macrophages in response to the invasion by various pathogens and other inflammatory stimuli.

- Cytokines stimulate the circumventricular organs near the optic chiasm, activating phopholipase A_2, and the cyclooxygenase pathway, increasing prostaglandin E_2.
- Prostaglandin E_2 crosses the blood-brain barrier and stimulates the neurons in the anterior hypothalamus.

BENEFITS AND HARMFUL EFFECTS OF FEVER

Benefits of Fever
- Serves as a warning sign for the onset of infection.
- Inhibits the growth of some viruses, bacteria, fungi, and parasites.
- Enhances the ability of macrophages and neutrophils to kill foreign pathogens and to improve cell-mediated immune function.

Harmful Effects of Fever
- Patients with heart disease, danger of cardiac ischemia fever
  ○ Increases heart rate
  ○ Increases cardiac oxygen demands
- Patients with severe pulmonary disease unable to compensate for the increased oxygen demands.
- Elderly patients can develop confusion and lethargy.
- Children can suffer from seizures in association with high fever.
  ○ No proof that reducing fever prevents febrile seizures.

TREATMENT OF FEVER
- Treat the underlying cause of the fever.
- Role of lowering body temperature remains controversial.
- Direct cooling of the body using ice, cold water, or cooling blanket not recommended.
  ○ Considered only in conjunction with medicines that reset the thermal set point.
  ○ Otherwise induces chills and shivering, increasing patient discomfort.
- Antipyretics probably warranted in:
  ○ Patients with heart disease
  ○ Patients with severe pulmonary disease
  ○ Elderly patients with mental dysfunction in association with fever
- The pharmacologic agents to reset the thermal set point all equally effective.
  ○ Inhibit prostaglandin synthetase activity and reduce prostaglandin E_2 production
  ○ Aspirin—avoid in children because of the increased risk of Reye's syndrome (results in hepatic and renal failure)
  ○ Nonsteroidal anti-inflammatory drugs (NSIDs)—avoid in patients with ischemic heart disease. Have been associated with coronary artery vasoconstriction
  ○ Acetaminophen—avoid in patients with serious underlying liver disease
- Administer antipyretic agents on a regular basis until the primary cause of fever has been treated.
  ○ Avoid repeated shifting of the thermal set point and recurrent shivering and chills caused by prn dosing.

FEVER OF UNDETERMINED ORIGIN (FUO)

HIGHLIGHTS

- FUO is a distinct clinical entity with a specific definition.
- Clinicians tend to overtest in this condition.
- After routine testing, additional tests should be ordered following Sutton's law: Go for "where the money is"; i.e., direct testing to explore specific abnormalities.
- Antibiotics are contraindicated in FUO.

POTENTIAL SEVERITY

- A chronic disorder that requires a thoughtful diagnostic approach.

DEFINITION OF FUO

- An illness that has lasted at least 3 weeks.
  - 3 weeks or longer excludes self-limited viral illnesses.
- Fever of over 101 °F or 38.3 °C on several occasions.
  - Eliminates persons who have a slightly higher core temperature set point and an exaggerated diurnal temperature variation.
- No diagnosis after routine workup for 3 days in hospital or after 3 or more outpatient visits.

OTHER IMPORTANT POINTS ABOUT DIAGNOSIS OF FUO

- Must document true fever.
  - Patient should measure both 6 A.M. and 6 P.M. temperature to rule out an exaggerated circadian rhythm.
  - An electronic thermometer should always be used to exclude factitious fever (see below).
- Exact pattern of fever usually not helpful. Exceptions:
  - Cyclic neutropenia
    - A defect of bone marrow stem cells that results in neutropenia every 21 days.
    - Neutrophils nadir associated with fever.
    - Weekly peripheral white blood cell counts with differential recommended for diagnosis.
  - Malaria
    - Periodic fever in *Plasmodium vivax*, *P. ovale*, and *P. malaria*.
    - Takes 1–2 weeks to synchronize the lysis of red blood cells by the trophozoites.
    - Once synchronized, red blood cell lysis occurs in 2–3-day intervals.
    - Associated with high fever, sweats, chills, and malaise.
  - Hodgkin's disease
    - Stage B Hodgkin's disease; abnormal T cells intermittently release pyrogens.
    - Fever develops at irregular intervals, followed by periods of normal body temperature.
      - Called Pel-Ebstein fever

CAUSES OF FUO

- Three major categories ("the big three")
    1. Infections
    2. Neoplasms
    3. Autoimmune disorders
- Miscellaneous etiologies, six diseases ("the little six") most common
    1. Granulomatous diseases
    2. Regional enteritis
    3. Familial Mediterranean fever (FMF)
    4. Drug fever
    5. Pulmonary emboli
    6. Factitious fever

INFECTIOUS CAUSES OF FUO

- Epidemiology important: The most common cause of FUO in patients < 65 years.
- Animal exposure, insect bites, outdoor camping, travel, and exposure to infected humans.
- Abdominal abscess, miliary tuberculosis, and disseminated fungal infections can be fatal.
- Prior antibiotic administration interferes with diagnosis.
- Most common infectious causes include:
    1. Abscesses
        ○ Abdominal abscesses most common.
        ○ May persist for prolonged periods before being diagnosed.
        ○ Improvements in imaging techniques have improved our ability to locate and drain.
    2. Osteomyelitis
        ○ Vertebra, mandible, and sinuses most common.
        ○ Bone scan is particularly helpful in identifying such infections.
    3. Subacute bacterial endocarditis
        ○ An audible murmur usually present.
        ○ Hold blood cultures for 2–3 weeks to grow fastidious slow-growing pathogens such as the HASEK organisms.
        ○ Draw large volumes of blood for culture (10 cc/culture) to improve the sensitivity of blood cultures.
        ○ Transesophageal echocardiography improves the ability to identify vegetations.
        ○ SBE is now a less common cause of FUO owing to improved culture techniques and echocardiography.
        ○ Administration of antibiotics reduces the utility of blood cultures. Must discontinue for 7–10 days before blood cultures become sensitive.
    4. Biliary system infections. Patients often have no right upper quadrant pain and no right upper quadrant tenderness.
    5. Subacute pyelonephritis can have prolonged fever in the absence of dysuria, frequency, or flank pain.

6. Miliary tuberculosis must always be considered (see Chap. 4).
   ○ Potentially lethal disease
   ○ Most common in:
     ▪ The elderly
     ▪ Immunocompromised patients, particularly HIV patients and patients on high-dose glucocorticoids
   ○ Bone marrow culture helpful in making this diagnosis.
   ○ CXR: micronodular (millet seed) interstitial changes, may be absent in the elderly.
   ○ If suspected, antituberculous therapy should be initiated promptly or the patient will deteriorate over 2–3 weeks and die.
7. Spirochetes (see Chap. 13). Leptospirosis is difficult to diagnose. Consider if:
   ○ Appropriate epidemiology (animal, contaminated soil or water exposure)
   ○ Conjuctival suffusion
   ○ Aseptic meningitis
   ○ Liver enzyme abnormalities and renal dysfunction
   ○ Lyme disease and relapsing fever are due to other spirochetes that less commonly cause FUO
8. Brucellosis (see Chap. 13). Consider if:
   ○ Animal exposure, particularly the skinning of wild boar
   ○ Ingestion of unpasteurized cheese
9. Rickettsial infections, intracellular infections difficult to diagnose (see Chap. 13). Consider if:
   ○ History of camping, hunting, or other outdoor activities in areas endemic for these infections.
   ○ Tickborne; however a history of tick bite is not always obtained.
10. Chlamydia, another intracellular pathogen
    ○ *C. psittaci* can result in a mononucleosis-like syndrome. Usually contracted from birds, including pigeons, members of the parrot family (parakeets, macaws, and cockatoos), finches (canaries, goldfinches), and poultry.
11. Epstein-Barr virus and cytomegalovirus cause a mononucleosis syndrome (see Chap. 15).
    ○ Sore throat
    ○ Lymphadenopathy and splenomegaly
    ○ Prolonged fever
12. Fungi: cryptococcosis and histoplasmosis the two most common fungal diseases reported.
13. Parasites can cause prolonged fever (see Chap. 12).
    ○ Malaria (nonfalciparum forms)
    ○ Toxoplasmosis
    ○ Trypanosomiasis

NEOPLASTIC CAUSES OF FUO

• In elderly patients neoplasia is the most frequent cause of FUO.
• The most common neoplasms to cause FUO include:
   1. Lymphomas most common
      ○ Pel-Ebstein fever, and, when present, raises the possibility of Hodgkin's lymphoma.
      ○ Patients with non-Hodgkin's lymphoma may also present with fever.
      ○ Fever can be high and mimic sepsis.

2. Leukemia, particularly in the elderly during the aleukemic or the preleukemic phase.
   ○ May have little or no evidence of leukemia on peripheral smear.
3. Hypernephroma was noted to cause FUO in older series.
   ○ In a large series of patients with hypernephroma this solid tumor was rarely associated with fever.
4. Hepatoma is the most common solid tumor to cause FUO; tumors that metastasize to liver rarely cause fever.
5. Atrial myxoma is a rare disorder associated with fever.
   ○ Can mimic subacute bacterial endocarditis.
   ○ Small pieces of the atrial tumor embolize, causing small infarcts similar to bacterial endocarditis.

AUTOIMMUNE DISEASES

- Systemic lupus erythematosis (SLE) now an uncommon cause of FUO.
  ○ Antinuclear and anti-DNA markers are sensitive tests.
  ○ Readily identify cases of SLE within 3 weeks.
- Most common autoimmune diseases to cause FUO are:
  1. Still's disease or adult juvenile rheumatoid arthritis. Key features:
     ○ Usually seen in younger patients
     ○ Evanescent macular rash
     ○ Arthralgias and sore throat
     ○ High fevers accompanied by a high peripheral white blood cell count
       ▪ Frequently causes the physician to begin antibiotic therapy.
       ▪ Fever fails to subside after initiation of antibiotics.
     ○ There is no specific test for Still's disease. Findings suggesting the disease:
       ▪ Serum ferritin levels markedly elevated
       ▪ High ESR
     ○ Diagnosis is presumptive.
  2. Polymyalgia rheumatica and temporal arteritis
     ○ Seen in elderly patients
     ○ Proximal muscle weakness
     ○ High ESR
     ○ Temporal headaches can accompany polymyalgia rheumatica.
       ▪ Visual complaints are common, can lead to blindness
       ▪ Headache
       ▪ Diagnosis by temporal artery biopsy
  3. Polyarteritis nodosa
     ○ A multisystemic disease
       ▪ Fever and malaise and weight loss
       ▪ Gastrointestinal symptoms secondary to mesenteric artery involvement
       ▪ Nephritis
       ▪ Peripheral neuropathy
       ▪ Skin rash
       ▪ Arthritis may be polyarticular and often asymmetric
     ○ Laboratory tests nonspecific
       ▪ High ESR
       ▪ Leukocytosis
       ▪ Low serum complement
     ○ Diagnosis based on arterial biopsy

4. Hypersensitivity angiitis
   ○ Palpable petechial skin lesions
   ○ Diagnosis by skin biopsy
5. Mixed connective tissue disease
6. Subacute thyroiditis
   ○ May present with prolonged fever
   ○ Thyroid is often tender
   ○ Elevated serum antithyroid antibodies
7. Kikuchi's disease or histiocytic necrotizing lymphadenitis
   ○ Self-limited autoimmune disorder
   ○ Occurs in young Asian females
   ○ Associated with generalized lymphadenopathy
   ○ Diagnosis by lymph node biopsy

MISCELLANEOUS DISEASES (THE LITTLE 6)

1. Granulomatous diseases of unclear etiology
   ○ Presents with fever and malaise
   ○ Generally involves the liver
     ▪ LFTs: mild abnormalities in alkaline phosphatase
     ▪ Liver biopsy reveals granulomas
2. Regional enteritis
   ○ May present with prolonged fever in the absence of gastrointestinal complaints.
   ○ Contrast studies of the GI tract recommended to exclude this diagnosis.
3. Familial Mediterranean fever (FMF)
   ○ A genetic disorder; a family history is critical in raising this possibility.
   ○ Recurrent serositis primarily of the abdominal cavity
   ○ Can also result in pleuritis, and pericarditis
4. Drug fever
   ○ One of the most frequently encountered causes of FUO (see Table 3-1).
   ○ The antiseizure medication dilantin one of the most frequent offenders.
   ○ Other frequent medications associated with fever:
     ▪ Quinidine
     ▪ Procaine amide
     ▪ Penicillins
   ○ All medications should be discontinued or switched in cases of FUO.

TABLE 3-1
DRUGS CAUSING FUO

Antihistamines	INH
Barbiturates	Nitrofurantoin
Chlorambucil	Penicillins
Dilantin	Procaine amide
Hydralazine	Quinidine
Ibuprofen	Salicylates
Iodides	Thiouracil
Aldomet	Mercaptopurine

5. Pulmonary emboli
   - Prolonged bed rest increases the risk.
   - Small embolli may not result in respiratory complaints and may present as fever.
   - Needs to be excluded in all patients with FUO, who are at increased risk for thrombophlebitis.
6. Factitious fever
   - Manipulating the mercury thermometer was a common strategy in old series of FUO. No longer possible with electronic thermometers
   - Now induced by self-injection of saliva or stool causing polymicrobial bacteremia
   - Most common in females
   - A history of health care training should raise suspicion,
     - Particularly if the patient takes great interest in her/his illness
     - A medical textbook at the bedside highly suspicious
   - Diagnosis: a search of the patient's room seeking a syringe used for self-injection.

HISTORY IN FUO

- History can play a critical role, needs to be very complete.
- Review of symptoms (ROS) should be periodically updated.
- Repeated questioning important because symptoms are often transient and may be overlooked by the patient.
- Past medical history (PMH) often helpful.
  - History of tuberculosis exposure or a positive PPD should be included.
- Family history (FH) must also be thoroughly reviewed to exclude genetic disorders such as cyclic neutropenia and familial Mediterranean fever.
- Epidemiology history: Needs to include:
  - Animal exposure (pets, other domestic as well as wild animals)
  - Home environment
  - Occupational exposure
- Travel history; inquire about travel to areas endemic for:
  - Malaria
  - Other parasites
  - Typhoid
  - Coccidioidomycosis and histoplasmosis
  - Tick-borne illnesses
- Important to list all medications
  - Include over-the-counter and natural organic remedies

PHYSICAL EXAM IN FUO

- Careful repeat physical examination is frequently helpful.
- Focus on:
  - Skin exam, looking for:
    - Embolic or vasculitic lesions
    - Evidence of physical manipulation
    - Nail beds; small emboli can become trapped in the distal capillaries of the fingers and toes resulting in small splinter-shaped infarcts.
  - Joint motion and the presence of effusions
  - Careful eye exam looking for:
    - Conjunctival petechiae or conjunctivitis
    - Punctate corneal lesions
    - Uveitis, optic nerve changes, retinal or choroidal abnormalities
  - Palpation of all lymph nodes repeatedly
    - Record consistency, size, and tenderness.
    - Palpate femoral, axillary, epitrochlear, supraclavicular, and neck regions.
  - Cardiac exam, repeat daily, listening for:
    - Cardiac murmurs
    - Pericardial rubs
  - Abdominal exam daily, looking for:
    - New masses
    - Localized tenderness
    - Hepato- or splenomegaly

LABORATORY STUDIES IN FUO

- See Figure 3-1 for algorithm that guides the initial workup.
- Table 3-2 lists the basic preliminary tests recommended for FUO.
- Clinicians err on the side of excessive and uninformative testing.
- A cookbook approach subjects the patient to undue costly testing and stress.
- Tailor the diagnostic workup to the abnormalities detected by history and physical findings.
- Apply Sutton's law: Go to "where the money is."
  1. Skin tests
     - An intermediate-strength PPD in all patients with FUO without a previously documented positive PPD.
       - Anergy panel is no longer recommended.
       - Malnourished chronically ill patients may have a false-negative PPD.
     - Histoplasmosis and coccidioidomycosis skin tests not generally recommended.
       - Biopsies and cultures preferred.

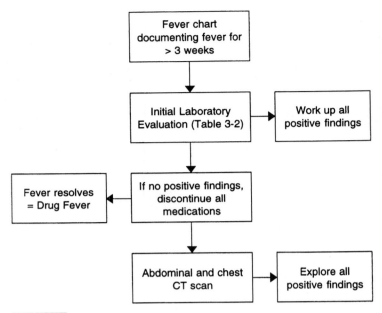

FIGURE 3-1
Algorithm for Initial Work up of FUO

TABLE 3-2
PRELIMINARY TESTS RECOMMENDED FOR FUO

1. Complete history
2. Careful physical exam
3. CBC with differential
4. Giemsa and Wright stain blood smears
5. Liver function tests
6. ANA and rheumatoid factor
7. ESR
8. Urinalysis
9. Blood cultures
10. Urine culture
11. PPD skin test
12. CXR
13. Upper GI with small bowel follow-through
14. Renal and gallbladder ultrasound

2. Cultures
   - Blood cultures
     - Yield for subacute bacterial endocarditis maximized by drawing three blood cultures (see Chap. 7).
     - No more than 6 blood cultures should be drawn.
     - Can repeat periodically or if there is a significant change in the fever pattern.
     - All blood cultures should be held for 3 weeks to detect fastidious slow-growing bacteria.
   - Urine culture, multiple cultures should be obtained to detect tuberculosis.
   - Sputum cultures
     - Obtain in patients with respiratory complaints or CXR abnormalities.
   - Bone marrow culture
     - Obtain in patients undergoing bone marrow biopsy for marrow analysis.
   - CSF culture
     - Obtain in cases with specific neurological complaints.
   - All biopsy specimens need to be cultured.
   - For all culture samples obtain:
     - Aerobic
     - Anaerobic
     - Mycobacteria
     - Fungal cultures
     - Consider viral cultures if cytomegalovirus or Epstein-Barr virus is suspected.
3. Smears
   - Peripheral blood smears using Giemsa and Wright stains for making the diagnosis of:
     - Malaria
     - Trypanosomiasis
     - Relapsing fever
   - Peripheral white blood cell count and differential cell count
     - Viral illnesses have:
       - Lower peripheral white blood cell count and a predominance of lymphocytes and monocytes.
       - Epstein-Barr virus, often atypical lymphocytes and monocytes.
       - Still's disease patients and those with acute bacterial infections have an elevated peripheral white blood cell count with a predominance of neutrophils and band forms.
       - Patients with cyclic neutropenia have fever at the time when their total neutrophil count is low.
   - CSF India ink smear and cryptococcal antigen
     - Very helpful in making the diagnosis of cryptococcal meningitis
     - Except in patients with HIV, a rare cause of FUO
   - Stool smears for ova and parasites
     - Less helpful
     - Gastrointestinal parasites rarely present as FUO

4. Other peripheral blood tests
   - Antibody titers to specific pathogens
     - Useful when specific pathogens are part of the differential diagnosis
     - A rising antibody titer is required to prove active infection
       - Two samples need to be drawn separated by 3–4 weeks.
       - A single titer simply demonstrates a past history of exposure.
     - Most useful in cytomegalovirus, Epstein-Barr virus, Toxoplasma, Rickettsia, Chlamydia, and Brucella infections
   - Antibody titers to human tissue
     - Considered in the majority of cases of FUO in order to diagnose connective tissue disease
     - Tests to include:
       - Antinuclear antibodies (ANA)
       - Anti-DNA antibodies
       - Rheumatoid factor
       - Immune complexes
   - An erythrocyte sedimentation assay (ESR) should be performed in all cases of FUO.
     - Very high ESR in polymyalgia rheumatica/temporal arteritis and Still's disease.
     - Normal ESR virtually excludes the above diagnoses as well as subacute bacterial endocarditis.
5. Imaging studies
   - Tests commonly performed during the initial diagnostic workup: All patients with FUO should have a:
     - Chest X-ray looking for:
       - Mediastinal enlargement (suggestive of lymphoma)
       - Micronodular interstitial changes (millet seed pattern, suggestive of miliary tuberculosis)
       - Nodular lesions or infiltrates (can be seen in many infectious diseases, connective tissue diseases, and neoplasms)
     - Air sinus films or sinus CT scan, required to exclude occult sinus infection and tooth abscess
     - Upper gastrointestinal barium study with small bowel follow-through to exclude regional enteritis
     - Ultrasound of the gallbladder and/or oral cholecystogram to exclude cholecystitis or an enlarged gangrenous gallbladder
     - Barium enema in older patients; however, yield of this procedure is likely to be low in FUO
     - Intravenous pyelogram often performed to exclude:
       - Renal tuberculosis
       - Renal stones
       - Polycystic kidney disease
       - Renal cell carcinoma
     - Joint X-rays in patients with persistent joint complaints
   - Test that should be ordered depending on the patient's symptoms and signs:
     - Radionuclide scans in patients with suspected chronic infection to localize the site of infection
       - Gallium scan accumulates in areas of inflammation, many false positives

- Indium white blood cell scan more specific and has a higher positive yield for identifying occult intra-abdominal infection than abdominal CT scan.
- [(18)F]fluorodeoxyglucose (FDG) accumulates in areas of inflammation and in malignant tumors.
    ◦ Gallium and indium scans require scanning over 24–36 hours.
    ◦ FDG positron emission tomography (PET) scan is completed within a few hours.
    ◦ In preliminary studies the FDG test was more sensitive and specific than gallium scan.
- Technetium scan is the most sensitive and specific for:
    ◦ Osteomyelitis
    ◦ Tumor metastasis to bone (exceptions: prostate cancer and multiple myeloma)

- Total-body CT scan
    - An expensive test
    - Commonly performed in patients without specific complaints despite prolonged observation
    - Up to a 10% yield
    - Helpful in identifying abdominal abscesses, mediastinal nodes, as well as defects in abdominal organs
    - If preliminary testing proves unrevealing, should be considered.
- Ultrasound tests
    - Cardiac echo
        ◦ Consider in patients with a heart murmur and persistent fever
        ◦ Transesophageal echo, the test of choice
            - > 90% sensitivity for detecting cardiac vegetations
            - Helpful in detecting myocardial abscess and atrial myxoma
    - Lower abdomen for:
        ◦ Cases where pelvic lesions are suspected.
        ◦ Abdominal CT is not as sensitive in this region because of reflection artifacts generated by the pelvic bones.

6. Invasive procedures
    ◦ Recommended if all noninvasive tests negative
        - Liver biopsy to exclude granulomatous hepatitis. Laparascopic guided biopsy improves yield.
        - Bone marrow aspiration and biopsy detects:
            - Leukemia in its early stages
            - Stage IV lymphoma
            - Important to appropriately culture (see above)
            - Disseminated infections often seed the bone marrow
                ◦ Tuberculosis
                ◦ Histoplasmosis
                ◦ Coccidioidomycosis
                ◦ Other fungal and mycobacterial infections
    ◦ Invasive procedures that depend on positive diagnostic findings, history, and physical findings
        - Temporal artery biopsy in elderly patient with a high ESR and persistent fever
            - Skip lesions are common in temporal arteritis.
            - A long sample of the temporal artery should be obtained and multiple arterial sections examined.

- Laparotomy was frequently recommended in early series; now laparoscopy is the diagnostic alternative.
  - With the advent of new abdominal imaging techniques now rarely performed.
  - May be considered in selected cases.
  - Processing of abdominal specimens should include cultures of all biopsy specimens as well as Brown-Brenn, Ziehl-Neelsen, methenamine silver, PAS, and Dieterle silver stains in addition to routine hematoxylin and eosin staining.
  - Frozen sections for immunofluorescence staining.
  - Save the remaining tissue block for additional future studies.
- When symptoms, signs, or a specific diagnostic abnormality is found, all other scheduled diagnostic tests should be delayed and Sutton's law applied.
- When in doubt about performing additional tests, tincture of time often proves the wisest course of action.
- Over time the patient's fever may spontaneously resolve or new manifestations may develop helping to identify the etiology of fever.

TREATMENT OF FUO

- Antipyretics can be administered in most cases of FUO once true fever has been documented.
  - May relieve some of the patient's symptoms as the diagnostic workup is pursued.
  - Aspirin, NSIDs, or acetomenophen must be administered at the proper time interval to maintain therapeutic levels and avoid repeated shifting of the thermal set point.
- Antibiotics are contraindicated until a specific diagnosis has been made.
  - In the majority of cases antibiotic treatment will have no effect.
  - Empiric antibiotics may mask the manifestations of the infection and delay diagnosis and treatment.
- Glucocorticoids may be given if a connective tissue is the most likely explanation for FUO.
  - Effective for treating temporal arteritis and polymyalgia rheumatica
  - May be helpful in Still's disease
  - Are used for specific complications in lupus erythematosus
  - Will markedly exacerbate bacterial, mycobacterial, fungal, and parasitic infections
  - Empiric glucocorticoids should be considered only if infection has been convincingly ruled out
  - Prolonged glucocorticoid treatment is associated with many side effects
    - Cushingoid faces
    - Osteoporosis
    - Aseptic necrosis of the hip
    - Diabetes mellitus
    - Opportunistic infections

PROGNOSIS

- Delay in diagnosis worsens the outcome in:
  - Intra-abdominal abscess
  - Miliary tuberculosis
  - Disseminated fungal infections
  - Pulmonary emboli
- 5-year mortality of only 3% in patients without a diagnosis in whom the above diseases have been carefully excluded.
- Prognosis somewhat worse in the elderly patient because of the increased risk of malignancy.
- Additional diagnostic study is not warranted after an FUO diagnostic battery has been completed and serious life-threatening diseases have been excluded.
- If fever persists 4–6 additional months, a complete series of diagnostic studies should then be repeated.

FUO IN THE HIV-INFECTED PATIENT

- Primary HIV infection can present with prolonged fever and should be considered as a cause of FUO in patients with the appropriate risk profile (see Chap. 17).
  - Serum markers are negative in the early stages of HIV infection.
  - Quantitative PCR for HIV is the diagnostic test of choice.
- Fever is also common manifestation of opportunistic infection in the later stages of HIV infection. The most common causes of FUO in AIDs patients, in order of frequency:
  - Mycobacterial infections (*M. tuberculosis*, *M. avium intracellulare*, other atypical mycobacteria)
  - Other bacterial infections
  - Cytomegalovirus
  - Pneumocystis
  - Toxoplasmosis
  - Cryptococcus
  - Histoplasmosis
  - Consider visceral leishmaniasis in HIV patients coming from endemic areas
- Noninfectious causes of fever in HIV patients include:
  - Non-Hodgkin's lymphoma
  - Drug fever
- Additional tests warranted in the HIV patient with prolonged fever include:
  - Mycobacterial blood culture
  - Cryptococcal serum antigen
  - Cytomegalovirus serum antigen
  - Bone marrow culture and histopathology for disseminated histoplasmosis

FEVER IN SURGICAL INTENSIVE-CARE AND MEDICAL INTENSIVE-CARE PATIENTS

- One of the most common problems encountered by the infectious disease consultant
  1. Consider wound infection in the postoperative patient.
     - ○ Examine all wounds for purulent discharge, erythema, edema, and tenderness.
     - ○ Group A streptococci develops in the immediate postoperative period (24–48 hours).
       - ▪ Can present with septic shock and severe bacteremia
       - ▪ May be only minimal purulence at the operative site
       - ▪ A Gram stain of serous exudate usually demonstrates Gram-positive cocci in chains.
     - ○ *Staphlococcus aureus* most common in the later postoperative period.
     - ○ Other nosocomial pathogens also cause wound infection in the later postoperative period
       - ▪ Pseudomonas
       - ▪ Klebsiella
       - ▪ *E. coli*
     - ○ Appropriate antibiotic therapy is generally guided by culture and Gram stain
     - ○ Empiric antibiotic therapy should include Gram-positive and Gram-negative coverage.
  2. Intra-abdominal abscess is a common cause of fever in patients who have suffered bowel perforation.
     - ○ Abdominal CT scan should be ordered to exclude this possibility.
  3. Bronchitis and pneumonia
     - ○ Intubation allows bacteria colonizing the nasopharyrnx to gain entry into the bronchi and pulmonary parenchyma.
     - ○ Sputum Gram stain is critical for differentiating colonization from true infection (see Chap. 1 and Chap. 4).
       - ▪ Infection suggested by:
         - • Gram stain showing:
           - ○ Presence of single organism on Gram stain
           - ○ Greater than 10 neutrophils per high-power field
         - • New infiltrate on chest X-ray
         - • Decrease in arterial pO_2
     - ○ Sputum culture identifies the offending organism as well its sensitivities to antibiotics.
  4. Intravascular device infection
     - ○ Intensive-care-unit patients often have multiple intravenous catheters in place as well as an arterial line.
     - ○ At the onset of new fever examine all intravenous and arterial lines for:
       - ▪ Erythema and warmth
       - ▪ Exudate
     - ○ Replace all lines in the patient who has developed shock.
     - ○ Empiric antibiotic coverage should be instituted to cover:
       - ▪ *S. aureus*
       - ▪ *S. epidermidis*
       - ▪ Gram-negative rods

- ○ Vancomycin and a third-generation cephalosporin is often used, but must be individualized to take into account:
    - Prevailing bacterial flora in each intensive-care unit
    - The history of antibiotic usage in the patient
5. Urinary tract infection
    - ○ Prolonged bladder catheterization is common in ICU patients.
        - Within 30 days nearly all patients, despite a closed urinary collecting system, will develop urinary tract infections (see Chap. 9).
    - ○ Urinalysis and urine culture are part of the fever workup in all patients with urinary catheters.
6. Air sinus infections
    - ○ Nasogastric tubes and nasotracheal intubation block the ostea draining the air sinuses and can lead to sinusitis and fever.
    - ○ Sinus CT scan is recommended as part of the fever workup.
    - ○ Therapy should include removing the tube from the nasal passage and appropriate antibiotic coverage should be instituted (see Chap. 5).
7. Noninfectious causes of fever
    - ○ Pulmonary emboli may present with fever.
    - ○ Drug fever
        - ICU patients usually are receiving a large number of medications and are at higher risk of developing drug fever.
        - Review all medications and discontinue or change any potential offending medications as possible.
    - ○ Sterile hematoma
        - Usually causes persistent low-grade fever.
        - Identify by CT scan.
        - Usually does not require drainage, but often takes time to fully resorb.
- Overall management of fever in the ICU patient
    - ○ Requires a systematic diagnostic approach.
    - ○ Judicious use of antibiotics. Avoid unnecessarily prolonged periods on broad-spectrum antibiotics.
        - Leads to the selection of highly resistant bacterial pathogens
        - Predisposes to candidemia
        - Increased risk of *C. difficile* colitis
    - ○ Streamline empiric antibiotic coverage once culture data are available.
    - ○ Close communication between the ICU staff and infectious disease consultant is critical to achieve the best care for the febrile ICU patient.

REFERENCES

Arch-Ferrer JE, Velazquez-Fernandez D, Sierra-Madero J, Lopez-Karpovitch X, Angeles-Angeles A, et al: Laparoscopic approach to fever of unknown origin. *Surg Endosc* 2003; 17:494–97.

Blockmans D, Knokaert D: Clinical value of [(18)F]fluordeoxyglucose positron emission tomography for patients with fever of unknown origin. *Clin Infect Dis* 2001; 32:191–96.

Larson EB, Featherstone HJ, Petersdorf RG: Fever of undetermined origin: Diagnosis and follow-up of 105 cases, 1970–1980. *Medicine (Baltimore)* 1982; 61:269–92.

Marik PE: Fever in the ICU. *Chest* 2000; 117:855–69.

Mayo J, Collazos J, Martinez E: Fever of unknown origin in the setting of HIV infection: Guidelines for a rational approach. *AIDS Patient Care STDS* 1998; 12:373–78.

Mert A, Ozaras R, Tabak F, Bilir M, Ozturk R, et al: Fever of unknown origin: A review of 20 patients with adult-onset Still's disease. *Clin Rheumatol* 2003; 22:89–93.

Petersdorf RG, Beeson PB: Fever of unexplained origin: Report of 100 cases. *Medicine* 1961; 40:1–30.

Vanderschueren S, Knockaert D, Adriaenssens T, Demey W, Durnez A, et al: From prolonged febrile illness to fever of unknown origin: The challenge continues. *Arch Intern Med* 2003; 163:1033–41.

4

PULMONARY INFECTIONS

ACUTE PNEUMONIAS

HIGHLIGHTS

- Pneumonia is one of the most common and severe infections.
- Pneumonia is classified by the pace of illness, constellation of symptoms and signs, and whether or not the infection was acquired in the hospital.
- When pneumonia is being considered, a chest X-ray should always be ordered.
- Sputum Gram stain should always be ordered with sputum culture.
- Specific clinical findings allow risk stratification of patients with community-acquired pneumonia.
- Empiric antibiotic regimens are helpful in guiding therapy and have improved outcome.
- Preventive vaccination with pneumococcal vaccine is safe, efficacious, and underutilized.

POTENTIAL SEVERITY

- Acute pneumonia is a potentially life-threatening illness.
- Requires rapid diagnosis and treatment, < 4 hours from presentation to treatment.
- A delay in antibiotic treatment increases the risk of a fatal outcome.

GENERAL CONSIDERATIONS

PREVALENCE

- 2 million to 3 million cases of pneumonia develop annually in the United States.
- 500,000 hospitalizations and 45,000 deaths per year
- 258 persons per 100,000
- Over age 65 years 962 per 100,000 (1/100) require hospitalization for pneumonia.

PATHOGENESIS AND PATHOLOGY

- Tracheobronchial tree is normally sterile.
- Protective mechanisms that prevent pathogens from gaining entry:
    1. Turbinates and hairs in the nasal passages trap foreign particles.
    2. Epiglottis covers the trachea and prevents secretions or food from entering the trachea.
    3. Mucin is secreted by the tracheobronchial tree.
        ○ Mucin contains antibacterial compounds, including:
            ▪ IgA antibodies
            ▪ Defensins
            ▪ Lysozyme and lactoferrin
        ○ Mucin is sticky and traps bacteria or other foreign particles.
    4. Cilia lining the inner walls of the trachea and bronchi beat rapidly and act as a conveyer belt to move mucin out of the tracheobronchial tree to the larynx.
    5. Cough reflex quickly removes large volumes of fluid or large particles that gain access to the trachea.
    6. Neutrophils and alveolar macrophages that ingest and kill infecting organisms enter the alveoli if pathogens reach this site. Immunoglobulins and complement are also present.
    7. The lymphatic channels adjacent to the alveoli serve to drain the alveolar space and transport fluid, macrophages, and lymphocytes to the mediastinal lymph nodes.
- Bacterial pathogens usually gain entry into the lung by:
    ○ Aspiration of mouth flora
    ○ Inhalation of small aerosolized droplets ($< 3 \mu m$ in diameter)
- Bacterial invasion results in a series of inflammatory responses.
    1. Outpouring of edema fluid into the alveoli
        ○ Serves as an excellent culture medium for further bacterial growth.
        ○ Spreads to adjacent alveoli through the pores of Kohn and via terminal bronchioles.
        ○ Results in the centrifugal spread of infection.
        ○ Coughing and the physical motion of respiration further enhance spread.
    2. Polymorphonuclear leukocytes (PMN) and some red blood cells then accumulate in the alveolar space, forming a zone of consolidation.
    3. Later macrophages enter the lesions and assist PMN in clearing the infection.
- Pathogens demonstrate marked differences in the invasiveness and ability to destroy lung parenchyma.
    ○ *S. pneumoniae* causes minimal tissue necrosis and little or no scar formation. Full recovery of pulmonary function is the rule.
    ○ *S. aureus* releases multiple proteases that permanently destroy tissue.
    ○ Gram-negative rods and aneaerobic bacteria also permanently destroy tissue.

PREDISPOSING FACTORS

- Viral upper respiratory infection the most common predisposing event.
    ○ Damages the bronchial epithelium and cilia.
    ○ Low viscosity exudate carries nasopharyngeal bacteria into the lungs.
- Smoking damages the bronchial epithelial cells and impairs mucociliary function.
- Congenital defects
    ○ Patients with Kartagener's syndrome have defective ciliary function
    ○ Cystic fibrosis results in highly viscous mucus.
- Drugs: alcohol, sedatives, and anesthetics depress coughing and epiglottis function.

- Elderly have:
  - Impairments in swallowing function
  - Reduced humoral and cell-mediated immunity
- Immunocompromised patients
  - Organ transplant patients on immunosuppressive agents
  - AIDs patients
- Chronic diseases
  - Multiple myeloma
  - Diabetes mellitus
  - Chronic renal failure
  - Sickle cell disease
- Cold weather
  - Cold, dry weather alters the viscosity of mucous and impairs bacterial clearance.
  - People tend to remain indoors enhancing person-to-person spread of respiratory infections.

ETIOLOGIES OF ACUTE PNEUMONIA

1. *S. pneumoniae* is the most common cause of acute pneumonia (40%).
2. Atypical pneumonia can be caused by:
   - *Mycoplasma pneumoniae*
   - *Chlamydia pneumoniae*
   - Respiratory viruses (influenza, adenovirus, parainfluenza, and RSV)
3. Rarer causes of community-acquired pneumonia
   - *H. influenzae*—more common in smokers
   - *S. aureus*—after influenza, very severe
   - *Legionella pneumophila*
   - Aspiration—mouth flora (anaerobes)
4. Nosocomial—usually Gram-negative organisms: Klebsiella, Pseudomonas, or *S. aureus*
   - Hospitalized (often intubated)
   - Elderly in nursing homes
   - Patients with cystic fibrosis, HIV, alchoholics

SYMPTOMS AND SIGNS

- Pneumonias are classified by:
  1. Pace of illness
     - Acute—symptoms develop over 24–48 hours.
     - Chronic—symptoms progress over 3 weeks or longer.
  2. Specific constellations of symptoms
     - Typical—rapid onset, more severe symptoms, productive cough, dense consolidation on CXR
     - Atypical—somewhat slower onset, less severe symptoms, nonproductive cough, patchy interstitial pattern on CXR
  3. Environment where the pneumonia was acquired
     - Community acquired—patient not recently ($\geq$ 14 days) in the hospital or chronic care facility
     - Nosocomial—patient in the hospital at the time the infection developed

- Certain key clinical characteristics are helpful in guiding the physician in determining the most likely etiologies (see Table 4-1).
  1. Cough—frequency, production of sputum, color and thickness of sputum
     - Nonproductive cough, or a cough productive of scanty sputum, suggests atypical pneumonia.
     - Rusty-colored sputum suggests *S. pneumoniae*.
     - Thick red currant jelly sputum found in *Klebsiella pneumoniae*.
     - Green-colored sputum found in patients with *H. influenzae* and *Pseudomonas aeruginosa* pneumonia.
     - Frank hemoptysis seen in cavitary tuberculosis, lung abscess, and lung carcinoma.
     - There is considerable overlap in the sputum characteristics and these observations cannot be considered specific.
  2. Chest pain—pain on deep inspiration, usually sharp = pleural involvement.
     - Diaphragm inflammation can cause pain that mimics cholecystitis or appendicitis and precipitate exploratory laparotomy.
     - Seen in *S. pneumoniae*, *S. aureus*, *S. pyogenes*, anaerobes, as well as coxsackievirus and echovirus.
  3. Rigors—a bed-shaking, teeth-chattering chill
     - One rigor in *S. pneumonia*
     - > one in *S. aureus*, *Klebsiella* spp, *S. pyogenes*, and anaerobes
     - *H. influenzae* rarely causes rigors
  4. Shortness of breath—a worrisome symptom
     - Suggests poor alveolar oxygen exchange, indicative of severe infection.
     - May be due to pleuritic chest pain rather than poor gas exchange.
  5. Epidemiology—travel history, animal exposure, exposure to people with respiratory illnesses, occupation and sexual history
     - Animal exposure including contact with wild game, birds, bats, and rodents (see Chap. 13).
     - Exposure to outside air-conditioning units or construction sites should be identified; increases the risk of Legionnaire's disease.
     - Travel to the Southwest raises concerns about coccidiomycosis.
     - Travel to the Ohio River valley increases the risk of histoplasmosis.
     - History of exposure to family members or friends with respiratory illnesses.

TABLE 4-1

CLINICAL CHARACTERISTICS OF ACUTE COMMUNITY-ACQUIRED
PNEUMONIA CLASSIFIED BY ETIOLOGY

Etiologic Agent	Classic Symptoms	Typical CXR findings
S. pneumoniae	Rusty-colored sputum, rigors, pleuritic chest pain	Lobar infiltrate, air bronchograms
Aspiration pneumonia	After loss of consciousness, poor gag, abnormal swallowing, foul-smelling sputum	Dense consolidation RLL > LLL, posterior segment of upper lobes, later lung abscess and empyema
Actinomycosis	Poor dental hygiene, spontaneous fistula formation, sulfa granules	Same distribution as aspiration; pleural involvement common
Nocardiosis	Associated with inhalation of soil particles, often immunocompromised host, can mimic lung Ca with brain metastasis	Multiple abnormalities, including cavitary disease, nodules, diffuse infiltrate, can be associated with brain abscess
H. influenzae	More gradual onset smokers with COPD	Lobar or patchy infiltrates
S. aureus	Follows influenza pneumonia, rapidly progressive acute disease	Bronchopneumonia, lung abscess, pneumothorax, and empyema
Legionella pneumophila	Nonproductive cough, GI symptoms, confusion	Lobar pneumonia, cavities in immunocompromised
Atypical pneumonia	Mild to moderate symptoms, nonproductive cough, pulmonary exam often normal	Patchy lower-lobe bronchopneumonia

PHYSICAL EXAMINATION

- Vital signs help determine the severity of illness. Bad prognostic findings:
    - A respiratory rate of > 30 breaths/minute
    - A systolic blood pressure of < 90 mm Hg
    - A pulse of > 125
    - A temperature of < 35 °C or > 40 °C
- Depressed mental status is also a poor prognostic sign.
- Ear, nose, and throat examination—look for herpes labialis, which may reactivate as a consequence of the stress of the primary illness.
- Neck stiffness in association with depressed mental status may indicate the development of bacterial meningitis.
- Pulmonary auscultation often fails to detect the extent of infection.
    - Asymmetry of chest movements, movement diminished on the side with pneumonia.
    - Rales and rhonchi.
    - Bronchial breath sounds and E-to-A changes (egophony) suggest consolidation.
    - Dullness to percussion also found in consolidation. In association with decreased breath sounds suggests a pleural effusion.
    - A "leathery" friction rub may be heard over areas of pleural inflammation.
- Physical examination is unreliable for making the diagnosis of pneumonia.

LABORATORY FINDINGS

- Chest X-ray (CXR) must be performed when pneumonia is being considered.
- Radiologic pattern can serve as a rough guideline as to possible etiologic agents.
- Five classic patterns have been described:
    1. Lobar pneumonia
        - A homogeneous radiologic density that involves a distinct anatomic segment of the lung (see Fig. 4-1).
        - Most commonly seen in *S. pneumoniae*, *H. influenzae*, and Legionella.
    2. Bronchopneumonia
        - Patchy infiltrate involving multiple areas of the lung which are not confined by the pulmonary fissures (see Fig. 4-2).
        - Most commonly observed with *S. aureus*, Gram-negative bacilli, Mycoplasma, Chlamydia, and respiratory viruses.
    3. Interstitial pneumonia
        - Caused by inflammation of the lung interstitium.
        - A fine, diffuse granular infiltrate.
        - Seen with influenza and cytomegalovirus (CMV), *Pneumocystis carinii*, and miliary tuberculosis (often micronodular).
    4. Lung abscess
        - Areas of necrosis lead to loss of lung tissue and formation of cavities.
        - Fluid-filled cavities usually not apical, found in anaerobic pulmonary infections and *S. aureus*.
        - Apical cavities without fluid are most commonly caused by *M. tuberculosis* and atypical mycobacteria (see Fig. 4-3).
    5. Nodular lesions
        - Histoplasmosis, coccidiodomycosis, and cryptococcosis can form multiple or single nodular lung lesions.
        - Hematogenous pneumonia due to right-sided endocarditis form "cannonball" lesions that can mimic metastatic carcinoma.

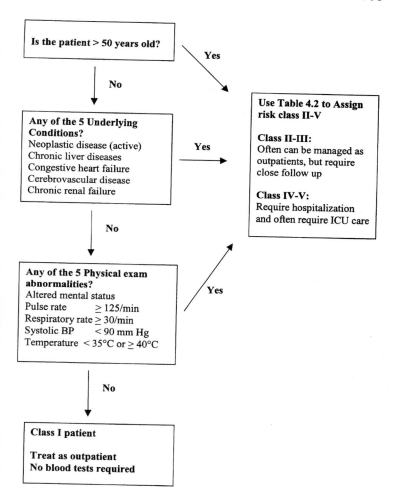

FIGURE 4-1

Utilizing PORT prediction rules for management of community-acquired pneumonia. Adapted from Fine MJ, Aubie TE, Yealy DM, et al: *N Engl J Med* 1997; 336:243–50.

TABLE 4-2
PORT ASSESSMENT OF RISK FACTORS IN COMMUNITY-ACQUIRED PNEUMONIA*

Risk Categories	Points	% Mortality
Class I	Absence of all predictors	0.1
Class II	< 70	0.6
Class III	71–90	0.9
Class IV	91–130	9.3
Class V	> 130	27.0

Risk Factors	Points
Demographic factors	
Age, men	Age (years)
Age, women	Age (years–10)
Nursing home resident	10
Coexisting disease	
Neoplastic disease	30
Chronic liver disease	20
Congestive heart failure	10
Cerebrovascular disease	10
Chronic renal disease	10
Physical findings	
Altered mental status	20
Respiratory rate ≥ 30/min	20
Systolic BP < 90 mm Hg	20
Temperature < 35°C or ≥ 40°C	15
Pulse ≥ 125 beat/min	10
Laboratory and CXR findings	
Arterial blood gas pH < 7.35	30
Blood urea nitrogen ≥ 30 mg/dL	20
Sodium < 130 mmol/L	20
Glucose > 250 mg/dL	10
Hematocrit < 30%	10
Arterial oxygen partial pressure < 60 mm Hg or O_2 sat < 90%	10
Pleural effusion	10

*Adapted from Fine MJ, Aubie TE, Yealy DM, et al: *N Engl J Med* 1997; 336:243–50.

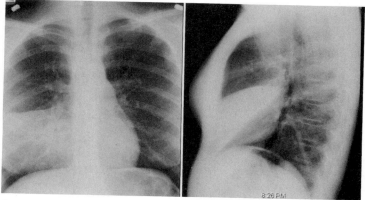

A

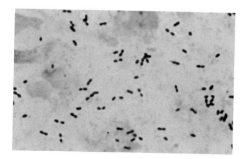

B

FIGURE 4-2

Lobar pneumonia due to *Streptococcus pneumoniae.* (A) Chest X-ray demonstrating a classic right middle lobe infiltrate. (Courtesy of Dr. Pat Abbitt, University of Florida College of Medicine.) (B) Sputum Gram stain showing *S. pneumoniae.* Note that the Gram-positive diplococci come to a slight point at each end, explaining the term "lancet-shaped."

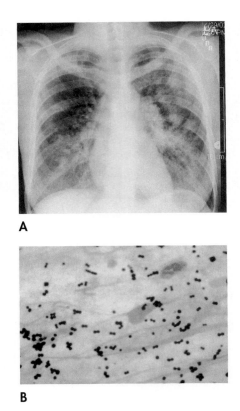

A

B

FIGURE 4-3

Bronchopneumonia due to *Staphylococcus aureus*. (A) Chest X-ray demonstrating diffuse macronodular infiltrates of both lung fields in a classic bronchopneumonia pattern. (Courtesy of Dr. Pat Abbitt, University of Florida College of Medicine.) (B) Sputum Gram stain showing large Gram-positive cocci in clusters and tetrads.

- Typical X-ray findings may not be observed in immunocompromised patients, including transplant patients, neutropenic patients, and patients with AIDS.
- The role of high-resolution chest CT scan is evolving. Helpful for:
  - Clearly demonstrating interstitial infiltration
  - Determining the exact anatomy of pulmonary cavities, nodules, and pleural fluid collections
- Patients with an infiltrate who are Class I in the PORT classification require no additional tests (see PORT classification below).
- Additional tests are required for more severely ill patients being considered for hospitalization.
  - A complete blood cell and differential count. Bad prognostic findings:
    - Peripheral WBC < 6,000/mm^3
    - Hct < 30%, usually indicative of chronic underlying disease

- ○ Blood oxygenation
  - ▪ If O_2 saturation is at all depressed, an arterial blood gas should be obtained.
  - ▪ Bad prognostic findings include:
    - • Systemic acidosis, pH < 7.35
    - • $PO_2 < 60$ mm Hg
- ○ Metabolic panel. Bad prognostic findings:
  - ▪ Blood urea nitrogen > 30
  - ▪ Serum sodium < 130 mEq/L
  - ▪ Serum glucose > 250 mg/dL
- ○ Two blood cultures should be drawn prior to the institution of antibiotics. Positive in 1–16% of cases of community-acquired pneumonia.
- • Sputum Gram stain
  - ○ The acquisition of sputum should be supervised to assure that the patient coughs deeply and brings up the sample from the tracheobronchial tree.
  - ○ Adequacy of the sample should be determined by low-power microscopic analysis of the sputum Gram stain.
    - ▪ > 10 squamous epithelial cells per low-power field (lpf) indicates significant contamination from the nasopharynx.
    - ▪ > 25 PMN/lpf strong evidence that the sample originated from the tracheobronchial tree.
  - ○ Gram stain can be helpful in differentiating normal flora (mixed Gram-positive and Gram-negative rods and cocci) from the offending pathogen.
    - ▪ Predominance of a single type of bacteria suggests it is the primary pathogen.
      - • Example: > 10 lancet-shaped Gram-positive diplococci per high-power field strong evidence for *S. pneumoniae* (85% specificity, 65% sensitivity) (see Fig. 4-1).
  - ○ Must assess the adequacy of decolorization.
    - ▪ In ideally stained regions, the nucleus and cytoplasm of PMN should be Gram-negative and a mixture of Gram-positive and Gram-negative organisms seen.
    - ▪ A Gram-positive nucleus indicates underdecolorization.
    - ▪ Presence of only Gram-negative bacteria, including cocci, suggests overdecolorization.
  - ○ Gram stain is helpful for assessing the inflammatory response.
    - ▪ Many PMN suggests a bacterial etiology.
    - ▪ Predominance of mononuclear cells is more consistent with Mycoplasma, Chlamydia, or viral infection.
- • Sputum culture
  - ○ Less helpful than Gram stain because contaminating normal flora frequently overgrow, preventing identification of the true pathogen.
  - ○ Rapid processing has been shown to increase the yield for *S. pneumoniae*. Sputum cultures are falsely negative approximately half the time.
  - ○ Sputum should never be cultured in the absence of an accompanying Gram stain.
  - ○ Primarily useful for determining the antibiotic sensitivity of potential pathogens.
  - ○ The combination of sputum Gram stain and antibiotic-sensitivity testing may allow the clinician to narrow the spectrum of antibiotic coverage and reduce the likelihood of selecting for highly resistant pathogens.
  - ○ In the intubated patient sputum culture alone should never be the basis for initiating antibiotic therapy. Sputum culture is almost always positive and often simply represents colonization rather than true infection (see Chap. 1).

- The polymerase chain reaction (PCR) is being used to amplify specific strands of DNA from pathogens.
  - Likely to be helpful in identifying organisms that normally are not part of the mouth flora, and that are difficult to culture:
    - *L. pneumophila*
    - *M. pneumoniae*
    - *C. pneumoniae*
    - *P. carinii*
- Urinary antigen for *L. pneumophila* serogroup 1 (the most common pathogenic serogroup) should be performed when Legionella pneumonia is a consideration (see below).
  - Moderately sensitive and highly specific.
  - A positive test is diagnostic; a negative test does not exclude the diagnosis.
- More invasive procedures usually are only required in the immunocompromised patient (see Chap. 16).
  - Fiberoptic bronchoscopy with protected brushing or lavage is usually sensitive and specific.
    - Quantitative cultures: growth of $> 10^3$–10^4/ml indicates infection.
  - Lavage of a lung segment with sterile fluid samples a larger volume of lung.
    - Useful for diagnosing *Pneumocystis carinii* pneumonia, mycobacterial infections, and cytomegalovirus.

DECIDING ON HOSPITALIZATION

- Pneumonia Patient Outcome Research Team (PORT) criteria allow objective assessment of the potential severity of pneumonia (see Table 4-2).
- PORT Class I can be treated as an outpatient. These patients are:
  - ≤ 50 years of age
  - Lack any of the five important comorbid conditions (neoplastic disease, liver disease, congestive heart failure, cerebrovascular diseases, or renal disease)
  - Normal mental status
  - Normal or only mildly deranged vital signs, and normal mental status (see Fig. 4-4)
- PORT Class II and Class III usually do not require hospitalization, but warrant close follow-up.
- PORT Class IV–V should always be hospitalized and usually need to be placed in an intensive-care unit.

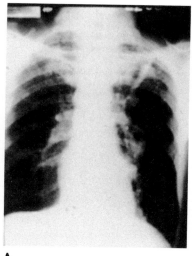
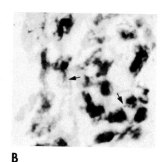

A   **B**

FIGURE 4-4
Bilateral apical infiltrates due to *Mycobacterium tuberculosis*. (A) Chest X-ray demonstrating bilateral upper lobe cavitary lesions. (B) AFB sputum smear showing small beaded-appearing acid-fast bacilli.

EMPIRIC TREATMENT AND OUTCOME

- Antibiotics are the mainstay of treatment and should be given within 4 hours (see Table 4-3).
  - Antibiotics should not be delayed because of difficulties with sputum collection.
  - Delays in antibiotic therapy have been associated with increased mortality.
- For ambulatory patients two alternatives are first-line therapy
  - A macrolide
    - Azithromycin
    - Clarithromycin
    - Erythromycin is the least expensive macrolide, but has:
      - A higher incidence of gastrointestinal complaints
      - Poor coverage for *H. influenzae*
  - A fluoroquinolone with good Gram-positive activity
    - Gatifloxacin
    - Moxifloxacin
    - Levofloxacin
    - Potential concerns about using fluoroquinolones as first-line therapy
      - Very broad-spectrum coverage is often not necessary.
      - Many experts are concerned about the development of resistance to fluoroquinolones.
    - Reserve for:
      - Older patients with underlying disease who have a higher incidence of Gram-negative pneumonia
      - Areas where high-level penicillin-resistant *S. pneumoniae* is common

TABLE 4-3
EMPIRIC TREATMENT OF PNEUMONIA (IDSA, 2003)

Drug	Dose	Relative Efficacy	Comments
Community-acquired outpatient			
Clarithromycin	500 mg po BID	First line	Low serum levels, high levels in macrophages, preferred for *H. influenzae*
Azithromycin	500 mg po followed by 250 mg po QD	First line	
Erythromycin	500 mg QID	First line	GI toxicity is common
Gatifloxacin	400 mg po QD	First line	Levofloxacin-resistant *S. pneumoniae* reported in Canada. Preferred for nursing home residents
Levofloxacin	500 mg po QD		
Moxifloxacin	400 mg po QD		
Doxycycline	100 mg po BID	First line	A bacteriostatic agent
Amoxicillin-clavulinate	875/125 po BID	Alternative	Useful if *S. pneumoniae* or *H. influenzae* suspected
2nd-generation cephalosporin		Alternative	Useful if *S. pneumoniae* or *H. influenzae* suspected
Cefuroxime	500 mg po BID		
Cefpodoxime	400 mg po BID		
Cefprozil	500 mg po BID		
Community-acquired inpatient			
Ceftriaxone (or)	1 gm IV or IM QD	First line	Add vancomycin if penicillin-resistance *S. pneumoniae* suspected
Cefotaxime (+)	1 gm IV Q8H		
Macrolide (+)	(same doses as above)		
Vancomycin (if severely ill)	1 gm IV Q12H		

110

		Alternatives	
Fluoroquinolone alone			
Gatifloxacin	400 mg IV QD		If severely ill, first-line regimen is preferred
Levofloxacin	500 mg IV QD		
Aspiration (community)			
Penicillin G	2 million IV Q4H	First line	Covers usual mouth flora
Clindamycin	600 mg IV Q8H	First line	Shown to be slightly more effective than PCN for lung abscess
Aspiration (in hospital)			
Ceftriaxone +	1 gm IV QD	First line	Regimen used by the author
metronidazole	500 mg IV Q8H		
Fluoroquinolone +	(same doses as above)	First line	
metronidazole	500 mg IV Q8H		
Piperacillin-tazobactam	3 /0.375 gm IV Q6H	Second line	Requires a large fluid load
Ticarcillin-clavulinate	3.1 gm IV Q4–6H		

- CXR is not helpful in monitoring improvement. Radiographic changes often persist for weeks despite clinical improvement. Can be used in combination with CT scan to assess the development of complications such as:
  - Progression of infiltrates
  - Pneumothorax
  - Cavitation
  - Empyema
  - Adult respiratory distress syndrome (ARDS)
- In hospitalized patient with acute community-acquired pneumonia, recommended empiric therapy
  - Cefotaxime or ceftriaxone (covers *S. pneumoniae*, *H. influnezae*, *S. aureus*, *Klebsiella* spp., some Gram negatives, and aerobic mouth flora).
  - Combined with a macrolide, erythromycin, azithromycin, or clarithromycin (covers Legionella, Mycoplasma, Chlamydia).
  - Once culture results, antibiotic susceptibilities, and clinical response can be determined, antibiotics can be adjusted.
  - If aspiration pneumonia is suspected, metronidazole can be added.
  - In the severely ill patient in whom highly resistant *S. pneumoniae* is suspected, vancomycin may be administered.
- The appropriate duration of treatment has not been systematically studied.
  - For *S. pneumonia*, generally treat for 72 hours after the patient becomes afebrile.
  - For infections with bacteria that cause necrosis of lung (*S. aureus*, Klebsiella, and anaerobes), therapy should probably be continued for ≥ 2 weeks.
  - For *Mycoplasma pneumonae*, *Chlamydia pneumoniae*, and Legionella in the immunocompetent patient, 2 weeks is generally recommended.
- Switch to oral antibiotics when:
  - The gastrointestinal tract is functioning normally.
  - The patient is able to take by mouth.
  - The patient's clinical condition is improving.
    - Two consecutive normal temperatures within 8 hours
    - Improved cough
    - Improved WBC
  - Usually occurs within 3 days
- When switching to oral antibiotics:
  - Utilize an oral preparation from the same antibiotic class as the intravenous preparation.
  - If not possible, utilize an oral medication with a similar spectrum of activity.
- Hospital discharge can be recommended if the patient has < 2 of the following characteristics indicating continued instability:
  - Temperature $> 37.8°C$
  - Respiratory rate > 24/minute
  - Heart rate > 100/minute
  - Systolic blood pressure < 90 mm Hg
  - Oxygen saturation $< 90\%$
  - Inability to maintain oral intake
  - Altered mental status

OUTCOME

- 45,000 deaths per year in the United States.
- 2–30% overall mortality in hospitalized patients.
- Higher mortality associated with:
  - >65 years old (150–250 deaths per 100,000)
  - Underlying diseases. Statistically significant increases in mortality have been associated with 5 conditions:
    1. Neoplastic disease
    2. Liver disease
    3. Congestive heart failure
    4. Cerebrovascular disease
    5. Renal disease

SPECIFIC CAUSES OF ACUTE COMMUNITY ACQUIRED PNEUMONIA

- Great overlap among the clinical manifestations of the pathogens that cause acute community-acquired pneumonia.
- Constellations of symptoms, signs, and laboratory findings serve to narrow the possibilities.
- The ability to focus on a few pathogens, or identify a specific pathogen, allows the clinician to:
  - Better predict the clinical course of pneumonia.
  - Narrow antibiotic coverage.

STREPTOCOCCUS PNEUMONIAE

Pathogenesis
- Pathogenic strains contain a thick capsule.
  - Prevent PMN binding and block phagocytosis.
  - Certain capsular types more effectively resist phagocytosis and are more likely to cause disease.
    - Capsular types 1, 3, 4, 7, 8, and 12 in adults.
    - Capsular types 3, 6, 14, 18, 19, and 23 in children.
    - Type 3 has the thickest polysaccharide capsule and is the most virulent strain, being associated with the worst prognosis.
  - Opsonins attach the bacterium to PMN and macrophage receptors, enhancing phagocytosis.
    - Immunoglobulins link the bacterium through Fc receptors.
    - Complement product C3b links through complement receptors.
- Other virulence factors
  - Enhance adherence to epithelial cells.
  - Resist phagocytosis.
  - Activate complement.
  - Does not produce significant quantities of proteases.
    - Disease manifestations are primarily the consequence of the host's inflammatory response.
    - Permanent tissue damage is rare, and spread across anatomic boundaries, such as lung fissures, is uncommon.

Prevalence and Predisposing Factors

* Most common etiology of acute community-acquired pneumonia (up to 2/3 of the cases where a specific pathogen is identified).
* Predisposing factors
  * Hypogammaglobulinemia and multiple myeloma
  * Deficiencies in complement (C1, C2, C3, C4)
  * Patients with HIV infection have defects in antibody production.
  * Splenic dysfunction greatly increases the risk of overwhelming *S. pneumoniae* sepsis
  * Chronic diseases
    * Cirrhosis
    * Nephrotic syndrome
    * Congestive heart failure
    * Chronic obstructive pulmonary disease
    * Alcoholism

Unique Clinical Characteristics

* Very abrupt onset
* Begins with a single severe rigor
* Rusty-colored sputum due to capillary leakage of blood into the alveolar space
* Pleuritic chest pain as a consequence of the frequent spread of infection to the peripheral lung and pleura

Diagnosis

* Sputum Gram stain
  * > 10 Gram-positive lancet-shaped diplococci/hpf (85% specificity, 65% sensitivity) (see Fig. 4-1).
  * Pneumococci within the cytoplasm of a PMN strongly support invasive infection.
* Sputum culture
  * Like *S. viridens*, demonstrates alpha (green) hemolysis on blood agar plates. *S. viridens* frequently overgrows *S. pneumoniae*.
    * Optochin disk inhibits *S. pneumoniae* growth but not *S. viridens*.
  * Catalase negative, bile soluble.
  * A positive sputum culture in the absence of a positive Gram stain or a positive blood culture does not prove infection.
    * *S. pneumoniae* can be present as normal mouth flora in up to 60% of healthy people.
* Blood cultures
  * Positive in up to 25% of patients with pneumococcal pneumonia.
  * Positive blood culture in combination with the appropriate symptoms and CXR findings = true infection.
    * Even in the absence of a positive sputum Gram stain
* Urine test for pneumococcal polysaccharide antigen available
  * This test is unable to differentiate between nasopharyngeal colonization and active infection.

- Chest X-ray
  - ○ Single area of infiltration involving one or more segments of a single lobe most common (see Fig. 4-1).
  - ○ Classic lobar radiologic pattern most common.
    - ▪ Respects the confining fissures of the lung and rarely extends beyond these boundaries.
  - ○ Air bronchograms are found in the minority of cases.
  - ○ Up to 40% have pleural fluid detected.
    - ▪ Volume of fluid is too small to sample by thoracentesis.
    - ▪ If antibiotic treatment is prompt, only a small percentage go on to develop true empyema.
  - ○ Despite rapid defervescence and the resolution of all symptoms, X-ray changes often persist for 4–6 weeks.

Treatment
- Increased prevalence of penicillin-resistant strains
  - ○ In the early antibiotic era *S. pneumoniae* was highly sensitive to penicillin (MIC < 0.06 μg/ml).
  - ○ Now in the United States:
    - ▪ 25–35% demonstrate intermediate resistance (MIC 0.1–1 μg/ml).
    - ▪ A small percentage demonstrate high-level resistance (MIC ≥ 2 μg/ml).
  - ○ In some areas of Europe and South Africa higher percentages of highly resistant strains have been observed.
  - ○ In the Netherlands and Germany, where strictly limited antibiotic usage is the standard of care, the prevalence of resistant strains is lower.
- Treatment of intermediate-resistant strains
  - ○ The decrease in the affinity of penicillin-binding proteins in these strains can be overcome by raising the concentration of penicillin.
  - ○ Standard doses of penicillin as well as third-generation cephalosporins ceftriaxone and cefotaxime (MIC ≤ 1 μg/ml) are effective **except for CNS infections**.
  - ○ Amoxicillin is more active than penicillin V-K and is the preferred oral antibiotic.
- Treatment for high-level penicillin resistance
  - ○ Usually resistant to:
    - ▪ Tetracyclines
    - ▪ Macrolides
    - ▪ Clindamycin
    - ▪ Imipenam
  - ○ Sensitive to:
    - ▪ Fluoroquinalones possessing good Gram-positive activity (levofloxacin, gatifloxacin, and moxifloxacin)
      - • Several cases of pneumonia due to levofloxacin-resistant *S. pneumoniae* have been reported.
      - • Overall percentage of pneumococcal strains resistant to fluoroquinolones remains low.
      - • Fluoroquinolones are not approved for CNS infections.
    - ▪ Vancomycin has excellent activity against all resistant strains.

Outcome
- 20–40% mortality in the preantibiotic era
- 5% in the antibiotic era
- Outcome is adversely influenced by:
  - Age; patients > 65 years old and infants have a worse outcome
  - Delayed treatment
  - Infection with capsular types 2 or 3
  - Involvement of more than one lobe of the lung
  - WBC of < 6,000
  - Bacteremia, as well as shock or the development of meningitis
  - Jaundice
  - Pregnancy
  - Presence of other underlying diseases (heart disease, cirrhosis, diabetes)
  - Alcohol intoxication
  - 3-fold increase in mortality for penicillin-resistant pneumococci
  - 7-fold for ceftriaxone-resistant pneumococci

Prevention
- Mortality during the first 36 hours of hospitalization has not changed despite the use of antibiotics.
- Vaccination recommended to:
  - Prevent early mortality
  - Reduce the incidence of *S. pneumoniae* infection (both penicillin-sensitive and -resistant strains)
- Strongly recommended for patients:
  - With chronic illnesses
  - Over the age of 65 years
- Specific antibodies directed against the bacterial cell wall confer protection by allowing PMN and macrophages to quickly ingest the invading pathogen.
  - May prevent or reduce the severity of disease.
- Polyvalent vaccine containing antigens to 23 capsular types is available.
- Efficacy
  - Approximately 60% reduction of bacteremia in immunocompetent adult.
  - Efficacy decreases with age and is not measurable in immunocompromised patients.
- The vaccine has proved to be safe and inexpensive, and should be widely used.

ASPIRATION PNEUMONIA
- Suspect in patients with:
  - A recent history of depressed consciousness
  - A poor gag reflex or an abnormal swallowing reflex
    - The elderly patient who has suffered a stroke is particularly susceptible to aspiration.
- Three major syndromes are associated with aspiration:
  1. Chemical burn pneumonitis
     - Aspiration of the acidic contents of the stomach.
       - Causes a chemical burn of the pulmonary parenchyma.
       - Aspiration of large quantities of fluid can result in the immediate opacification of large volumes of lung.
       - Acid damage causes pulmonary capillaries to leak fluid, release of cytokines, and infiltrate with PMN and can cause noncardiogenic pulmonary edema or ARDS.
       - Onset of symptoms occurs immediately after aspiration.

2. Bronchial obstruction due to aspiration of food particles
   ○ Results in mechanical obstruction.
   ○ Interferes with ventilation and the patient becomes immediately tachypneic.
3. Pneumonia due to a mixture of anaerobic and aerobic mouth flora
   ○ Onset several days after the aspiration of mouth flora.
   ○ Patients with severe gingivitis have higher colony counts of bacteria in their mouth and are at higher risk.
   ○ Necrosis of tissue is common, resulting in lung abscess formation.
   ○ Infection often spreads to the pleura, resulting in empyema, pleural effusions filled with bacteria, and PMN.
   ○ Bronchopleural fistula
     ▪ Develop as a result of necrosis of the pleural lining and lung parenchyma and the formation of a fistula tracking from the bronchus to the pleural space.
     ▪ Prolongs hospitalization and eventually may require surgical repair.

Diagnosis of Bacterial Aspiration Pneumonia

• Sputum often foul smelling as a result of the high numbers of anaerobic bacteria.
• Sputum Gram stain and cultures
   ○ Community-acquired aspiration
     ▪ Gram stain: many PMN and a mixture of Gram-positive and Gram-negative organisms.
     ▪ Culture grows normal mouth flora.
   ○ Hospital-associated aspiration
     ▪ Gram stain: predominance of Gram-negative rods or Gram-positive cocci in clusters.
     ▪ Culture: Often grows antibiotic-resistant Gram-negative organisms as well as S. aureus.
• CXR reveals infiltrates in the dependent pulmonary segments.
   ○ Aspiration in the upright position infiltrates found in:
     ▪ Lower lobes.
     ▪ Right lower lobe more common than the left because the right bronchus takes off from the trachea at a straighter angle than the left mainstem bronchus.
   ○ When aspiration occurs in the recumbent position, infiltrates occur in:
     ▪ Superior segments of the lower lobes.
     ▪ Posterior segments of the upper lobes usually become opacified.

Treatment (see Table 4-3)

• Community-acquired
   ○ Clindamycin and penicillin equally effective
     ▪ Both kill aerobic and anaerobic mouth flora.
     ▪ In cases where lung abscess has developed, clindamycin has been shown to be slightly superior.
• Nosocomial
   ○ Third-generation cephalosporin combined with metronidazole
   ○ Alternatives
     ▪ Semisynthetic penicillin combined with a β-lactamase inhibitor (ticarcillin-clavulinate or piperacillin-tazobactam)
     ▪ Carbapenem (imipenam or meropenem)
• Foreign-body aspiration requires bronchoscopy to remove the foreign material from the tracheobronchial tree.

ACTINOMYCOSIS

- Microaerophilic or anaerobic Gram-positive bacteria
  - Takes up Gram stain poorly
  - Branching forms
  - Modified acid-fast negative
- Infection usually associated with poor oral hygiene.
- Disease is most commonly caused by *Actinomyces israelli.*
- Pulmonary infection often indolent and slowly progressive.
  - Often breaks through fascial planes.
  - Causes pleural infection, resulting in a thickened pleura, empyema, and fistulous tracks.
  - Forms "sulfur granules" that consist of clusters of branching Actinomyces filaments.
- Alert the microbiology laboratory if considering actinomycosis because the anaerobic culture needs to be held for a prolonged period.
  - Takes a minimum of 5–7 days for colonies to be identified.
  - Can take up to 4 weeks.
- Treatment must be prolonged.
  - High-dose intravenous penicillin (18–24 million units IV QD) is recommended for 2–6 weeks.
  - Followed by oral penicillin therapy for 6–12 months.
  - Therapy must be continued until all symptoms and signs of active infection have resolved.
  - Other antibiotics that have been successfully used include erythromycin, tetracyclines, and clindamycin.

NOCARDIA

- An aerobic Gram-positive filamentous bacterium that needs to be differentiated from Actinomyces.
- Nocardia is ubiquitous in the environment, growing in soil, organic matter, and water.
- Inhalation of soil particles leads to pneumonia.
- *N. asteroides* is the most common species to cause disease.
- Infects
  - Patients who are immunocompromised
    - Those with AIDS
    - Those with organ transplants
    - Alcoholics
    - Diabetics
    - HIV and organ transplant patients at risk of developing disseminated infection
  - Normal hosts, 40–50% of cases
  - Alveolar proteinosis is associated with higher risk
- Onset of pulmonary disease is highly variable, being acute in some cases and having a gradual onset in others.
- CXR may reveal cavitary lesions, single or multiple nodules, a reticular nodular pattern, interstitial pattern, or a diffuse parenchymal infiltrate.
- Pulmonary infection can seed the bloodstream and form brain abscesses.
  - Often mistaken for lung carcinoma with CNS metastasis.

- Diagnosis is made by sputum examination or lung or cerebral cortex biopsy.
  - ○ Gram stain demonstrates weakly Gram-positive branching filamentous forms.
  - ○ Acid fast on modified acid-fast stain, Actinomyces acid-fast negative.
  - ○ On tissue biopsy organisms are demonstrated on Brown-Brenn or methenamine silver stain.
  - ○ Alert the clinical microbiology laboratory to use selective media and hold the cultures for a prolonged time.
    - The organism is slow-growing.
    - Frequently overgrown by mouth flora on conventional plates.
- Treatment
  - ○ Nocardia are sensitive to sulfonamides and trimethoprim.
  - ○ Trimethoprim-sulfamethoxazole is generally accepted as the treatment of choice with a daily dose of 2.5–10 mg/kg of the trimethoprim component.
  - ○ High-dose therapy for at least 6 weeks followed by lower doses for 6–12 months.
  - ○ Other sulfonamide preparations when available are also effective (6–12 gm QD in 4–6 divided doses).
  - ○ Also sensitive to amikacin, imipenam, third-generation cephalosporins, minocycline, and dapsone. Only anecdotal case reports support their use.

HAEMOPHILUS INFLUENZAE

- Disease can be caused by both Group B and nontypable *H. influenzae.*
  - ○ Nontypable *H. influenzae* is more common in the elderly and in smokers with chronic obstructive pulmonary disease.
- Clinically similar to *S. pneumoniae*, except onset slower and rigors are rare.
- CXR can demonstrate lobar or patchy infiltrates.
- Sputum Gram stain reveals small Gram-negative pleomorphic coccobacillary organisms.
  - ○ Because of their small size and similar color to background material, this pathogen may be missed by the inexperienced diagnostician.
- Treatment
  - ○ For hospitalized patients intravenous ceftriaxone or cefotaxime is recommended.
  - ○ For oral antibiotic treatment amoxacillin-clavulinate is effective.
  - ○ Other oral antibiotics also are active against this organism.
    - Trimethoprim-sulfamethoxazole
    - Newer macrolides (azithromycin and clarithromycin)
    - Fluoroquinolones
    - Extended-spectrum cephalosporins (cefpodoxime, cefixime)

STAPHYLOCOCCUS AUREUS

- A rare cause of community-acquired pneumonia.
- A large Gram-positive aerobic coccus that grows readily on blood agar plates.
- Most commonly follows influenza infection (a marker for the onset of an influenza epidemic), seen in intraveous drug abusers, and in AIDs patients in association with *Pneumocystis carinii* pneumonia.
- Clinical manifestations
  - ○ Illness more severe than in other forms of pneumonia
    - High fever
    - Slow response to conventional therapy.

- ○ CXR (see Fig. 4-2) shows destructive bronchopneumonia that can be complicated by:
  - ▪ Lung abscesses
  - ▪ Pneumothorax
  - ▪ Empyema (seen in 10% of patients)
- Diagnosis is generally easy.
  - ○ Sputum Gram stain reveals sheets of PMN and an abundance of Gram-positive cocci in clusters and tetrads (see Fig. 4-2).
  - ○ Sputum culture readily grows *S. aureus*.
  - ○ Blood cultures may also be positive.
- The treatment of choice for methicillin-sensitive *S. aureus* is high-dose intravenous nafcillin or oxacillin (8–10 gm/day IV in Q4H dosing) and for MRSA vancomycin (1 gm IV Q12H).

LEGIONELLA PNEUMOPHILA

- An aerobic bacterium that fails to take up Gram stain
- Legionella spp. are found throughout the environment in standing water and soil. Infection due to the inhalation of:
  - ○ Water droplets contaminated with Legionella from:
    - ▪ Cooling towers
    - ▪ Showerheads
    - ▪ Less commonly, unsterilized tap water in respiratory therapy devices
  - ○ Soil during excavation of a contaminated area.
  - ○ Immunocompromised patients, smokers, and the elderly are at increased risk.
- Clinical manifestations are similar to those of other acute community-acquired pneumonias. Some unique features may include:
  - ○ Minimal sputum production
  - ○ Gastrointestinal symptoms
  - ○ Confusion
  - ○ Hyponatremia (noted in 1/3 of patients)
- CXR
  - ○ Most frequently demonstrates a lobar pneumonia.
  - ○ Cavitary lesions may be seen in the immunocompromised host.
  - ○ Small pleural effusions are commonly found.
- Diagnosis requires a high index of suspicion.
  - ○ Sputum Gram stain reveals only acute inflammatory cells.
  - ○ Culture sputum on buffered charcoal yeast extract agar with added suppressive antibiotics.
  - ○ Direct fluorescent antibody staining of the sputum has a low sensitivity (30–50%).
  - ○ Polymerase chain reaction amplification of Legionella DNA from sputum samples is available in some reference laboratories.
  - ○ Urinary antigen test is commercially available.
    - ▪ Moderately sensitive and highly specific.
    - ▪ The antigen is excreted early in the illness and persists for several weeks.
    - ▪ Detects only *L. pneumophila* serogroup 1, the most common cause of Legionella pneumonia in the United States (> 80% of cases).
    - ▪ A positive test is diagnostic, but a negative test does not exclude the diagnosis.

- Treatment
    - For hospitalized patients maximum doses of intravenous:
        - Azithromycin (500 mg IV QD)
        - A fluoroquinolone
            - Ciprofloxacin 400 mg IV Q12H
            - Levofloxacin 500 mg IV QD in patients
        - In transplant patients a fluoroquinolone is preferred because the macrolides interfere with cyclosporin or tacrolimus metabolism.
    - Duration of therapy
        - Immunocompetent patients
            - 5–10 days with azithromycin
            - 10–14 days with a fluoroquinolone
        - Immunocompromised patients therapy
            - 14–21 days to prevent relapse
- Mortality is high in legionnaires' disease.
    - 16–30% in community-acquired disease
    - Up to 50% in hospitalized patients

ATYPICAL PNEUMONIA

- Clinically different from bacterial pneumonia
    - Subacute in onset; usually 10 days of symptoms before seeking medical attention
    - Nonproductive cough
    - Clinical manifestations tend to be less severe
- Three primary causes
    1. *Mycoplasma pneumoniae*
        - Primarily seen in patients under age 40.
        - Seasonal, the highest incidence of Mycoplasma being in the late summer and early fall.
        - Clinical findings suggestive of mycoplasma:
            - Sore throat is usually a prominent symptom.
            - Bullous myringitis is seen in 5% of cases.
            - Tracheobronchits results in a hacking cough that is often worse at night and persists for several weeks.
            - Moist rales may be heard on examination.
            - CXR abnormalities classically are more extensive than predicted by physical examination, and show unilateral or bilateral patchy lower-lobe infiltrates in a bronchial distribution.
            - The clinical course is usually benign.
            - Peripheral WBC is usually < 10,000/mm^3.
            - Sputum Gram stain and culture reveal only normal mouth flora and a moderate inflammatory response.
        - Diagnosis
            - History and clinical manifestations make a presumptive diagnosis.
                - Epidemiological history of contact with a person having similar symptoms helpful.
            - There is no definitive test.
            - PCR of the sputum is under development.
            - Cold agglutinin titers of ≥ 1:64 support the diagnosis and correlate with severity of pulmonary symptoms.
            - Complement fixation antibody titers begin to rise 7–10 days after the onset of symptoms.

- ○ Therapy is empiric.
  - ▪ A macrolide (standard doses of azythromycin, clarithromycin, or erythromycin)
  - ▪ Doxycycline 100 mg po BID
  - ▪ Alternatively a fluoroquinolone can be administered.
  - ▪ The duration of treatment should be 2–3 weeks to prevent relapse.
2. *Chlamydia pneumoniae* (TWAR)
  - ○ 5–15% of cases of community-acquired pneumonia.
  - ○ Similar clinically to Mycoplasma.
    - ▪ Sore throat, hoarseness, and headache
    - ▪ Nonproductive cough
    - ▪ CXR similar to Mycoplasma
  - ○ No rapid diagnostic test is widely available.
  - ○ Treatment is empiric.
    - ▪ Doxycyline is considered the treatment of choice.
    - ▪ Macrolides and fluoroquinolones are also effective.
3. Respiratory viruses
  - ○ Influenza A and B
  - ○ Adenovirus
  - ○ Parainfluenza virus
  - ○ Respiratory syncytial virus: primarily infects young children, the elderly, and the immunocompromised host
  - ○ Clinical presentation
    - ▪ Nonproductive cough
    - ▪ Malaise and fever
    - ▪ Auscultatory findings are minimal
    - ▪ CXR: lower-lobe infiltrates
  - ○ Diagnosis
    - ▪ Viral cultures of the sputum or nasopharyngeal swab.
    - ▪ Rapid commercial tests (take 10–20 minutes) are available for detection of influenza (Quick View, Flu O1A, and Zstatflu).
      - • Sensitivity of 57–77%
      - • Can distinguish between type A and B.
  - ○ Treatment
    - ▪ If Influenza A virus is diagnosed, early treatment with amantadine or rimantadine is recommended.
    - ▪ For both A and B, neuramidase inhibitors have activity and may reduce the severity of influenza.
    - ▪ The influenza vaccine is safe and efficacious.
      - • Give annually in October through early November to:
        - ○ Patients ≥ 65 years
        - ○ Individuals with serious underlying diseases
        - ○ Nursing home residents
        - ○ Health care workers

NOSOCOMIAL PNEUMONIA

- • Accounts for 13–19% of all nosocomial infections.
- • The leading infectious-related cause of death in the hospital, mortality roughly one out of three cases.
- • The development of pneumonia in the hospital prolongs hospitalization by more than a week.

- Risk factors
  - Endotracheal intubation, increases risk by 20 ×, 1–3% incidence/day
  - Age > 70 years
  - Depressed mental status, particularly coma
    - Sedatives and narcotics depress epiglottal function.
  - Underlying diseases
  - Malnutrition
  - Metabolic acidosis
  - Corticosteroids and other immunosuppressants allow bacteria to more readily invade the lung parenchyma.
- Etiologies
  - Aerobic Gram-negative bacteria account for over half the cases of nosocomial pneumonia.
    - *E. coli*
    - Klebsiella
    - Serratia
    - Enterobacter
    - Pseudomonas spp.
  - Gram-positive bacteria
    - *S. aureus* is the most common Gram-positive pathogen, causing 13–40% of nosocomial pneumonias.
    - The risk *of S. aureus* is higher in patients who have wound infections or burns.
    - In patients intubated with head trauma and post neurosurgery.
  - Anaerobes are often isolated in nosocomial pneumonia, but are the primary agent in only 5% of cases.
  - *S. pneumoniae* rarely causes pneumonia in the patient who has been hospitalized for more than 4 days.
- Diagnosis of true pneumonia often difficult in the intubated patient.
  - Difficult to differentiate from:
    - Chronic bronchitis
    - Congestive heart failure
    - ARDS
  - Differentiating infection from colonization critical (see Chap. 1)
    - Colonization of the tracheobronchial tree will change within 3–5 days after initiation of antibiotics.
    - A change in the organisms growing on sputum culture is to be expected, and does not, by itself, indicate new infection.
    - Evidence supporting the onset of a new infection
      - A new fever or a change in fever pattern
      - Rise in the peripheral white blood cell count with a increase in the percentage of PMNs and band forms (left shift)
      - Gram stain demonstrating increased number of PMN in association with a predominance of bacteria that are morphologically consistent with the culture
      - Increased purulent sputum production from the endotracheal tube
      - Reduced arterial pO_2 indicating interference with alveolar-capillary oxygen exchange
      - Enlarging infiltrate on CXR
      - Indiscriminate modifications of antibiotic therapy eventually select for highly resistant pathogens that are difficult, or in some cases impossible, to treat.

- Treatment
  - Third-generation cephalosporin (ceftriaxone, cefotaxime, ceftizoxime, or ceftazidime)
  - Cefepime
  - Ticarcillin-clavulinate or piperacillin-tazobactam
  - Imipenam or meropenam
  - With or without an aminoglycoside (gentamicin, tobramycin, or amikacin)
  - If Pseudomonas aeruginosa is suspected, cefepime, imipenam, or meropenam preferred.
  - If *S. aureus* suspected, vancomycin should be added pending antibiotic sensitivities.
  - Specific anaerobic coverage is usually not required.

EMPYEMA

ETIOLOGIES

- Usually due to spread of pneumonia to the parietal pleura
- Over half of cases of empyema are associated with pneumonia.
- Most common pathogens
  - *S. pneumoniae*
  - *S. aureus*
  - *S. pyogenes*
  - Anaerobic mouth flora
- Empyema can complicate trauma and surgery. Usually caused by:
  - *S. aureus*
  - Aerobic Gram-negative bacilli
- In the immunocompromised patient most likely causes are:
  - Fungi
  - Gram-negative bacilli

PATHOPHYSIOLOGY

- Pleural fluid is deficient in the opsonins, IgG, and complement. If bacteria can find their way to this site, the fluid is very permissive for bacterial growth.
- PMN break down in this closed space and release lysosozyme, bacterial-permeability-increasing protein, and cationic proteins.
  - Slow the growth of bacteria, lengthening doubling times by 20–70-fold.
  - Slow growth of bacteria renders them less sensitive to the cidal effects of antibiotics.
- The pH of the empyema cavity is low, impairing white blood cell function and inactivating some antibiotics, in particular aminoglycosides.

CLINICAL MANIFESTATIONS

- Persistent fever despite appropriate antibiotic treatment for pneumonia
  - Often accompanied by chills and night sweats
- Pleuritic chest pain and shortness of breath
- Physical examination
  - Dull to percussion and decreased breath sounds
  - At the margin between the fluid and aerated lung, egophony as well as bronchial breath sounds is heard.

- Diagnostic tests
  - CXR detects fluid collections as small as 25 ml.
    - On lateral view, 200 cc of fluid is generally required to blunt the posterior costophrenic angle.
    - A lateral decubitus view can demonstrate layering of 5–10 ml of free fluid.
  - Ultrasound is useful for determining the dimensions of the effusion and for guiding thoracentesis.
  - Contrast-enhanced chest CT
    - Differentiates lung abscess from empyema
    - Demonstrates the full extent of the effusion and the degree of pleural thickening
  - Thoracentesis should be performed when empyema is being considered.
    - Ultrasound guidance is associated with decreased incidence of complicating pneumothorax.
    - Fluid should be analyzed for:
      - Cellular content
      - Gram stain, fungal stain, AFB stain
      - Aerobic and anaerobic cultures should be obtained.
      - If fluid is not overtly purulent, should also be analyzed for:
        - pH, glucose, LDH, and total protein
        - pH of <7.2, a glucose of <40 mg/dl, and an LDH of $\geq 1,000$ IU/L = empyema and requires drainage.

TREATMENT

- Antibiotic therapy for the offending pathogen of primary importance.
  - Coverage depends on the pathogen identified by sputum or pleural fluid Gram stain, and culture.
  - A prolonged course of antibiotics, 2–4 weeks, generally required.
- Thoracentesis
  - Parapneumonic effusions that move freely and are less than 1 cm in width on lateral decubitus do not require thoracentesis.
  - Larger collections or evidence that fluid does not flow freely warrants thoracentesis.
  - Chest tube is required if biochemical evidence for empyema is present.
  - Repeated thoracentesis is rarely successful in completely draining the pleural fluid.
  - Closed chest tube drainage for smaller effusion (occupying 20% of the hemithorax)
  - When fluid collects in $\geq 40\%$ of the hemithorax
    - Interventional radiology to precisely place French catheters at sites of loculation and to break up areas of adhesion under CT guidance.
    - If tube drainage proves ineffective after 24 hours, intrathoracic urokinase (125,000 units diluted in 50–100 cc of sterile normal saline) should be instilled, left for 2 or more hours, and then removed.
  - Surgery recommended if thoracentesis and urokinase are unsuccessful.
    - Video-assisted thoracoscopy usually preferred.
- Outcome
  - 8–15% mortality in young previously healthy patients
  - 40–70% mortality in the elderly and those with underlying disease
  - Worse prognosis in those infected with nosocomial pathogens and/or with polymicrobial infection
  - Delay in diagnosis and appropriate drainage increases the need for surgery

---

CHRONIC PNEUMONIAS

- Symptoms develop over weeks to months.
- A careful epidemiologic history and past medical history are very helpful.
- Tuberculosis is spread strictly from person to person and warrants respiratory isolation of all suspected cases.
- Acid-fast sputum smear is helpful in assessing infectiousness and the PPD is a useful screening tool for prophylaxis.
- Miliary tuberculosis must always be considered in the patient with failure to thrive.
- Multiple drugs should always be used to treat active tuberculosis in order to prevent the development of resistance.
- Atypical mycobacterial and fungal pulmonary infections are rare, but need to be considered in specific risk groups and in patients with the appropriate exposure histories.

TUBERCULOSIS

- Potential severity
  - Miliary form of disease can be fatal.
  - Maintain a high index of suspicion in immigrants, the indigent, the elderly, and patients with AIDS.

Microbiology and Pathogenesis

- Aerobic, nonmotile bacillus with a waxy lipid-rich outer wall containing high concentrations of mycolic acid.
- Waxy outer wall fails to take up Gram stain.
- Acid-fast-positive
  - Must be heated to melt the outer wall to allow penetration and binding of the red dye fuchsin.
  - Binds this dye with high affinity and resists acid-alcohol decolorization.
  - Small in size and appears beaded.
- High lipid content allows M. tuberculosis to:
  - Survive in the external environment, resist drying and many chemical disinfectants.
  - Resist killing by macrophages and PMN, and survive for many years within the body.
  - The waxy cell wall limits access to nutrients and slows the rate of growth to about 1/20th the growth rate of most conventional bacteria.
- Intracellular survival induces a profound chronic inflammatory response.
  - Takes approximately 1 month to develop.
  - Accumulation of the cell wall wax, cord factor, stimulates the formation of granulomas (clusters of epithelioid cells, giant cells, and lymphocytes).
  - Over time the centers of the granulomas become necrotic, forming cheesy debris termed caseous necrosis, the hallmark lesion of tuberculosis.
- Activates macrophages to produce multiple cytokines.
  - Interleukin-1 stimulates the hypothalamus to raise core body temperature, causing fever.
  - Tumor necrosis factor interferes with lipid metabolism and causes severe weight loss.

Epidemiology

- Humans are the only reservoir for *M. tuberculosis.*
- Person-to-person spread of infection via aerosolizing droplet nuclei that are dispersed by coughing or sneezing.
  - Increased numbers of particles found in patients with:
    - Laryngeal tuberculosis
    - AIDS
    - Large pulmonary cavities, which intermittently release large numbers of infectious particles
  - Repeated exposure and close contact are generally required to contract this disease.
  - Respiratory isolation and rapid treatment of infected persons are critical for preventing the spread of infection.
- Remains a leading cause of death worldwide despite the availability of antituberculous medications.
- Persons at increased risk:
  - Immigrants from developing countries, nearly 40% of cases in the United States
  - Single men
  - Alcoholics
  - Intravenous drug abusers
  - The urban poor (particularly the homeless)
  - Migrant farm workers
  - Prison inmates
  - HIV-infected patients
  - The elderly (more likely to develop secondary tuberculosis)
- A genetic predisposition in:
  - African Americans
  - Hispanics
  - Asian Pacific Islanders
  - Native Americans

Clinical Syndromes

Primary Tuberculosis

- Occurs when a patient inhales infectious *M. tuberculosis* droplets for the first time.
- A flu-like illness usually follows, but patients can also be asymptomatic.
- Within 4–8 weeks of exposure, a cell-mediated immune response develops.
  - Activated macrophages control the spread and growth of the organisms.
- Areas of fibrosis or calcification develop, called Ghon lesions.
  - In combination with hilar adenopathy is called a Ranke complex.
- Macrophages often gain access to the thoracic duct, enter the bloodstream, and spread throughout the body.
- *M. tuberculosis* survives best in regions with high oxygen tension:
  - Kidneys
  - Long bone epiphyses
  - Vertebral bodies
  - Apices of the lung, the regions of the lung with the highest oxygen content
  - Bacilli usually are not completely eradicated and can survive for decades, being held in check by the host immune response.

Miliary Tuberculosis

- Occurs when initial exposure to *M. tuberculosis* fails to induce cell-mediated immunity.
- Mycobacteria continue to multiply and disseminate, causing miliary tuberculosis.
- Patients at risk include:
  - The very young
  - The very old
  - Patients receiving immunosuppressants
  - Patients with HIV infection
  - Patients with underlying medical conditions, including alcoholism, malignancy, connective tissue diseases, renal failure, and pregnancy
- The absence of an underlying disease does not exclude the possibility of miliary tuberculosis.
- Clinical presentation
  - Children develop:
    - High fever and night sweats
    - Weight loss
    - Hepatosplenomegaly and lymphadenopathy
  - In adults, particularly the elderly, the symptoms and signs may be subtle:
    - Fever and night sweats
    - Malaise and anorexia
    - Weakness
    - Weight loss
    - Physical examination
      - Chronically ill patient with no specific findings.
      - Lymphadenopathy may be detected.
      - Funduscopic examination reveals choroid tubercles in up to 50%.
- Laboratory findings
  - Leukemoid reaction (extremely high white blood cell counts, 30–40,000 WBC).
  - Pancytopenia can also develop.
  - Liver function tests: An elevated alkaline phosphatase and moderate increase in transaminase values.
  - Low serum sodium (due to adrenal insufficiency or inappropriate antidiretic hormone secretion [SIADH])
  - Serum A.M. and P.M. cortisol levels should be measured to exclude adrenal insufficiency.
- CXR: Two thirds have small nodules (0.05–1 mm in diameter) that resemble millet seeds (the basis for the name miliary).
  - A negative CXR does not exclude the diagnosis, particularly in the elderly and in the HIV-infected.
  - ARDS may develop, causing complete opacification of the lungs.
- Diagnosis
  - The key to the diagnosis is a high index of suspicion.
  - Sputum smears are positive in the minority of patients.
  - Histopathology of enlarged lymph nodes, liver biopsy, and bone marrow (reveals granulomas and acid-fast bacilli), and culture.
  - Transbronchial biopsy can yield the diagnosis in large percentage of patients.
  - Blood cultures for mycobacteria should be drawn: commonly positive in AIDS patients.
  - If CNS symptoms are noted, a lumbar puncture should also be performed.

- Treatment
    - A delay in treatment can have fatal consequences.
    - Empiric antituberculous therapy should be initiated once cultures have been obtained.
    - A four-drug regimen of INH, rifampin, pyrazinamide, and ethambutol is the preferred regimen.
    - Patients usually defervesce within 7–14 days.

Secondary Tuberculosis
- Any condition that subsequently depresses cell-mediated immunity can free *M. tuberculosis* to grow and cause symptomatic secondary tuberculosis.
    - 10–15% of primary disease reactivates.
    - 1/2 of the cases reactivate within 2 years of exposure.
    - Most commonly occurs in the elderly.
    - In the United States, the majority of secondary cases occur in middle-aged adults (age 30–50 years).
- Clinical manifestations
    - Early in the course of reactivation, patients are often asymptomatic and reactivation is found only by CXR.
    - If undetected, symptoms slowly develop and worsen over several months.
        - Progressively worsening cough with sputum production
        - Low-grade fever and night sweats
        - Fatigue
        - Weight loss
    - Symptoms of more advanced disease include:
        - Hemoptysis (indicating erosion of a tuberculous cavity into an arteriole)
        - Pleuritic chest pain (suggesting pleural involvement and probable tuberculous pleural effusion)
    - Physical exam
        - Usually unrevealing
        - Despite extensive pulmonary disease auscultation may be normal
        - Posttussic rales may be heard (fine rales in the apices after full expiration followed by a cough and rapid inspiration)
        - Decreased breath sounds and dullness to percussion at one or both bases are present with tuberculous pleural effusions
    - CXR: apical cavitary lesions on CXR
        - Usually in the posterior segments of the upper lobes just below the clavicle.
        - Less frequently seen in the apex of the lower lobe, usually obscured by the heart shadow.
        - In HIV, CXR often does not show cavities.
        - All AIDS patients with pneumonia are considered to have tuberculosis until proven otherwise.
        - Apical lordotic view is often helpful in visualizing upper-lobe apical lesions.
    - Chest CT scan is helpful for assessing the extent of disease.
        - Air fluid levels are uncommon in tuberculous cavities.

Diagnosis
- Zeil-Nielson acid-fast sputum smear the classic method for diagnosis.
  - Morning sputum samples tend to have the highest yield.
  - A single negative smear does not exclude TB.
  - Three sputum smears are recommended, because in cavitary disease the release of infectious droplets is intermittent.
  - Negative smears do not definitively exclude tuberculosis.
    - Smear has a 60% sensitivity as compared to sputum culture.
    - To be smear-positive the sputum must contain 1×10^4 organisms per ml.
  - A fluorochrome stain using auramine-rhodamine is more sensitive and allows sputum to be examined at low magnification.
  - The number of organisms seen on smear directly correlates with infectiousness.
  - Cavitary disease is potentially very infectious.
    - Cavities may contain 10^9–10^{10} organisms. Patients with cavitary disease should be placed in respiratory isolation pending sputum AFB smears.
- PCR can effectively detect as few as 10 organisms in a clinical specimen.
  - Sensitivity and specificity are greater than 95% in smear-positive cases.
  - Specificity in smear-negative cases is also high.
  - False-negative and false-positive results are common in less experienced laboratories.
  - Recommended only to complement traditional methods.
  - Cannot differentiate killed from actively growing organisms in patients on antituberculous therapy.
- Culture remains the most accurate method for diagnosis.
  - In patients who fail to produce sputum, aspiration of the gastric contents in the morning prior to arising from bed is useful for obtaining samples for culture.
  - Blood cultures in which all cells are lysed to release intracellular mycobacteria may be positive in patients with suspected disseminated disease.
  - The bacterium grows at about 1/20th the rate of more conventional bacteria and takes 3–6 weeks to grow on Lowenstein Jensen media.
  - BACTEC radiometric culture system can detect mycobacteria metabolism within 9–16 days.
  - Drug susceptibilities can also be reliably tested using this method.

Treatment
- See Chapter 1 for the principles of antituberculous therapy.
- Prolonged therapy is required to kill dormant organisms in necrotic lesions.
- To prevent the development of resistance, therapy should always include two or more antituberculous medications.
  - 1×10^6 organisms are naturally resistant to INH.
  - Cavitary lesions containing 10^9–10^{10} organisms and therefore 100–1,000 organisms would be expected be INH resistant.
  - The probability of selecting for a resistant organism would be expected to be 1×10^{12} organisms ($10^6 \times 10^6$) for 2 drugs.

- Resistance to antituberculous drugs is a concern.
  - 10% INH resistance noted in large urban areas.
  - Multidrug-resistant tuberculosis (MDR-TB) indicates resistance to two or more drugs.
    - Early 1990s in the United States an increase in frequency observed. New York State 1991, 12.9% resistant to both INH and rifampin.
    - 1998 incidence of MDR-TB in New York City dropped to 2%.
    - Secondary resistance, i.e., the development of resistance while on therapy, is major problem for:
      - The homeless
      - Illicit drug users
      - AIDS patients
    - Outside the United States the percentage of strains that are resistant to INH and MDR varies widely.
      - INH resistance 7.5% worldwide. Higher levels in Asia, Africa, and Latin America.
      - Lower levels observed in Europe and Oceania.
      - Rates of secondary MDR-TB are high (13%) in countries where tuberculosis control programs have deteriorated (Latvia, South Korea, and Russia).
- Treatment recommendations
  - If drug-sensitive infection is likely:
    - INH, rifampin, pyrazinimide, and ethambutol or streptomycin × 2 months followed by INH, rifampin, and pyrazinimide × 4 months.
  - If MDR-TB is suspected:
    - Extensive susceptibility testing should be performed with decisions made with the assistance of an expert in the field.
    - Treatment should consist of at least three drugs to which the organism is proven to be susceptible.
    - Fluoroquinolones combined with aminoglycosides are particularly useful.
    - In the unreliable patient, directly observed therapy (DOT) should be instituted. Use DOT in all patients with INH- or rifampin-resistant organisms.

Prevention

- Identification of exposed individuals and preventing them from developing active disease is the major way to prevent person-to-person spread.
- PPD is a useful tool for accomplishing this task.
  - Subcutaneous injection of 0.1 ml. Examine the diameter of induration at 48–72 hours.
  - ≥ 10 mm induration, 90% are infected with tuberculosis.
  - > 15 mm induration, 100% are infected.
  - Indicates that sometime in the past the individual has been exposed to active tuberculosis, but does not indicate active disease.
  - Conversion from negative to positive, indicates exposure to tuberculosis during the time interval between the two tests.
- PPD not reliable in:
  - HIV patients with low CD4 counts
  - Patients receiving immunosuppressants
  - Patients with severe malnutrition

- INH prophylaxis, 300 mg po QD × 6 months if:
  - PPD conversion with less than 2-year interval, and a negative CXR
  - Positive PPD in high-risk patients
    - HIV-infected prophylaxis for 12 months
    - Known recent exposure to Tb
    - Chronic underlying disease
  - Positive PPD, abnormal CXR, and three sputums negative for AFB to exclude active disease
  - Positive PPD ≥ 15 mm and age < 35 years
  - Positive PPD ≥ 10 mm and age < 35 years who is an immigrant, medically underserved, or a resident of a long-term care facility

ATYPICAL MYCOBACTERIA

- Atypical mycobacteria are found throughout the environment in soil and water.
- Low virulence
  - Rarely cause pulmonary disease in otherwise healthy individuals.
  - Patients with underlying pulmonary disease can inhale these organisms and develop pneumonia.
- *M. avium* complex is the most common mycobacterium causing cavitary upper-lobe lesions.
  - Cavities somewhat smaller and thinner-walled than with *M. tuberculosis*.
  - Seen primarily in male smokers in their early 50s who abuse alcohol.
  - Women age 60 or older with no apparent underlying disease; involves the right middle lobe or lingula.
- *M. kansasii*, *M. fortuitum*, and *M. abscessus* can also cause chronic cavitary disease.
- Elaborate criteria for differentiating colonization from infection have been established.
- Therapy is prolonged and is based on sensitivity testing.
- Patients respond poorly to therapy and resection of the infected lung segment may be required for cure.
- Management of these patients is complex and requires the supervision of an experienced pulmonary or infectious disease specialist.

HISTOPLASMOSIS

Epidemiology
- Survives in moist soil in temperate climates
- Most commonly reported in the Ohio and Mississippi River valleys
- Infection usually develops after exposure to contaminated soil in association with:
  - Construction or excavation of contaminated soil
  - Cave exploration; dried bat guano contains high concentrations of infectious particles
  - Renovation of old buildings previously inhabited by birds or bats

Pathogenesis
- This fungus exists in two forms, as mycelia or yeast forms.
  - Mycelial form found in the moist soil of temperate climates existing as macroconidia (8–15 μm is size) and microconidia (2–5 μm).
  - Microconidia float in the air, and can be inhaled into the lung.

- ◦ When ingested by alveolar macrophages and neutrophils, mycelia transform to rounded, encapsulated yeast cells.
  - ◦ Upregulation of multiple genes, including a gene that increases production of a calcium-binding protein (may explain the calcifications in infected tissues)
- Yeast transported to hilar node where cell-mediated immunity develops within several weeks

Clinical Manifestations
- 90% are asymptomatic or develop a mild influenza-like illness after exposure.
- Active disease. Seen in the very young, the elderly, and in patients with compromised immune systems
- After 14 days' incubation, develop:
  - ◦ High fever, headache, nonproductive cough, and dull nonpleuritic chest pain.
  - ◦ CXR—patchy infiltrates later convert to "buckshot" calcifications.
  - ◦ Mediastinal lymphadenopathy may mimic lymphoma or sarcoidosis.
  - ◦ Progressive mediastinal fibrosis a rare complication.
  - ◦ Cavitary disease develops in 8% of cases, clinically similar to tuberculosis.
    - ▪ Males > 50 years old with COPD at higher risk
    - ▪ Spontaneous resolution occurs in 10–60% of cases.
- Disseminated disease in 10% of symptomatic primary disease
  - ◦ Increased likelihood in the very old, very young, AIDS patients, and immunosuppressed.
  - ◦ Meningitis with lymphs and low glucose may develop.
  - ◦ Reticulonodular pattern on CXR in most, but CXR normal in one third.
  - ◦ Mortality is high if treatment is not initiated.

Diagnosis
- Readily grows from sputum, tissue samples, and body fluids
  - ◦ Requires selective media (brain heart infusion with antibiotics and cyclohexamide)
  - ◦ Not a routine method, clinical microbiology must be notified
- Bronchoscopy improves yield (90% in HIV patients)
- Bone marrow positive in 50%
- Blood cultures—lysis centrifugation method positive in up to 50%
- Polysaccharide urine and serum antigen test most sensitive, positive:
  - ◦ 90% of disseminated disease
  - ◦ 40% cavitary disease
  - ◦ 20% acute pulmonary disease
- Histopathology—noncaseating or caseating granulomas
  - ◦ Silver stain best for identifying the yeast forms
  - ◦ Periodic acid-Schiff may identify organisms not seen on hematoxylin-eosin

Treatment
- Itraconazole the oral agent of choice. Recommended for treatment of:
  - ◦ Acute pulmonary disease that fails to improve over 7 days
  - ◦ Extensive mediastinal involvement
  - ◦ Progressive cavitary disease
- Amphotericin B used for more severe disease
  - ◦ Primary pulmonary disease if patient unable to take oral medications
  - ◦ Cavitary disease that fails to improve on itraconazole
  - ◦ Progressive disseminated disease

COCCIDIOMYCOSIS

Epidemiology
- *Coccidioides immitis* grows in soil (prefers dry, alkaline soil) in regions with hot summers and winters with few freezes.
- Primarily found in central California, southern Arizona, New Mexico, and Texas. Also found in Mexico, Central America, and South America.
- Contracted during the summer, dust storms, excavation, earthquakes.

Pathogenesis
- A dimorphic fungus, mycelial form called arthroconidia
- Inhaled arthroconidia transform to spherules (yeast forms) that release endospores
- Ingested by macrophages; transported to hilar lymph nodes, lymphatics, and bloodstream

Clinical Manifestations
- Approximately two thirds of patients exposed to arthroconidia have minimal symptoms.
- 7–21 days after inhalation, one third symptomatic: nonproductive cough, fever, pleuritic chest pain, shortness of breath, headache, and fatigue.
- Skin manifestations common: erythema nodosum, erythema multiforme, non-pruritic papular rash.
- Eosinophilia may be noted on peripheral blood smear.
- Abnormal CXR frequent: unilateral infiltrates, pleural effusions, hilar adenopathy.
- AIDS patients with CD4 < 100 mm^3 can disseminate causing diffuse lung opacification, meningitis, bone infection, arthritis.
- Chronic lung disease can lead to fibrosis, nodules, or cavities.
- Isolated pulmonary nodules are not calcified, and can be differentiated from neoplasm only by biopsy.
- Chronic pleural effusions most commonly develop in young, healthy, athletic males.

Diagnosis
- Travel to or past residence in an endemic area should alert the clinician to the possibility of coccidioidomycosis.
- Spherules may be seen on induced sputum or after bronchoscopy.
- Readily cultured on routine bacterial and mycology culture plates.
- Histopathology—noncaseating and caseating granulomas; silver stain best, not seen on Gram stain.
- Multiple serological tests available to measure IgG and IgM antibody titers.
  - IgM titer elevated in acute disease.
  - IgG often persists for years, rising titer ≥ 1:32 signals dissemination, falling titer indicative of a favorable prognosis.
  - Patients with no detectable lesions can have titers ≤ 1:8 for many years after exposure.

Treatment
- The majority of infections spontaneously resolve. Treatment usually reserved for disseminated disease (higher risk of dissemination in blacks, Filipinos, pregnant women, diabetics, and immunosuppressed patients, including those with AIDS).
- Amphotericin B for severe disease (0.7–1 mg/kg/day).

- Fluconazole (400–800 mg po QD) or itraconazole (200 mg po BID) for less severe disease.
- Treatment for a minimum of 6 months.
- Complement fixation IgG titers should decrease to a stable low titer.
- For meningitis, triazole therapy should be continued indefinitely.
- Surgery to resect expanding lung lesions, prevent bronchopleural fistula formation, and to correct life-threatening pulmonary hemorrhage.

REFERENCES

General

Baik I, Curhan GC, Rimm EB, Bendich A, Willett WC, Fawzi WW: A prospective study of age and lifestyle factors in relation to community-acquired pneumonia in US men and women. *Arch Intern Med* 2000; 160:3082–88.

Ben-David D, Rubinstein E: Appropriate use of antibiotics for respiratory infections: Review of recent statements and position papers. *Curr Opin Infect Dis* 2002; 15:151.

Fine MJ, Stone RA, Singer DE, et al: Processes and outcomes of care for patients with community-acquired pneumonia: Results from the Pneumonia Patient Outcomes Research Team (PORT) cohort study. *Arch Intern Med* 1999; 159:970–80.

Gilbert K, Gleason PP, Singer DE, et al: Variations in antimicrobial use and cost in more than 2,000 patients with community-acquired pneumonia. *Am J Med* 1998; 104:17–27.

Guthrie R. Community-acquired lower respiratory tract infections: Etiology and treatment. *Chest* 2001; 120:2021–34.

Mandell LA, Bartlett JG, Dowell SF, File TM, Jr., Musher DM, et a: Update of practice guidelines for the management of community-acquired pneumonia in immunocompetent adults. *Clin Infect Dis* 2003; 37:1405–33.

Mortensen EM, Coley CM, Singer DE, et al: Causes of death for patients with community-acquired pneumonia: Results from the Pneumonia Patient Outcomes Research Team cohort study. *Arch Intern Med* 2002; 162:1059–64.

Roson B, Carratala J, Verdaguer R, Dorca J, Manresa F, Gudiol F: Prospective study of the usefulness of sputum Gram stain in the initial approach to community-acquired pneumonia requiring hospitalization. *Clin Infect Dis* 2000; 31:869–74.

Pneumococcal Pneumonia

Bauer T, Ewig S, Marcos MA, Schultze-Werninghaus G, Torres A: *Streptococcus pneumoniae* in community-acquired pneumonia: How important is drug resistance? *Med Clin North Am* 2001; 85:1367–79.

Marrie TJ: Pneumococcal pneumonia: Epidemiology and clinical features. *Semin Respir Infect* 1999; 14:227–36.

Musher DM, Alexandraki I, Graviss EA, et al: Bacteremic and nonbacteremic pneumococcal pneumonia: A prospective study. *Medicine (Baltimore)* 2000; 79:210–21.

Hemophilus Influenzae Pneumonia

Sarangi J, Cartwright K, Stuart J, Brookes S, Morris R, Slack M: Invasive *Haemophilus influenzae* disease in adults. *Epidemiol Infect* 2000; 124:441–47.

Aspiration Pneumonia

Marik PE: Aspiration pneumonitis and aspiration pneumonia. *N Engl J Med* 2001; 344:665–71.

Legionnaires' Pneumonia
Akbas E, Yu VL: Legionnaires' disease and pneumonia: Beware the temptation to underestimate this "exotic" cause of infection. *Postgrad Med* 2001; 109:135–38, 141–42, 147.
Waterer GW, Baselski VS, Wunderink RG: Legionella and community-acquired pneumonia: A review of current diagnostic tests from a clinician's viewpoint. *Am J Med* 2001; 110:41–48.

Atypical Pneumonia
Marrie TJ, Peeling RW, Fine MJ, Singer DE, Coley CM, Kapoor WN: Ambulatory patients with community-acquired pneumonia: The frequency of atypical agents and clinical course. *Am J Med* 1996; 101:508–15.

Actinomycosis and Nocardiosis
Heffner JE: Pleuropulmonary manifestations of actinomycosis and nocardiosis. *Semin Respir Infect* 1988; 3:352–61.

Tuberculosis
Packham S: Tuberculosis in the elderly. *Gerontology* 2001; 47:175–79.
Small PM, Fujiwara PI: Management of tuberculosis in the United States. *N Engl J Med* 2001; 345:189–200.

Histoplasmosis
Gurney JW, Conces DJ: Pulmonary histoplasmosis. *Radiology* 1996; 199:297–306.

Coccidioidomycosis
Standaert SM, Schaffner W, Galgiani JN, et al: Coccidioidomycosis among visitors to a *Coccidioides immitis*–endemic area: An outbreak in a military reserve unit. *J Infect Dis* 1995; 171:1672–75.

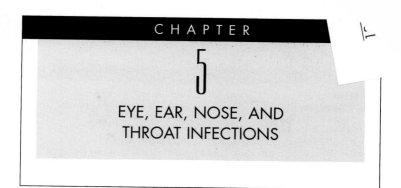

CHAPTER

5

EYE, EAR, NOSE, AND THROAT INFECTIONS

EYE INFECTIONS

HIGHLIGHTS

- Conjunctivitis is generally a self-limited mild disease that responds to topical therapy.
- Complaints of eye pain or visual loss suggest keratitis or endophthalmitis and warrant emergency evaluation by an ophthalmologist.
- The potential for permanent loss of vision is high in cases of endopthalmitis.

CONJUNCTIVITIS

- Potential severity: Usually rapidly responds to therapy and does not threaten vision.
- Tears contain antibacterial agents that protect against conjunctivitis.
- Bacterial conjunctivitis causes a thick purulent discharge.
  - Most common causes: *S. aureus*, *S. pneumoniae*, *H. influenzae*, and *Moraxella*.
  - *N. gonorrhoeae* causes a very severe conjunctivitis that can progress to keratitis.
  - Topical antibiotics are usually recommended.
- Viruses are the most common cause.
  - Bilateral involvement is the rule.
  - Result in serous exudate and follicle formation.
  - The disease is self-limited.
- Allergic conjunctivitis
  - Usually bilateral
  - Accompanied by itching

Diagnosis

- Cultures are not usually obtained in routine cases of conjunctivitis.
- In more severe cases conjunctival scrappings are obtained for culture and Gram stain.
  - PMNs are found in bacterial and chlamydial conjunctivitis.
  - Mononuclear cell exudate in viral conjunctivitis
  - Eosinophils in allergic conjunctivitis

137

Treatment
- For severe bacterial conjunctivitis and chlamydia conjunctivitis, systemic treatment is recommended.
- For milder forms, topical antimicrobial agents usually are sufficient.
  - Fluoroquinolones now preferred, cover both Gram-positive and Gram-negative organisms
  - Other topical drops include:
    - Gentamicin or tobramycin for Gram-negative infections
    - Polymyxin B/bacitracin, neomycin/polymyxin, polymyxin B-trimethoprim or erythromycin for Gram-positive infections

CORNEAL INFECTIONS

- Potential severity: Can cause blindness, and requires rapid treatment. Often requires management by an experienced ophthalmologist.
- All patients with significant corneal lesions should be referred to an ophthalmologist experienced in the management of keratitis.
- Risk factors:
  - Trauma to the eye
  - Contact lens abrasions
  - Eye surgery
  - Defective tear production can result in damage to corneal epithelium
  - Comatose patients receiving respiratory support with defective eye closure
  - Immunosuppression and diabetes mellitus
- Usually preceded by a break in the cornea (exceptions Neisseria, *Corynebacteria diphtheriae*, Listera, and Shigella)
- Clinical manifestations
  - The primary symptom of keratitis is eye pain, a foreign body sensation in the eye.
  - Vision is usually impaired as a consequence of corneal edema.
  - Photophobia and reflex tearing are also common.
  - Slit lamp examination allows identification of the corneal break.
  - Intraocular inflammation is common; severe inflammation can lead to the formation of a hypopyon (a collection of pus in the anterior chamber).
- Etiologies and unique characteristics
  - Bacterial infection is the leading cause of keratitis, accounting for 65–90% of cases.
    - *S. aureus* most common
    - *S. pneumoniae* causes a well-circumscribed ulcer with sharp margins.
    - *Pseudomonas aeruginosa* associated with hard contact lenses, very destructive, and causes severe eye pain
  - Herpes simplex causes distinct dendritic lesions that take up fluorescein. Consider in the hospitalized patient who develops a unilateral red eye.
  - Aspergillus usually follows eye injury with organic matter (tree branch).
  - Acanthamoeba occurs in contact lens wearers who use tap water with their cleaning solutions.

Diagnosis and Treatment
- Slit lamp examination is helpful in identifying potential causes.
- Corneal scrapings for culture if bacterial or fungal etiology is suspected.
  - Gram stain, Giemsa stain, and methenamine silver stain should be performed.
  - Aerobic bacteria grow readily on standard media within 48 hours.
  - Special processing may be required if Acanthamoeba, fungi, mycobacteria, or Chlamydia are the suspected pathogens.

- Viral keratitis can usually be diagnosed by appearance and generally does not require culturing.
- Treatment must be instituted emergently.
  - Patients often hospitalized for close observation.
  - Initially therapy can be based on Gram stain in 75% of patients.
  - Antibiotics are commonly given topically, and in some instances also subconjunctivally.
    - Eye drops need to be administered every half hour during the day and hourly during sleep for 7–10 days.
    - Subconjunctival injections should be repeated every 12–24 hours for a total of 3–6 doses.
  - Systemic therapy in addition to topical therapy is recommended for patients with imminent perforation.
  - Topical regimens include:
    - Topical fluoroquinolones recommended as empiric therapy for non-sight-threatening bacterial keratitis. 0.3% ofloxacin least toxic regimen, often combined with topical cephalothin.
    - Bacitracin 5000 U/ml and gentamicin (13 mg/ml) for *S. pneumoniae.*
    - Cephalothin (50 mg/ml) plus bacitracin for other Gram-positive cocci such as *S. aureus.*
    - Tobramycin (13.6–15 mg/ml) or gentamicin for Pseudomonas spp.; gentamicin for other Gram-negative bacilli.
    - Amphotericin B (1.5–3 mg/ml) plus flucytosine (1%) for yeast-like fungi.
    - Natamycin (5%) for hyphal fungi.
    - Neomycin (5–8 mg/ml) plus pentamidine isethionate (0.15%) for Acanthamoeba spp.
    - Trifluoridine ophthalmic solution or topical acyclovir is recommended for 7–10 days for herpes simplex keratitis. Oral acyclovir 400 mg po BID is often given for several months or in some cases for years, to prevent recurrence.

ENDOPHTHALMITIS

- Potential severity: An ocular emergency. A very serious infection that often leads to permanent visual impairment or blindness.
- An inflammatory disease involving the ocular chamber and adjacent structures. Involvement of all the ocular tissue layers and chambers is called panophthalmitis.
- Clinical manifestations
  - Eye pain, photophobia, reduced vision, and redness
  - In hematogenous spread, sudden onset of blurred vision without pain, photophobia, or redness
  - Fungal endophthalmitis symptoms and signs tend to be less severe. May only note blurry vision or spots in the visual field.
  - Exam:
    - Eyelid edema, chemosis of conjunctiva, moderate to severe anterior chamber inflammation with a hypopyon
    - Loss of the red reflex, retinal hemorrhages, and venous sheathing
    - Monitor the fundi in all patients with candidemia looking for:
      - Focal areas of inflammation
      - Gray-white fluffy exudates most characteristic

Etiologies and predisposing conditions

- Acute postoperative caused by endogenous flora, *S. epidermidis*, *S. aureus*, streptococcal spp.
- Posttraumatic results in mixed infections. *B. cereus* very aggressive. Fungal infections after injuries with organic material.
- Hematogenous form more commonly involves the right eye. Candida most common etiology, *B. cerius* in IV drug abusers.

Diagnosis

- Cultures and smears of the aqueous and vitreous (vitreous gives the highest positive yield). Conjunctival cultures often misleading.
- In suspected hematogenous endophthalmitis, blood, urine, and CSF cultures often reveal the etiologic agent.

Treatment

- Vitreous sampling should be followed by intravitreal antibiotic injection in patients with retained visual acuity.
- Vitrectomy can improve vision in patients with only light perception.
- Broad-spectrum antibiotic treatment is recommended (example, vancomycin 0.1 cc of a 10 mg/ml solution plus gentamicin 0.1 cc of a 1 mg/ml solution).
- Systemic therapy in cases of hematogenous endophthalmitis, but of no benefit in other forms of endophthalmitis.
- For Candida endophthalmitis intravenous amphotericin B, and in more severe cases, intravitreous amphotericin B (5–10 ug).
- About half of patients with endophthalmitis retain visual acuity of 20/400 or better. 1/10 patients requires enucleation.

THROAT INFECTIONS

HIGHLIGHTS

- Pharyngitis is often overtreated with antibiotics.
- Sore throat associated with drooling and difficulty breathing suggests epiglottitis, a condition associated with respiratory arrest.

PHARYNGITIS

- Potential severity: Usually a self-limited disease, with the exception of the rare life-threatening complication of peritonsillar abscess.
- Etiology
  - Viruses are most common, and include: rhinoviruses and coronaviruses (common cold viruses), adenovirus, herpes simplex, parainfluenza, influenza, coxsackievirus A, Epstein-Barr virus, cytomegalovirus, and HIV.
  - Bacterial
    - Group A streptococci
      - 50% of all cases of pharyngitis in children
      - 15% in adults
    - Other forms of streptococci, GpB and C
    - Mixed anaerobic flora can extend under the tongue and into the neck—called Vincent's angina.

- *Corynebacterium diphtheriae* a rare cause in the United States.
  - A grayish pseudomembrane develops that tightly adheres to the pharyngeal wall.
- *Neisseria gonorrhoeae* and *Treponema pallidum*; consider in sexually promiscuous patients.
- Mycoplasma and Chlamydia should be considered when pharyngitis is accompanied by pneumonia.

Clinical Manifestations and Diagnosis
- Bacterial pharyngitis suggested by:
  - Pharyngeal exudates
  - Tender adenopathy
  - Absence of rhinitis or cough
  - Fever
- Antigen tests allows rapid diagnosis of *S. pyogenes*.
  - >90% specificity
  - Only 60–95% sensitivity
  - Negative antigen test in association with physical findings consistent with bacterial pharyngitis warrants a throat culture.
- Peritonsillar abscess a rare complication
  - Consider if medial displacement of one or both tonsils.
  - Neck CT with contrast is the diagnostic procedure of choice.
  - Delay in appropriate surgical drainage can result in spread of infection to the retropharyngeal, pretracheal, and danger space, and can result in fatal purulent pericarditis (see Chap. 7).

Treatment depends on the etiology (see Table 5-1).
- Too often antibiotics are given for viral pharyngitis.
- Antibiotics should not be administered to the patient with a negative rapid antigen test and physical findings suggestive of viral pharyngitis.
- Oral penicillin VK × 10 days or a single injection of long-acting benzathine penicillin (1.2 million units IM) recommended for proven *S. pyogenes*.
- Erythromycin × 10 days is recommended for penicillin-allergic patients.
- Eradication of the *S. pyogenes* markedly reduces the incidence of poststreptococcal glomerulonephritis and rheumatic heart disease.

Epiglottitis
- Potential severity: An infectious disease emergency because of the risk of a fatal respiratory arrest.
- Now more common in adults owing to use of *H. influenzae* vaccine in children.
- Sore throat associated with difficulty swallowing and drooling followed by difficulty breathing.
  - Respiration is often tentative
  - Inspiratory stridor
- Indirect laryngoscopy: swollen cherry-red epiglottis.
- Lateral neck X-ray demonstrates the enlarged epiglottis.
- Respiratory arrest is a danger, and pediatric patients should be electively intubated. (Respiratory arrest in children is associated with an 80% mortality.)
- *H. influenzae* is the most common. *S. pneumonia*, other streptococcal spp, and *Staphylococcus aureus* have been reported in adults.
- Intravenous ceftriaxone or cefotaxime for 7–10 days is the treatment of choice (see Table 5-1).

TABLE 5-1
ANTIBIOTIC THERAPY FOR EAR NOSE AND THROAT INFECTIONS

Drug	Dose	Relative Efficacy	Comments
Pharyngitis			
Viral most frequent	Avoid antibiotics		
Penicillin V-K	500 mg po QID × 10 days		Administer only if proven *S. pyogenes* infection
Benzathine penicillin	1.2 million units IM × 1		
Erythromycin	500 mg QID × 10 days		For PCN-allergic patients
Epiglottitis			
Ceftriaxone (or)	1 gm IV or IM QD	First line	Intubation recommended for children
Cefotaxime	1 gm IV Q8H		
Malignant otitis externa			
Ciprofloxacin	500 mg IV Q12h	First line	Prolonged therapy × 6 weeks
Ceftazidime	2 gm IV Q8H		
Cefepime	2 gm IV Q12H		
Otitis media			
Amoxicillin (or)	500 mg po TID	First line	Amoxicillin more cost effective; if no improvement, switch to amoxicillin-clavulinate
Amoxicillin-clavulinate	875/125 mg po BID	First line	If failure to improve on amoxicillin, also can use one of these regimens
2nd-generation cephalosporin			
Cefuroxime	500 mg po BID		
Cefpodoxime	400 mg po BID		
Cefprozil	500 mg po BID		

Mastoiditis (acute)

Ceftriaxone (or)	1 gm IV or IM QD	First line	Therapy × 3–4 weeks
Cefotaxime	1 gm IV Q8H		

Mastoiditis (chronic)

Piperacillin-tazobactam	3 /0.375 gm IV Q6H		Polymicrobial including anaerobes. Intraoperative
Ticarcillin-calvulinate	3.1 gm IV Q4–6H		cultures helpful
Imipenam	500 mg IV Q6H		

Sinusitis (outpatient)

Amoxacillin-clavulinate	875/125 mg po BID	First line	
Cefuroxime	400 mg po BID	First line	
Gatifloxacin	400 mg po QD	Second line	Danger of selecting for resistant *S. pneumoniae*, use for
Levofloxacin	500 mg po QD		the PCN-allergic
Moxifloxacin	400 mg po QD		

Sinusitis (inpatient)

Ceftriaxone (or)	1 gm IV or IM QD	First line	
Cefotaxime (+)	1 gm IV Q8H		
Metronidazole (+)	500 mg IV Q8H		
Nafcillin or Oxacillin	2 gm IV Q4H		

143

EAR INFECTIONS

HIGHLIGHTS

- With the exception of diabetics and immunocompromised hosts, external otitis media can be treated topically.
- Otitis media most commonly occurs in children, and warrants antibiotic treatment when fluid is detected behind the eardrum.
- Mastoiditis is a severe complication of otitis media that can lead to brain abscess and septic lateral sinus thrombosis, and requires intervention by an ENT specialist.

OTITIS EXTERNA

- Potential severity: In the normal host usually an annoying, but not serious, disease; however, in the diabetic or immunocompromised host can be life-threatening.
- Due to trapped water in the external ear.
- Symptoms: local itching and pain.
- Physical findings include redness and swelling of the external canal. Tenderness of the pina is often noted.
- Caused by Gram-negative bacilli, *Pseudomonas aeruginosa* most common.
- Malignant otitis externa
  - Occurs in diabetics and immunocompromised patients
  - Can infect the base of the skull
  - Multiple cranial nerves can be damaged, including cranial nerves 7, 9, 10, and 12
  - Can be fatal
  - Requires prolonged antipseudomonal antibiotic therapy

Treatment
- For standard otitis externa:
  - Polymyxin drops combined with hydrocortisone (corticosporin otic drops) or an oral fluoroquinolone (ciprofloxacin 500 mg BID) combined with topical hydrocortisone.
- For malignant otitis externa:
  - Systemic therapy for Pseudomonas (ciprofloxacin, ceftazidime, or cefepime) must be instituted for a minimum of 6 weeks and necrotic tissue surgically debrided (see Table 5-1).

OTITIS MEDIA

- Potential severity: Rapid treatment and close follow-up reduce the risk of serious complications. Delay in therapy can lead to potentially fatal complications.
- Due to obstruction of the eustachian tube in association with a viral URI. More common in children who have narrow eustachian tubes.
- Ear pain, ear drainage, and occasionally hearing loss. Less common symptoms: fever, vertigo, nystagmus, and tinnitus.
- Infants may present with irritability and diarrhea.
- Diagnosis is made by demonstrating the presence of fluid behind the tympanic membrane. Redness of the tympanic membrane is not specific.

- *S. pneumoniae*, *H. influenzae*, and *Moraxella catarrhalis* most common causes.
- Amoxacillin to start followed by amoxacillin-clavulinate or cefuroxime if no response within 72 hours (see Table 5-1).

MASTOIDITIS

- Potential severity: A rare disease that can lead to fatal complications.
- A complication of otitis media.
- Swelling, redness, and tenderness can develop directly behind the ear in the area of the mastoid bone.
- Readily diagnosed by mastoid X-rays.
- Treatment similar to otitis media; however, antibiotic therapy must be prolonged for 3–4 weeks.
- Chronic mastoid infections can be associated with Gram-negative aerobic bacteria.
- Can lead to:
  ○ Brain abscess
  ○ Septic lateral sinus thrombosis
- Surgical drainage required if an abscess forms within the mastoid or temporal lobe or if septic lateral sinus thrombosis develops.

SINUS INFECTION

HIGHLIGHTS

- Often difficult to differentiate viral from bacterial sinusitis.
- Prolonged symptoms, associated with more severe pain and purulent drainage, warrant antibiotic treatment. However, the efficacy of amoxacillin-clavulinate has been called into question.
- Infections of the ethmoid, frontal, and sphenoid sinuses can result in severe neurologic complications,

POTENTIAL SEVERITY:

- Delays in therapy can result in spread of infection outside of the air sinus and result in fatal complications.

PREDISPOSING FACTORS

- Viral upper respiratory infections cause inflammation of the sinuses and the production of serous exudate; 0.5–1% of viral upper respiratory infections progress to bacterial sinusitis.
- Anatomic obstruction
- Septal deformities and nasal polyps
- Foreign bodies
- Chronic adenoiditis
- Intranasal neoplasms
- Indwelling nasal tubes interfere with normal drainage of the sinus ostia.
- Nasal allergies

- Dental abscesses of the upper teeth can spread to the maxillary sinuses and can result in recurrent bacterial sinusitis.
- Genetic disorders
  ○ Cystic fibrosis (associated with abnormal viscous mucous)
  ○ Kartagener's syndrome (causing defective mucous cell ciliary function)

CLINICAL MANIFESTATIONS

- Symptoms
  ○ Pressure sensation and headache.
  ○ Retro-orbital and hemicranial headache suggests sphenoid sinusitis.
  ○ Purulent foul-smelling, bad-tasting drainage (most helpful).
- Signs
  ○ Fever is rare in adults.
  ○ Sinus tenderness elicited in maxillary and frontal, but not sphenoid, sinusitis.
  ○ Transillumination helpful for maxillary and frontal sinusitis.
  ○ Look for purulent drainage from the ostia and posterior nasopharynx (most helpful).
  ○ Hypo- or hyperesthesia of the ophthalmic and maxillary branches of the Vth cranial nerve found in maxillary, ethmoid, and sphenoid disease.

DIAGNOSIS

- Peripheral white blood cell count is often within normal limits.
- Nasopharyngeal cultures are not helpful.
- A limited CT scan of the sinuses is preferred over routine sinus X-rays in sphenoid, ethmoid, and frontal sinusitis. Positive radiographic findings (see Fig. 5-1).
  ○ Sinus opacification
  ○ Air fluid levels and/or mucosal thickening (≥ 8 mm)
  ○ CT allows assessment of bony erosions and extension beyond the sinuses

COMPLICATIONS

Ethmoid Sinusitis
- Infection can easily spread medially through the lamina papyracea to cause:
  ○ Preorbital cellulitis
  ○ Orbital cellulitis
  ○ Orbital abscess
  ○ Septic cavernous sinus thrombosis (rare)
- Orbital cellulitis must be differentiated from septic cavernous sinus thrombosis.
  ○ Orbital cellulitis is unilateral, cavernous sinus thrombosis bilateral.
  ○ Cavernous sinus disease is associated with:
    ▪ Papilledema
    ▪ Vth nerve deficits
    ▪ CSF pleocytosis.
    ▪ Orbital CT scan with contrast delineates the extent of infection.
  ○ Surgical drainage of the sinus recommended if there is loss of visual acuity, proptosis, or ophthalmoplegia.

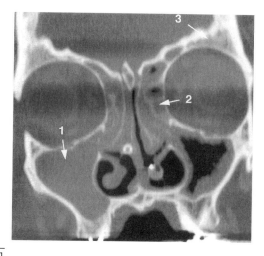

FIGURE 5-1

Pansinusitis. CT scan, coronal view of the air sinuses. 1. Maxillary sinus 2. Ethmoid sinus 3. Frontal sinus. Note the marked opacification of the right maxillary (left side of figure) and marked mucosal thickening of the left maxillary sinus. Both ethmoid sinuses are opaque as are the frontal sinuses. (Courtesy of Dr. Ilona Schamalfus, University of Florida College of Medicine.)

Frontal Sinusitis
- Infection can spread anteriorly and cause Pott's puffy tumor.
- Infection can spread posteriorly and cause epidural, subdural, or brain abscess.
- Posterior spread leads to severe headache, but frontal cerebral cortex lesions are usually neurologically silent.
- Contrast-enhanced CT scan is recommended for diagnosis.

Sphenoid Sinusitis
- The most dangerous form of sinusitis
- Most patients require hospitalization and intravenous antibiotics
- Close to many vital neurologic structures
- Complications:
  - Septic cavernous sinus thrombosis (a leading cause)
    - Impairment of III, IV, VIth nerve causing ophthalmoplegia
    - Vth nerve dysfunction, ophthalmic and maxillary branches (hypo- or hyperesthesia)
    - Proptosis and chemosis
    - Bacterial meningitis
    - Pituitary abscess formation
  - CT scan with contrast defines the sites of involvement, including cavernous sinus thrombosis. MRI also useful for the diagnosis of cavernous sinus thrombosis.
  - Surgical drainage of the sphenoid sinus often required to prevent spread outside the sinus walls.

Microbiology
- *S. pneumoniae* and *H. influenzae* most common, anaerobes seen in adults and in chronic disease, *S. aureus* in sphenoid disease
- Gram-negatives (*P. aeruginosa*) in AIDS patients
- Fungi (Aspergillus) in neutropenic patients

Treatment (see Table 5-1 for dosing)
- Nasal decongestants are helpful.
  - Neo-Synephrine nose drops, 1/4–1/2%, Q4H are effective.
  - Treatment for longer than 3–4 days results in tachyphylaxis or rebound nasal congestion.
  - Pseudoephedrine may unduly dry out the nasal passages and increase the viscosity of the nasal discharge.
- The threshold for antibiotic treatment should be low; however, definitive proof of bacterial sinusitis is often lacking, making treatment trials suspect.
  - Amoxicillin-clavulinate, the efficacy of treatment with this antibiotic, has been questioned in a placebo-controlled trial.
  - Cefuroxime axitel
  - Fluoroquinolones (concerns about resistance)
  - Azithromycin equivalent to amoxicillin-clavulinate with reduced diarrhea
  - Amoxicillin no longer recommended for initial therapy
- Patients with frontal, ethmoid, or sphenoid sinus infection
  - Usually hospitalized
  - Intravenous antibiotics (oxacillin + third-generation cephalosporin + metronidazole)

REFERENCES

Eye Infections

Benson WH, Lanier JD: Current diagnosis and treatment of corneal ulcers. *Curr Opin Ophthalmol* 1998; 9:45–49.

Callegan MC, Engelbert M, Parke DW II, Jett BD, Gilmore MS: Bacterial endophthalmitis: Epidemiology, therapeutics, and bacterium-host interactions. *Clin Microbiol Rev* 2002; 15:111–24.

Durand ML, Heier JS: Endophthalmitis. *Curr Clin Top Infect Dis* 2000; 20:271–97.

Sheikh A, Hurwitz B: Topical antibiotics for acute bacterial conjunctivitis: A systematic review. *Br J Gen Pract* 2001; 51:473–77.

Shields SR: Managing eye disease in primary care. Part 2. How to recognize and treat common eye problems. *Postgrad Med* 2000; 108:83–86, 91–96.

Pharyngitis

Ebell MH, Smith MA, Barry HC, Ives K, Carey M: The rational clinical examination: Does this patient have strep throat? *JAMA* 2000; 284:2912–18.

Hayes CS, Williamson H, Jr: Management of Group A beta-hemolytic streptococcal pharyngitis. *Am Fam Physician* 2001; 63:1557–64.

Otitis Media

Schwartz LE, Brown RB: Purulent otitis media in adults. *Arch Intern Med* 1992; 152:2301–4.

Stool S, Carlson LH, Johnson CE: Otitis media: Diagnosis, management, and judicious use of antibiotics. *Curr Allergy Asthma Rep* 2002; 2:297–303.

Sinusitis
Bucher HC, Tschudi P, Young J, Periat P, Welge-Luussen A, et al: Effect of amoxicillin-clavulanate in clinically diagnosed acute rhinosinusitis: A placebo-controlled, double-blind, randomized trial in general practice. *Arch Intern Med* 2003; 163:1793–98.
Erkan M, Aslan T, Ozcan M, Koc N: Bacteriology of antrum in adults with chronic maxillary sinusitis. *Laryngoscope* 1994; 104: 321–24.
Henry DC, Riffer E, Sokol WN, Chaudry NI, Swanson RN: Randomized double-blind study comparing 3- and 6-day regimens of azithromycin with a 10-day amoxicillin-clavulanate regimen for treatment of acute bacterial sinusitis. *Antimicrob Agents Chemother* 2003; 47:2770–74.
Lew D, Southwick FS, Montgomery WW, Weber AL, Baker AS: Sphenoid sinusitis. *N Engl J Med* 1983; 309:1149–54.
Tami TA. The management of sinusitis in patients infected with the human immunodeficiency virus (HIV). *Ear-Nose-Throat-J* 1995; 74: 360–63.
Varonen H, Kunnamo I, Savolainen S, Makela M, Revonta M, et al: Treatment of acute rhinosinusitis diagnosed by clinical criteria or ultrasound in primary care: A placebo-controlled randomised trial. *Scand J Prim Health Care* 2003; 21:121–26.
Wald ER, Milmoe GJ, Bowen A, Ledesma-Medina J, Salamon N, Bluestone CD: Acute maxillary sinusitis in children. *N Engl J Med* 1981; 304:749–54.
Young J, Bucher H, Tschudi P, Periat P, Hugenschmidt C, et al: The clinical diagnosis of acute bacterial rhinosinusitis in general practice and its therapeutic consequences. *J Clin Epidemiol* 2003; 56:377–84.

Complications of ENT Infections
Ramsey PG, Weymuller EA: Complications of bacterial infection of the ears, paranasal sinuses, and oropharynx in adults. *Emerg Med Clin North Am* 1985; 3(1): 143–60.
Southwick FS: Septic thrombophlebitis of major dural venous sinuses. *Curr Clin Top Infect Dis* 1995; 15:179–203.

6

CENTRAL NERVOUS SYSTEM INFECTIONS

HIGHLIGHTS

- Bacterial meningitis usually causes generalized headache and stiff neck followed by lethargy and progression to coma.
- Viral meningitis presents with similar complaints, but does not cause changes in mental status.
- When considering the diagnosis of meningitis, a lumbar puncture should be performed before CT scan in the absence of focal deficits or papilledema (exception: the HIV patient, who more commonly has a space-occupying lesion).
- Encephalitis can present similarly to meningitis, but stiff neck is usually less prominent or absent. Hallucinations and seizures are more common.
- MRI is the most helpful test for diagnosing encephalitis and brain abscess.

POTENTIAL SEVERITY

Often life-threatening illnesses. Infections of the central nervous system are infectious disease emergencies and require immediate treatment.

BACTERIAL MENINGITIS

EPIDEMIOLOGY AND ETIOLOGY (SEE TABLE 6-1)

- Primarily a disease of adults
- Four major pathogens are associated with community-acquired disease:
  1. *S. pneumoniae*
     - Most common etiology
     - Follows bacteremia from ear, sinus, or lung infection.
     - Also associated with chronic CSF leaks.
  2. *N. meningitidis*
     - Begins with colonization of the nasopharynx.
     - Sporadic cases associated with terminal complement defects.
     - Epidemics due to person-to-person spread; occur in crowded environments such as dormitories and military training camps.

TABLE 6-1
BACTERIAL ETIOLOGIES OF MENINGITIS IN ADULTS

	Community	Nosocomial
S. pneumoniae	38%	8%
Gram-negative bacilli	4%	38%
N. meningitidis	14%	1%
Listeria	11%	3%
Streptococci	7%	12%
Staph. aureus	5%	9%
H. influenzae	4%	4%

3. *Listeria monocytogenes*
   - Occurs in neonates, pregnant women, and immunocompromised patients.
   - Contracted by eating contaminated refrigerated foods:
     - Unpasteurized soft cheeses and improperly processed dairy products
     - Defectively processed hot dogs and fish
4. *H. influenzae*
   - Was the most common form of meningitis in children.
   - Now rare following widespread administration of *H. influenzae* B vaccine.
- Other forms of bacterial meningitis:
  - In neonates
    - Gram-negative bacilli
    - Group B Streptococcus meningitis
  - Nosocomial meningitis
    - Usually associated with neurosurgery and/or placement of a ventriculostomy tube
    - Gram-negative bacilli: *E. coli* and Klebsiella spp. most common
    - *S. aureus*
    - Enterococci
    - *S. epidermidis*
    - *B. subtilis* and corynebacteria

PATHOGENESIS
- Mechanisms by which bacteria gain entry into the subarachnoid space and CSF
  - Hematogenous spread most common, gain entry via large venous channels. Primary foci of infection leading to bacteremia:
    - Nasopharyngeal colonization (*N. meningitidis*)
    - Otitis media (*S. pneumoniae*, *H. influenzae*)
    - Air sinus infection (*S. pneumoniae*, *H. influenzae*)
    - Pneumonia (*S. pneumoniae*)
    - Bacterial endocarditis (*S. aureus*)
    - Asymptomatic gastrointestinal infection (*Listeria monocytogenes*)
  - Direct spread from the nasopharynx due to a CSF leak caused by a cribiform plate defect or basilar skull fracture
  - Direct spread from a brain abscess or air sinus infection
- Rapid growth in the CSF because the blood-brain barrier blocks entry of immunoglobulins and complement

- Inflammation damages the blood-brain barrier, increasing permeability, allowing entry of serum protein, and impairing glucose transport.
- Progressive cerebral edema, increased CSF pressure, and decreased cerebral blood flow lead to irreversible ischemic damage.

CLINICAL MANIFESTATIONS OF BACTERIAL MENINGITIS

- Upper respiratory or ear infection interrupted by the abrupt onset of meningeal symptoms:
  ○ Generalized, severe headache (not relieved by over-the-counter pain medications)
  ○ Neck stiffness (inflammation of the meninges causes spasm of the neck muscles)
  ○ Vomiting (due to brain stem irritation and elevated CSF pressure)
  ○ Depression of mental status (lethargy, confusion, disorientation)
- Abnormal physical findings
  ○ Positive Brudzinki (resistance to neck flexion) and Kernig's (straight leg raise causes neck pain) signs
  ○ Papilledema on funduscopic exam
    ▪ Rare in meningitis
    ▪ More commonly found in patients with brain abscess or brain tumor
  ○ Abnormal ear exam (*S. pneumoniae* or *H. influenzae*)
  ○ Pharyngeal erythema (*N. meningitidis*)
  ○ Clear nasal discharge due to CSF leak (*S. pneumoniae*) often stops at the time of presentation owing to increased inflammation and edema at the site of leakage.
  ○ Petechial or purpuritic skin lesions
    ▪ *N. meningitidis* most common
    ▪ Also seen with rickettsial infection, echovirus, *S. aureus*, and asplenic sepsis
  ○ Abnormal neurological exam
    ▪ Abnormal mental status
      • Severity of mental status changes correlates with poorer prognosis
      • Assess response to voice, superficial and deep pain
    ▪ Focal findings (suggests a space-occupying lesion)
- The very young and very old do not present with these classic symptoms and signs.
  ○ Elderly often more insidious onset
    ▪ Fever and alterations in mental status
    ▪ Meningeal signs are less commonly reported, and many elderly patients have neck stiffness as a consequence of osteoarthritis, an old cerebrovascular accident, or Parkinson's disease.
  ○ Neonates and infants usually present with:
    ▪ Fever and irritability
    ▪ No history is obtainable
    ▪ Lumbar puncture part of the fever workup

DIAGNOSIS

- If meningitis is a consideration, a lumbar puncture must be performed.
  ○ Lumbar puncture should be performed before CT scan if:
    ▪ No focal neurologic deficits
    ▪ No papilledema

TABLE 6-2
CSF PROFILES

Type of Infection	WBC's	Glucose (nl 2/3 of serum)	Protein
Untreated bacterial	Polys	Low (often $<$ 25 mg%)	Elevated (150–1000 mg%)
TB Fungi bacterial Treated	Lymphs	Low	Moderately elevated (80–500 mg%)
Viral	Lymphs	Normal (low in early mumps)	Moderately elevated (usually $<$ 150 mg%)
Parameningeal infection (brain abscess)	Polys or lymphs	Normal	Normal or slight elevation

- L.P. findings
  - Measure CSF opening pressure, often elevated in bacterial meningitis.
  - CSF formula is very helpful in deciding whether or not the patient has bacterial meningitis (see Table 6-2). Bacterial meningitis has:
    - $>$ 90% PMN (exception Listeria)
    - Elevated CSF protein (usually 150–1000 mg/dl)
    - Low CSF glucose, $<$ 2/3 the serum value ($<$ 25 mg/dl, poor prognosis in pneumococcal meningitis)
    - CSF Gram stain positive in $>$ 75% of cases (exception Listeria, 25%)
    - Blood and CSF cultures allow antibiotic sensitivity testing.
    - CSF PCR may allow more rapid diagnosis in the near future.
  - CT scan is too often ordered prior to performing the lumbar puncture, needlessly delaying the appropriate diagnostic study.
    - One major exception is the patient with AIDS.
      - Should have a CT scan prior to L.P.
      - High frequency of cortical space-occupying lesions

TREATMENT (SEE FIG. 6-1)

- Antibiotics should be given within 30 minutes if bacterial meningitis suspected.
- Blood cultures should be drawn and antibiotics given **prior** to CT scan.
- Maximal doses of antibiotics must given because of limited passage through the blood-brain barrier.
- Empiric antibiotic therapy (see Table 6-3)
  - Community-acquired, 3 months-50 years: ceftriaxone or cefotaxime
    - If severely ill, add vancomycin
    - $>$ 50 years or immunocompromised, add ampicillin

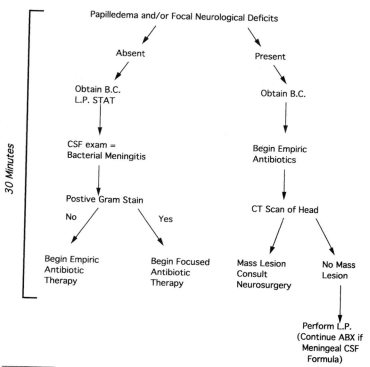

FIGURE 6-1

Initial management of suspected bacterial meningitis. (Adapted from Mandell GL, et al: *Principles and Practice of Infectious Diseases*. Philadelphia: Churchill Livingston, 2000.)

- Penicillin-resistant *S. pneumoniae* a major concern.
    - For intermediate resistant stains (penicillin MIC 0.1–1 μg/ml), vancomycin is preferred.
    - High-level penicillin-resistant *S. pneumoniae* (penicillin MIC > 2 μg/ml) also requires vancomycin. If receiving dexamethasone, consider adding rifampin.
- Nosocomial—vancomycin and ceftazidime or cefepime. If methicillin-sensitive *S. aureus* cultured, switch to oxacillin or nafcillin.
- Aminoglycosides, erythromycin, clindamycin, tetracyclines, and first-generation cephalosporins do not cross the blood-brain barrier. Systemic administration not effective for treating meningitis.
- Dexamethasone (10 mg Q6H IV in adults) give 30 minutes before antibiotics in:
    - Children; shown to be efficacious in *H. influenzae*
    - In adults, associated with a significant reduction in morbidity and mortality without increasing the risk of GI bleeding
- Maintain ventilation, prevent increase in pCO_2 or decrease in pO_2.
- Avoid hypotonic solutions.
- Consider mannitol or glycerol for increased CSF pressure.
- Antiseizure medications after first seizure.

TABLE 6-3
ANTIBIOTIC TREATMENT FOR BACTERIAL MENINGITIS

Organism	Antibiotic	Dose	Alternative
S. pneumoniae (PCN MIC < 0.1 ug/ml)	Penicillin	20–24 mil. units/day (divided Q4H)	Chloramphenicol 4–6 g/day (divided Q6H)
	Ceftriaxone	2–4 g/day (divided Q4H)	
	Cefotaxime	12 g/day (divided Q12H)	
S. pneumoniae (MIC ≥ 0.1 ug/ml)	Vancomycin ± rifampin	2 g/day (divided Q12H)	Chloramphenicol
N. meningitidis	Penicillin	20–24 mil. units/day (divided Q4H)	Ceftriaxone
			Cefotaxime
L. monocytogenes	Ampicillin ± gentamicin	12 g/day (divided Q4H) 4–8 mg intrathecal 5 mg/kg/day systemic	Trimethoprim-sulfa 15–20 mg/day (trimethroprim) (divided Q6H)
H. influenzae	Ceftriaxone	2–4 g/day (divided Q12H)	Chloramphenicol
	Cefotaxime	12 g/day (divided Q6H)	
Enterobacteriaceae	Ceftriaxone ± gentamicin	2–4 g/day (divided Q12H) 4–8 mg intrathecal 5 mg/kg/day systemic	Aztreonam 6–8 g/day (divided Q6H)
	Cefotaxim ± gentamicin	12 g/day (divided Q6H)	Trimethoprim-sulfa
Pseudomonas aeruginosa	Ceftazidime + gentamicin	6–12 g/day (divided Q8H) 4–8 mg intrathecal 5 mg/kg/day systemic	Antipseudomonal penicillin 18–24 g/day (divided Q4H) + gentamicin
S. aureus (methicillin sensitive)	Naficillin or Oxacillin ± rifampin	9–12 g/day (divided Q4H) 9–12 g/day (divided Q4H) 1,200 mg/day (divided Q12H)	Vancomycin + rifampin Trimethoprim-sulfa + rifampin
S. aureus (methicillin resistant)	Vancomycin + rifampin	2 g/day (divided Q12H) 1,200 mg/day (divided Q12H)	
S. epidermidis	Vancomycin + rifampin	2 g/day (divided Q12H) 1,200 mg/day (divided Q12H)	

156

COMPLICATIONS

- Mortality is high:
  - Listeria, 26%
  - *S. pneumoniae*, 19%
  - *N. meningitidis*, 13%
  - *H. influenzae*, 3%
- Permanent sequelae are common
  - Children
    - Mental retardation
    - Hearing loss
    - Seizure disorders
    - Cerebral palsy
  - Adults
    - Hydrocephalus
    - Cerebellar dysfunction
    - Paresis
    - Seizures
    - Hearing loss

PREVENTION

- Vaccines efficacious:
  - *S. pneumoniae*: 23-valent vaccine, safe, inexpensive. Recommended if:
    - ≥ 65 years old
    - Chronic cardiovascular disease
    - Pulmonary or liver disease
    - Diabetes mellitus
    - Sickle cell disease
    - Asplenia
  - *H. influenzae*: PedvaxHIB vaccine safe and inexpensive
    - All children 2–4 months of age
    - Highly efficacious, has dramatically reduced *H. influenzae* meningitis
  - *N. meningitidis*: quadravalent meningococcal vaccine serogroups A, C, Y, and W135, misses group B. Recommended for:
    - Military recruits
    - College students
    - Patients with asplenia
    - Patients with terminal complement defects
    - Travelers going to areas where the prevalence of meningococcal disease is high

CHEMOPROPHYLAXIS

- *H. influenzae*: Rifampin (adult dose, 600 mg po QD × 4) within 6 days for:
  - Household contacts with unvaccinated child under 2 years of age
  - Children under 2 years of age exposed in a day care center
- *N. meningitidis*: Single dose of ciprofloxacin (adult dose 500 mg po) within 5 days for:
  - Household contacts
  - Day care contacts
  - Persons exposed to index case's oral secretions

OTHER FORMS OF MENINGITIS

VIRAL MENINGITIS

- Potential severity: A self-limited disease that does not cause significant morbidity or mortality.
- The most common form of meningitis; etiologies include:
  - Enteroviruses, echovirus, and coxsackievirus most frequent, summer and early fall
  - Mumps in the nonimmune; may be no parotid gland swelling, ages 5–9 years
  - Herpes simplex type II primary disease; also cause of Mollaret's recurrent meningitis
  - Epstein-Barr virus and cytomegalovirus, rare
  - Lymphocytic choriomeningitis excreted in rhodent urine, rare
  - HIV infection, can be the initial presentation of infection
- Primary clinical manifestations
  - Headache and photophobia, stiff neck
  - No loss of consciousness
  - Conjunctivitis, maculopapular, and rarely petechial rashes with echovirus
- CSF (see Table 6-2)
  - Predominance of lymphs, rarely PMNs early
  - Normal glucose
  - Mild protein increase
- Diagnosis
  - PCR not commercially available
  - Stool culture for enterovirus may be performed
  - Diagnosis usually presumptive
- Treatment
  - Observation
  - Antibiotics if PMNs in CSF pending bacterial cultures
  - Self-limited disease lasting 7–10 days

TUBERCULOUS MENINGITIS

- Potential severity: A potentially fatal infection that is often initially misdiagnosed
- Usually develops during miliary tuberculosis
- No pulmonary disease is evident in 50% of adults
- Clinically similar to other forms of meningitis
  - A basilar process involving the pons and optic chiasm
  - III, IV, and VI cranial nerve deficits may be found
  - Can cause noncommunicating hydrocephalus
  - Development of coma a bad prognostic sign
- CSF usually obeys the 500 rule
  - < 500 WBC, usually lymphs, but may have PMNs early in the disease
  - Protein < 500 mg/dl
  - Glucose often < 45 mg/dl
- Culture large volumes of CSF
  - AFB smear + 1/3
  - PCR sensitive
- CT or MRI with contrast may reveal rounded densities indicative of tuberculomas, basilar arachnoid inflammation, and hydrocephalus.
- PPD often positive, but negative test does not exclude
- Fatal if not treated within 5–8 weeks

- Treatment with INH, rifampin, and pyrazinamide
- A glucocorticoid (60 mg prednisone QD in adults and 1–3 mg/kg in children) is recommended in patients with hydrocephalus to reduce basilar inflammation.

CRYPTOCOCCAL MENINGOENCEPHALITIS

- Potential severity: A life-threatening illness with symptoms that often wax and wane leading to delays in diagnosis and treatment
- Pathogenesis
  - Transmitted by pigeon excreta
  - Inhaled
    - Infects the lung
    - Enters the bloodstream
    - Seeds the meninges and brain
  - Yeast-like fungus with several important virulence factors
    - Thick, negatively charged polysaccharide capsule that is immunosuppressive
    - Melanin provides protection against oxidants.
    - Mannitol may induce cerebral edema and inhibit phagocyte function.
- Primarily infects immunocompromised hosts
  - Infections in normal hosts are also reported.
  - The most common form of meningitis in AIDS patients (see Chap. 17)
- Clinical manifestations
  - Waxing and waning symptoms and diagnosis often delayed for ≥ 1 month
  - Headache most common
  - Personality change, confusion
  - Stiff neck is uncommon
  - Papilledema in 1/3, usually secondary to hydrocephalus
  - Cranial nerve deficits: III, IV, VI, and VIII, due to basilar inflammation
- L.P. required for diagnosis
  - Elevated CSF pressure common, owing to obstructive hydrocephalus
  - 20–200 WBC/mm^3, predominance of mononuclear cells
  - Mildly elevated protein
  - Moderately depressed glucose
  - Positive India Ink preparation, 25–50%
  - Positive cryptococcal antigen
  - Culture usually positive in 5–7 days
- CT scan or MRI with contrast may show:
  - Hydrocephalus
  - Cerebral edema
  - Ring-enhancing lesions (cryptococcomas)
- Treatment with:
  - Amphotericin B (0.5–0.7 mg/kg/day) and flucytosine (100–150 mg/kg/day given in 4 divided doses × 2 weeks)
  - Followed by fluconazole (400 mg po QD) for 3–6 months
- Mortality 25–30%, worse prognosis if:
  - CSF: + India Ink prep
  - CSF antigen > 1:32
  - WBC < 20/mm^3
  - Increased opening pressure, common
  - An extraneural infection

VIRAL ENCEPHALITIS

- Potential severity: An acute and severe illness associated with a high mortality
- Three major categories of viral encephalitis, based on their routes of spread
  - Mosquito-borne—arboviruses
    - Occur in the summer months when mosquitoes are active.
    - In addition to humans, often infect birds and horses.
    - Crows are very susceptible to West Nile virus.
    - Public health officials frequently set out sentinel chickens in areas heavily infested with mosquitoes.
    - The different arboviruses tend to be associated with outbreaks in specific areas of the country, and have somewhat different host preferences (see Table 6-4).
  - Animal to human—rabies virus
    - A very deadly form of encephalitis
    - Spread by animal bites, most commonly bats
  - Human to human—herpes simplex-1, mumps, measles, varicella zoster; less commonly, EBV, CMV, and enteroviruses
- Symptoms primarily due to cortical dysfunction
  - Hallucinations, repetitive higher motor activity such as dressing and undressing
  - Seizures
  - Severe headache
  - Ataxia
  - Development of coma is associated with a poor prognosis.
- Rabies causes distinct syndromes
  - Hydrophobia
  - Rapid, short respirations
  - Hyperactivity and autonomic dysfunction
  - Less commonly ascending paralysis

DIAGNOSIS OF ENCEPHALITIS

- Often presumptive, requires acute and convalescent serum
- CSF
  - < 500 WBC/mm^3 primarily lymphocytes, PMN may be seen early in the infection.
  - Mildly increased protein
  - RBCs in herpes simplex-1
  - CSF PCR for herpes simplex very helpful, culture rarely positive
- MRI/CT scan
  - MRI is preferred, detects smaller lesions
  - Temporal lobe abnormalities found in herpes simplex-1
- EEG localized temporal lobe abnormalities in herpes simplex-1, may find frontal slowing in West Nile encephalitis
- Brain biopsy if temporal lobe abnormalities and no improvement on acyclovir

TREATMENT

- The only treatable form is herpes simplex.
- Acyclovir (10 mg/kg Q8H IV × 14–21 days) usually initiated empirically
- Intravenous immunoglobulin (IVIG) may be helpful in West Nile virus.

TABLE 6-4
ENCEPHALITIS CAUSED BY ARBOVIRUSES

Disease	Virus	Location	Hosts	Clinical
Eastern equine encephalitis	Alphavirus	Eastern U.S., Canada, Central and South America, Caribbean, Guyana	Birds, horses	Severe disease, high mortality
Western equine encephalitis	Alphavirus	U.S., Canada, Central and South America, Guyana	Birds, small mammals, snakes, horses	Mild disease, primarily in children
Venezuelan equine encephalitis	Alphavirus	Northern South America, Central America, Florida, Texas	Horses, rodents, birds	Febrile illness, encephalitis uncommon
St. Louis encephalitis	Flavivirus	Western, central and southern U.S., Central and South America, Carribean	Birds	Attacks those over 50
West Nile encephalitis	Flavivirus	Entire United States	Birds (Crows)	Usually mild disease, in elderly severe disease
Japanese encephalitis	Flavivirus	Japan, Siberia, Korea, China, SE Asia, India	Birds, pigs, horses	Can cause severe encephalitis
California group encephalitis	Bunyavirus	U.S., Canada	Small mammals	School-age children, permanent behavior changes

OUTCOME

- Varies depending on the agent.
  - Herpes simplex type I has a mortality of 50–60%.
    - Early treatment reduces mortality.
  - Rabies nearly 100%
  - Arboviruses prognosis varies with:
    - Patient's age
    - Extent of cortical involvement
    - Specific agent
      - Eastern equine encephalitis most virulent, 70% mortality.
      - Western Equine and West Nile encephalitis are usually mild and often subclinical; however, in the elderly and immunocompromised host can be severe life-threatening diseases.
      - Venezuelan equine encephalitis usually mild.
      - Japanese encephalitis varies in severity.

PREVENTION

- Avoid mosquito bites during epidemics.
- For suspected rabies:
  - Wash wound with a 20% soap solution and irrigate with a virucidal agent such as povidone-iodine solution.
  - Rabies immune globulin (20 IU/kg) should be injected around the wound and given intramuscularly.
  - Several safe and effective antirabies vaccines are available. The vaccine should be given on days 0, 3, 7, 14, and 28.

BRAIN ABSCESS

Potential severity: Often subacute in onset, but may be life-threatening if improperly managed. Early neurosurgical consultation is of critical importance.

PATHOGENESIS

- Two major pathways:
  - Direct spread from:
    - Middle ear (spreads to the inferior temporal lobe and cerebellum)
    - Frontal sinus or ethmoid sinuses (spreads to the frontal lobes)
    - Dental infection (usually spreads to the frontal lobes)
    - Facial trauma can be followed by brain abscess
    - Complication of a neurosurgical procedure. May be delayed, symptomatic infection occurring 3–15 months after surgery
  - Hematogenous spread from infections arising in the:
    - Lung, chronic infection
    - Skin
    - Pelvis and other intra-abdominal sites
    - Less commonly due to:
      - Bacterial endocarditis
      - Bacteremia after esophageal dilatation
      - Cyanotic heart disease (when these patients develop headache, brain abscess must be excluded)
- No primary site or underlying condition identified in 20–40%

- Abscesses develop at the gray-white matter junction.
  - Locations: frontal or temporal > fronto-parietal > parietal > cerebellar > occipital
  - Three pathologic stages (earliest to latest)
    - Cerebritis (acute inflammation and edema)
    - Necrosis, develops in 2–3 weeks
    - Fibrotic capsule formation

MICROBIOLOGY

- Anaerobes—from mouth flora, pelvis, and gastrointestinal tract
  - Bacteroides (may include *B. fragilis*)
  - *Prevotella melaninogenica*
  - Propionibacterium, Fusobacteria, Eubacterium, Veillonella
  - Actinomyces
- Aerobic Gram-positive cocci
  - *Streptococcus milleri* (has protease activity and a predisposition to form abscesses)
  - Microaerophilic streptococci
  - *Staphylococcus aureus* (associated with endocarditis, trauma, neurosurgery)
  - Viridans streptococci
- Gram-negative rods rare
  - Pseudomonas species
  - *Haemophilus aphrophilus* and *Actinobacillus actinomycetemcomitans*
  - Klebsiella
- In immunocompromised host consider:
  - Toxoplasmosis
  - Nocardia
  - Fungal—Aspergillus, *Cryptococcus neoformans*, and *Coccidiodides immitis*
  - AIDS (see Chap. 17)
    - Toxoplasmosis most common
    - Tuberculomas or cryptococcoma
    - Progressive multifocal leukoencephalopathy (PML)
    - *Listeria monocytogenes*
    - Salmonella
    - Candida, Histoplasma, and Aspergillus
    - CNS lymphoma can mimic brain abscess
- In immigrants, consider cysticercosis

CLINICAL SYMPTOMS AND SIGNS

- Symptoms initially nonspecific and delay in diagnosis is common (2 weeks)
  - Severe headache is often localized to the site of the abscess
  - Neck stiffness noted in occipital brain abscess or after rupture into the ventricle
  - Alterations in mental status
    - Inattentiveness
    - Lethargy
    - Coma (a bad prognostic sign)
  - Vomiting associated with increased CSF pressure

- Physical findings often minimal
  - Fever not present in half of patients
  - Focal neurologic findings late and depend on the location of the abscess (see Table 6-5)
  - Papilledema, a late manifestation, seen in 25%
  - VIth and IIIrd nerve deficits due to increased CSF pressure
  - Seizures most common in association with frontal brain abscess

DIAGNOSIS

- Focal symptoms or neurologic signs as well as papilledema = possible space-occupying lesion
  - Lumbar puncture is contraindicated
  - Associated with 15–30% risk of brain stem herniation
- Blood cultures and empiric antibiotics should be initiated
- CT scan (see Fig. 6-2) or MRI with contrast should then be performed
  - MRI is preferred over CT scan
    - More sensitive for detecting early cerebritis
    - Detects smaller lesions (1 mm resolution)
    - More accurately estimates the extent of central necrosis, ring enhancement, and cerebral edema
    - Visualizes the brain stem; bony reflections cause interference with CT scan

TABLE 6-5
NEUROLOGIC MANIFESTATIONS OF BRAIN ABSCESS

Location	Neurologic Deficits
Temporal	Wernicke's aphasia, homonymous superior quadranopsia, mild contralateral facial muscle weakness
Frontal	Drowsy, inattentive, disturbed judgment, mutism, seizures, + grasp, suck, and snout reflexes; contralateral hemiparesis when abscess is large
Parietal	Impaired position sense, two-point discrimination and stereognosis; focal sensory and motor seizures, homonymous hemianopsia, impaired optikokinetic nystagmus
Cerebellar	Ataxia, nystagmus (coarser on gaze toward the lesion); ipsilateral incoordination of arm and leg movements with intention tremor; rapid progression (usually not encapsulated)
Brain stem	Facial weakness and dysphagia, multiple other cranial nerve palsies, contralateral hemiparesis

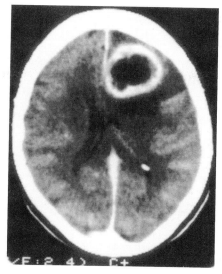

FIGURE 6-2

CT scan with contrast of brain abscess. Note the large ring-enhancing lesion in the left frontal cortex associated with the marked edema and obliteration of the lateral ventricle.

- Antibiotic therapy must be prolonged (6–8 weeks), and use highest doses of:
  - Penicillin, covers mouth flora
  - Metronidazole, concentrates in abscesses and kills all anaerobes (intralesional concentrations reach 40 µg/ml)
  - Ceftriaxone or cefotaxime, covers Gram-positive and Gram-negative aerobes
    - If Pseudomonas is possible, replace with ceftazidime or cefepime.
  - Nafcillin or oxacillin for abscess following head trauma, neurosurgery, or *S. aureus* bacteremia; if high risk of MRSA, cover with vancomycin.
- Neurosurgery usually required for culture and drainage. Always consult neuro-surgery.
  - Needle aspiration usually preferred (less collateral damage)
  - Open resection recommended after head trauma and with fungal abscess
  - Observation in cases of early cerebritis with frequent follow-up MRI or CT scan• Dexamethasone (10 mg IV followed by 4 mg Q6h) used when mass effect and depressed mental status. Avoid when possible.
  - Reduces contrast enhancement during imaging
  - Slows capsule formation and increases the risk of ventricular rupture
  - Reduces antibiotic penetration into the abscess
- Mortality ranges from 0 to 30%. Poor prognosis is associated with:
  - Rapid progression in the hospital
  - Coma on admission (60–100% mortality)
  - Rupture into the ventricle (80–100% mortality)
- Surviving patients have a high incidence of neurologic sequelae (30–60%) (re-current seizures most common, particularly with frontal abscess).

INTRACRANIAL EPIDURAL AND SUBDURAL ABSCESS

- Potential severity: Subdural abscess spreads rapidly. Emergency surgical drainage, is life-saving.
- Rare and usually result from spread of infection from a nidus of osteomyelitis following:
  ○ Neurosurgery
  ○ Air sinus infection (in particular the frontal sinus)
  ○ Less commonly, an infected middle ear or mastoid
- *S. aureus* common; otherwise the microbiology is similar to that of brain abscess.
- Epidural abscess forms between the skull and dura.
  ○ The dura is normally tightly adherent to the skull.
  ○ Infection usually remains localized.
  ○ Progresses slowly
  ○ Requires surgical drainage
- Subdural abscess spreads quickly.
  ○ Patient usually appears acutely ill and septic.
  ○ Often mimics meningitis
    ▪ Severe headache, often local
    ▪ Nuchal rigidity is common.
  ○ Within 24 hours seizures and focal neurological deficits
  ○ L.P. contraindicated; CT scan or MRI emergently
  ○ Requires immediate surgical drainage
  ○ Mortality 14–18%

SPINAL EPIDURAL ABSCESS

- Potential severity: Often subacute in onset. Development of motor weakness indicates imminent spinal cord infarction and requires emergency surgical drainage.
- The spinal canal has both an anterior and posterior epidural space containing fat and small vessels.
- The spinal epidural space can become infected by:
  ○ Spread of infection from osteomyelitis or disk space infection
  ○ Spinal surgery or epidural catheter placement
  ○ Hematogenous spread following skin and soft tissue infection, urinary tract infection, and IV drug abuse

SYMPTOMS AND SIGNS

- Low back pain and fever
- Localized spinous process tenderness in posterior epidural abscesses
- Radicular pain caused by compression of the nerve roots
  ○ Accompanied by lower motor neuron deficits
    ▪ Decreased reflexes
    ▪ Loss of light touch and pain sensation in specific dermatomes
- Later, signs of cord compression accompanied by upper motor neuron deficits
  ○ Babinski reflex
  ○ Hyperreflexia
  ○ Loss of motor function
  ○ Bladder dysfunction
  ○ Within 24 hours of onset, irreversible paraplegia may occur.
- In the patient with back pain and fever, always consider spinal epidural abscess.

DIAGNOSIS

- MRI with contrast is the diagnostic study of choice. Clearly delineates:
  - ○ Size of the abscess
  - ○ The degree of cord compression

MICROBIOLOGY

- *S. aureus* is cultured from over half of cases.
- Gram-negative aerobes are the second most frequent cause.
- Aerobic streptococci, *S. epidermidis*, and anaerobes also reported.
- *M. tuberculosis* most commonly being associated with tuberculous infection of the thoracic vertebra.

TREATMENT

- Emergency surgical drainage if signs of cord compression or significant compression on MRI.
- Prolonged antibiotic therapy (4–6 weeks) with nafcillin or oxacillin; metronidizole and ceftriaxone for empiric therapy pending cultures.

REFERENCES

Aronin SI, Peduzzi P, Quagliarello VJ: Community-acquired bacterial meningitis: Risk stratification for adverse clinical outcome and effect of antibiotic timing. *Ann Intern Med* 1998; 129:862–69.

Berger JR: Tuberculous meningitis. *Curr Opin Neurol* 1994; 7:191–200.

Carpenter JL: Brain stem abscesses: Cure with medical therapy, case report, and review. *Clin Infect Dis* 1994; 18:219–26.

Choi C: Bacterial meningitis in aging adults. *Clin Infect Dis* 2001; 33:1380–85.

de Gans J, van de Beek D: Dexamethasone in adults with bacterial meningitis. *N Engl J Med* 2002; 347:1549–56.

Dill SR, Cobbs CG, McDonald CK: Subdural empyema: Analysis of 32 cases and review. *Clin Infect Dis* 1995; 20:372–86.

Durand ML, Calderwood SB, Weber DJ, Miller SI, Southwick FS, Caviness VS, Swartz MN: Acute bacterial meningitis in adults: A review of 493 episodes. *N Engl J Med* 1993; 328:21–28.

Ely EW, Peacock JE, Jr, Haponik EF, Washburn RG: Cryptococcal pneumonia complicating pregnancy. *Medicine (Baltimore)* 1998; 77:153–67.

Gandelman-Marton R, Kimiagar I, Itzhaki A, Klein C, Theitler J, et al: Electroencephalography findings in adult patients with West Nile virus-associated meningitis and meningoencephalitis. *Clin Infect Dis* 2003; 37:1573–78.

Haley M, Retter AS, Fowler D, Gea-Banacloche J, O'Grady NP: The role for intravenous immunoglobulin in the treatment of West Nile virus encephalitis. *Clin Infect Dis* 2003; 37:88–90.

Hong DS, Jacobson KL, Raad, II, de Lima M, Anderlini P, et al: West Nile encephalitis in 2 hematopoietic stem cell transplant recipients: Case series and literature review. *Clin Infect Dis* 2003; 37:1044–49.

Hussein AS, Shafran SD: Acute bacterial meningitis in adults: A 12-year review. *Medicine (Baltimore)* 2000; 79:360–68.

Mackenzie AR, Laing RB, Smith CC, Kaar GF, Smith FW: Spinal epidural abscess: The importance of early diagnosis and treatment. *J Neurol Neurosurg Psychiatry* 1998; 65:209–12.

Mitchell DH, Sorrell TC, Allworth AM, et al: Cryptococcal disease of the CNS in immunocompetent hosts: Influence of cryptococcal variety on clinical manifestations and outcome. *Clin Infect Dis* 1995; 20:611.

Nussbaum ES, Rigamonti D, Standiford H, Numaguchi Y, Wolf AL, Robinson WL: Spinal epidural abscess: A report of 40 cases and review. *Surg Neurol* 1992; 38:225–31.

Odio CM, et al: The beneficial effects of early dexamethasone administration in infants and children with bacterial meningitis. *N Engl J Med* 1991; 324:1525–31.

Offenbacher H, Fazekas F, Schmidt R, et al: MRI in tuberculous meningoencephalitis: Report of four cases and review of the neuroimaging literature. *J Neurol* 1991; 238:340–44.

Raschilas F, Wolff M, Delatour F, Chaffaut C, De Broucker T, et al: Outcome of and prognostic factors for herpes simplex encephalitis in adult patients: Results of a multicenter study. *Clin Infect Dis* 2002; 35:254–60.

Rex JH, Larsen RA, Dismukes WE, Cloud GA, Bennett JE: Catastrophic visual loss due to *Cryptococcus neoformans* meningitis. *Medicine (Baltimore)* 1993; 72:207–24.

Rich PM, Deasy NP, Jarosz JM: Intracranial dural empyema. *Br J Radiol* 2000; 73:1329–36.

Saravolatz LD, Manzor O, VanderVelde N, Pawlak J, Belian B: Broad-range bacterial polymerase chain reaction for early detection of bacterial meningitis. *Clin Infect Dis* 2003; 36:40–45.

Seydoux C, Francioli P: Bacterial brain abscesses: Factors influencing mortality and sequelae. *Clin Infect Dis* 1992; 15:394–401.

Swartz MN, Dodge PR: Bacterial meningitis: A review of selected aspects. *N Engl J Med* 1965; 272:725, 779, 842, 898, 954, 1003.

7

CARDIOVASCULAR INFECTIONS

HIGHLIGHTS

- Infective endocarditis is usually preceded by valvular damage establishing a nidus of platelets and thrombi for bacterial adherence (called nonbacterial thrombotic endocarditis).
- Bacteria from the mouth, as well as enterococcus and *S. aureus*, are particularly adept at adhering to damaged valves.
- Patients usually present with fatigue and low-grade fever.
- Blood cultures are the mainstay of diagnosis and need to be separated in time.
- Antibiotic treatment needs to be prolonged and the threshold for surgery should be low.
- Intravascular device infections are increasing in frequency and warrant rapid diagnosis and treatment. Guidelines for the duration of therapy have been established.

INFECTIVE ENDOCARDITIS

Potential severity: Acute endocarditis is life-threatening and often requires surgical intervention. Subacute endocarditis is an indolent disease that can continue for months.

EPIDEMIOLOGY

- A rare disease; each primary physician is likely to see 1–2 cases/career.
- More common in men.
- Increasingly a disease of the elderly; in recent series over half of the patients with endocarditis were over the age of 50 years.

PATHOGENESIS AND PREDISPOSING RISK FACTORS

Host Factors
- Nonbacterial thrombotic endocarditis (NBTE) due to valve damage followed by platelet and fibrin deposition
- NBTE results from:
  ○ Rheumatic heart disease
  ○ Congenital heart disease (bicuspid valve and VSD)
  ○ Mitral valve prolapse
  ○ Degenerative valve disease (calcific aortic valve disease)
  ○ Prosthetic valve

- Venturi effect results in vegetation formation on the low-pressure side of high-flow valvular lesions
- Vegetations
  - After attachment, pathogenic bacteria induce platelet aggregation and form a dense platelet-fibrin complex
  - Protected environment that neutrophils cannot penetrate
  - Colony counts in vegetations are usually 10^9–10^{11} bacteria/g of tissue
  - Bacteria within the vegetations periodically lapse into a metabolically inactive, dormant phase
- Mitral valve > aortic valve > tricuspid valve (usually IV drug abusers)
  - Reflects the degree of sheer stress
  - Valves exposed to higher pressure subjected to greater stress; explains why most endocarditis is left-sided
- Patients with prosthetic valves are at higher risk; the artificial material serves as an excellent site for bacterial adherence.
- Patients who have recovered from infective endocarditis are at increased risk of developing a second episode.

Bacterial Factors
- Bacteria with high dextran content stick to NBTE more readily and also cause dental caries.
  - *S. viridans* is the leading cause of subacute bacterial endocarditis.
  - *S. bovis* also has high dextran content, associated with colonic carcinoma.
  - *Candida albicans* adheres well to NBTE; *C. krusei* adheres poorly.
- Causes of bacteremia that lead to infective endocarditis (see Table 7-1)
  - Dental manipulations (extraction and periodontal surgery), water picks
  - Tonsillectomy
  - Urology procedures (urethral dilatation, cystoscopy, and prostatectomy)
  - Other procedures are associated with a lower incidence of bacteremia.
    - Pulmonary procedures (rigid bronchoscopy, intubation)
    - GI procedures (upper GI endoscopy, sigmoidoscopy, colonoscopy)

ETIOLOGIES OF INFECTIVE ENDOCARDITIS (SEE TABLE 7-2)
- Native valve endocarditis
  - Streptococci most common
    - *S. viridans* most common
    - *S. faecalis* and *S. faecium* (enterococcus)
    - *S. bovis* (associated with colonic cancer)
  - *S. aureus* second most common; increasing in frequency in the hospital setting
  - HACEK group uncommon, consider in culture negative cases (hold B.C. > 7 days)
    - *Hemophilus aphrophilus*
    - *Actinobacillus actinomycetemcomitans*
    - *Cardiobacterium hominis*
    - *Eikenella corrodens*
    - *Kingella kingae*
  - *Coxiella burnetti* (Q fever endocarditis), and Chlamydia spp. Very rare
  - In 3–5% of cases, cultures are repeatedly negative.

TABLE 7-1
CAUSES OF BACTEREMIA LEADING TO POTENTIAL ENDOCARDITIS

Procedure or Manipulation	% Positive Blood Cultures
Dental	
Dental extraction	18–85
Periodontal surgery	32–88
Chewing gum	15–51
Tooth brushing	0–26
Oral irrigation device	27–50
Upper airway	
Bronchoscopy (rigid scope)	15
Intubation/nasotracheal suction	16
Gastrointestinal	
Upper GI endoscopy	8–12
Sigmoidoscopy/colonoscopy	0–9.5
Barium enema	11
Liver Bx, percutaneous	3–13
Urologic	
Urethral dilatation	18–33
Urethral catheter	8
Cystoscopy	0–17
Transurethral prostatectomy	12–46

From Everett ED, Hirschmann JV: *Medicine* 1977; 56:61.

- ° Intravenous drug users
  - ▪ Most commonly caused by *S. aureus*
  - ▪ Gram-negative aerobic bacilli second most common, *Pseudomonas aeruginosa*
  - ▪ Fungi
  - ▪ Polymicrobial
- Prosthetic valve
  - ° Early: Nocoscomial pathogens—*S. aureus*, coagulase-negative Staphylococcus, Gram-negative bacilli and fungi
  - ° Late: (>2 months postop), mouth and skin flora—*S. viridans*, coagulase-negative Staphylococcus, *S. aureus*, Gram-negative bacilli and fungi

TABLE 7-2
MICROORGANISMS CAUSING INFECTIVE ENDOCARDITIS

Organism	% Native	iv drug user	Early PVE	Late PVE
Streptococcal spp.	60–80	15	<10	35
Viridans	30–40	5	<5	25
S. bovis	10	<5	<5	<5
S. faecalis (GpD)	5–18	8	<5	<5
Other	<5	<5	<5	<5
Staphylococcus spp.	20–35	50	50	30
Coagulase-positive	10–27	50	20	10
Coagulase-negative	1–3	<5	30	20
Gram-negative bacilli	<5	15	20	20
Miscellaneous bacteria	<5	5	5	5
HACEK group	<5	<1	<1	<5
Coryne- and propionibacteria	<1	<5	<5	<5
Anaerobes	<1	<1	<1	<1
Fungi	<5	5	5	5
Coxiella burnetii	<1	<1	<1	<1
Polymicrobial	<1	<5	<5	<5
Culture negative	3–5	3–5	<5	<5

Adapted from Schlant RC, Alexander RW, O'Rourke RA, Soonneblick EH (eds): *Hurst's The Heart*, 8th ed. New York: McGraw Hill, 1994, pp 1681–1709.

CLINICAL MANIFESTATIONS

Symptoms
- Usually begin 2 weeks after initial bacteremia
  - Diagnosis on average takes 5 weeks from onset of symptoms.
- Subacute bacterial endocarditis (SBE) most common and presents with:
  - Low-grade fever, 38°C range, may be accompanied by night sweats.
  - Fatigue, malaise, generalized weakness, anorexia, and weight loss, mimics cancer.
  - Myalgias and arthralgias may suggest a connective tissue disease.
  - Low back pain can be the initial primary complaint. Consider endocarditis, as well as epidural abscess and osteomyelitis, when back pain is accompanied by fever.
  - Systemic emboli can result in sudden hemiparesis or sudden limb pain due to tissue ishcemia.
- Acute onset of symptoms is rarer and indicates acute bacterial endocarditis (ABE).
  - High fever, 40°C range, associated with rigors.
  - Most commonly due to *S. aureus* or enterococcus and rarely *S. pneumoniae*.
  - Higher likelihood of serious cardiac and extravascular complications.
  - Rapid diagnosis and treatment are mandatory to reduce valvular destruction and embolic complications.

Physical Findings

- Fever is the rule and is detected in 95% of patients.
- A cardiac murmur is heard in nearly all patients.
  - Absence of a murmur should call into question the diagnosis of infective endocarditis.
  - Classic changing murmur is rare, may occur with rupture chordae tendinae.
  - New aortic regurgitation is a bad prognostic sign and is often followed by congestive heart failure.
  - A new aortic regurgitant murmur is due to infective endocarditis until proven otherwise.
- Embolic phenomena are found in over 50% of cases (see Fig. 7-1).
  - Petechiae—most common in conjunctiva; clusters can be found anywhere.
  - Splinter hemorrhages—linear streaks found under nails
  - Osler nodes—painful raised lesion in the pads of the fingers or toes, evanescent
  - Janeway lesions—painless or sometimes painful, red hemorrhagic macules, persistent, most common in acute endocarditis due to *S. aureus*
  - Roth spots, retinal hemorrhage with a clear center; flame-shaped hemorrhages more common
- Splenomegaly can be found; left upper quadrant tenderness can occur with embolic infarction.
- Check all pulses as a baseline, because of the risk of obstructive emboli.
- Perform a thorough neurologic exam; a sudden embolic stroke can develop.
  - Confusion, severe headache, or focal neurologic deficits warrant a head CT scan or MRI with contrast.
  - Need to exclude embolic infarction, intracerebral hemorrhage, or brain abscess.

Laboratory Findings

- Anemia of chronic disease found in 70–90% of subacute cases
  - Normocytic normochromic red cell morphology
  - Low serum iron and low iron-binding capacity
- Normal peripheral WBC, unless myocardial abscess or acute disease
- Manifestations of chronic antigenemia, mimics a connective tissue disorder
  - Elevated ESR and C-reactive protein
  - Positive rheumatoid factor
  - Elevated immunoglobulins, cryoglobulins, and immune complexes
  - Decreased complement
  - Hematuria and proteinuria
- CXR may be abnormal
  - Circular, cannonball-like lesions in embolic right-sided endocarditis
  - Pulmonary edema pattern secondary to left-sided CHF
- EKG—monitor closely
  - Conduction defects can progress to complete heart block
  - Indicative of myocardial abscess

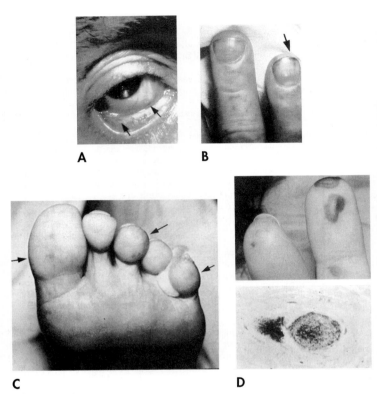

A

B

C

D

FIGURE 7-1

Embolic lesions in infective endocarditis. (A) Conjunctival hemorrhages: Arrows point to two discrete linear hemorrhages. (B) Nail bed splinter hemorrhage: Multiple petechiae are seen on both fingers. Arrow points to a splinter hemorrhage underlying the nail bed. (C) Osler nodes: Arrows point to subtle discolorations of the pads of the toes. These sites were raised and tender to palpation. (D) Janeway lesions: Top: Painless hemorrhagic lesions are seen. Bottom: Biopsy of a typical lesion shows thrombosis and intravascular Gram-positive cocci. Culture was positive for *S. aureus*.

DIAGNOSIS

- Blood cultures documenting constant bacteremia with endocarditis-associated pathogen
  - Blood cultures need to be spaced at least 15 minutes apart, 3 over 24 hours for SBE.
  - Large volumes (at least 10 ml) of blood need to be added to blood cultures because of the lower numbers of bacteria in the bloodstream.
  - Sensitivity of blood cultures is excellent, 85–95% on the first blood culture and 95–100% with a second blood culture.
  - Notify the microbiology laboratory to hold blood cultures for 4 weeks.
    - Laboratories routinely discard blood cultures after 7 days.
    - Slow-growing HACEK group members may take 4 weeks to grow.
  - Previous antibiotics interfere with blood cultures.
    - False-negative blood cultures persist for ≥ 7 days after an antibiotic is given.
    - In cases of SBE, antibiotics should be withheld until the blood cultures are confirmed to be positive.
- Documentation of endocardial involvement by echocardiography
  - Allows detection of vegetations, assessment of valve function, myocardial contractility, and chamber volume
  - Transesophageal echo (TEE) is preferred over transthoracic echo (TTE). More sensitive for detecting:
    - Vegetations (94–100% vs. 44–63% sensitivity for TTE); can detect vegetations smaller than 3 mm
    - Extravalvular extension of infection (87% vs. 28% sensitivity)
    - Valve perforations (95% vs. 45% sensitivity)
- Duke criteria are helpful for making the clinical diagnosis of infective endocarditis in the absence of pathologic tissue (see Table 7-3).
  - Definite infective endocarditis = 2 major criteria, or 1 major and 3 minor criteria, or 5 minor criteria
  - Possible infective endocarditis = 1 major and 1 minor criterion or 3 minor criteria

COMPLICATIONS

- 60% of patients suffer one complication, 25% two, and 8% three or more.
- Cardiac complications occur in up to half of patients.
  - Congestive heart failure usually due to valve regurgitation
  - Myocardial abscess
    - Associated with leukocytosis and persistent fever
    - Conduction defects on EKG suggestive
      - Abscess in the aortic ring can spread to the conduction system.
  - Myocardial infarction a rare complication of aortic disease
- Systemic emboli
  - Two-thirds go to the cerebral cortex, right side > left side.
  - Limb emboli cause sudden pain.
  - Splenic and renal infarction can also occur.
  - Right-sided endocarditis results in pulmonary emboli.

TABLE 7-3
MODIFIED DUKE CRITERIA FOR INFECTIVE ENDOCARDITIS

Major criteria

1. (+) Blood cultures with typical endocarditis-associated organisms including *S. aureus*
   —2 separate (+) B.C
   (or)
   —Persistent (+) BC (2 positive over 12 hours apart or 3 or the majority of >4 BC pos. over 1 hour)
2. Evidence of endocardial involvement
   (+) echo (patients with possible IE, a TEE is recommended)
   (or)
   —New regurgitant murmur
3. + Q fever serology (antiphase I IgG > 1:800) or single BC + *Coxiella burnetii*

Minor criteria

1. Predisposing heart condition
2. Fever ≥ 38°C
3. Vascular phenomenon
4. Immunologic phenomenon
5. Single positive BC with typical organism
6. (The previous minor criteria of suspicious lesion on TTE eliminated)

Definite infective endocarditis =

—2 major
—1 major and 3 minor
—5 minor

Possible infective endocarditis =

—1 major and 1 minor
—3 minor

From Li JS, et al: *Clin Infect Dis* 2000; 30:633–38.

- Neurological complications develop in 25–35% of patients.
  - Embolic stroke (most common with fungi and HACEK group)
  - Mycotic aneurysms
    - Middle cerebral artery most common location
    - *S. aureus* the usual cause
    - Because of the risk of intracerebral hemorrhage, anticoagulants should be avoided in cases of infective endocarditis.
  - Encephalopathy, meningitis, and brain abscess

- Renal complications
  - Serum creatinine > 2 mg/dl develops in 1/3 of patients. Higher risk in:
    - The elderly
    - Patients with thrombocytopenia
  - Renal failure can be caused by:
    - Membranoproliferative glomerulonephritis
      - Due to immune-complex deposition
      - Accompanied by hematuria, red cell casts, and mild proteinuria
      - Rapidly improves with antibiotic therapy
    - Interstitial nephritis
    - Embolic damage

TREATMENT (SEE TABLE 7-4)

- Cidal antibiotics must be used, and therapy must be prolonged.
  - Therapy 4–6 weeks except for uncomplicated *S. viridans* with penicillin or ceftriaxone combined with low-dose gentamicin; effective in 2 weeks.
  - Therapy must be guided by MIC and MBC values and synergy testing.
    - Serum cidal levels of 1:8–1:32 have been associated with cure.
  - Synergistic therapy not shown to be of benefit for *S. aureus.*
- β-lactam antibiotics are preferred over vancomycin whenever possible.
  - Vancomycin associated with failures rates of up to 40% in *S. aureus* endocarditis
  - Cephalosporins are not effective in enterococcal endocarditis; ampicillin or penicillin in combination with gentamicin recommended. In the elderly may be able to shorten gentamicin treatment to 2–3 weeks to minimize toxicity.
  - Cefazolin not recommended for *S. aureus* endocarditis because of the risk of type A β-lactamase producing strain that can inactivate this drug.
- Antibiotics alone rarely sterilize prosthetic valves.
  - Deposition of biofilm on the prosthetic material
  - Valve often has to be replaced.
  - Some success with coagulase-negative cocci using vancomycin, gentamicin, and rifampin
- Tricuspid endocarditis
  - Nafcillin or oxacillin plus tobramycin $\times$ 2 weeks effective, except for HIV-infected patients
  - Oral ciprofloxacin plus rifampin $\times$ 4 weeks may also be effective.

TABLE 7-4
ANTIBIOTIC THERAPY FOR INFECTIVE ENDOCARDITIS

Drug	Dose	Relative Efficacy	Comments
Acute, empiric	Duration 4–6 weeks unless otherwise noted		
Vancomycin (+)	1 gm IV Q12H		Vancomycin more slowly cidal. Whenever possible use an alternative
Ampicillin (+)	2 gm IV Q4H		
Gentamicin	1 mg/kg IV Q8H		
Culture negative			
Ampicillin (+)	2 gm IV Q4H		
Gentamicin	1 mg/kg IV Q8H		
Prosthetic, empiric			
Vancomycin (+)	1 gm IV Q12H		
Gentamicin (+)	1 mg/kg IVQ8H		
Rifampin	600 mg po QD		
S. viridans			
Penicillin G (or)	2–3 million units IV Q4H	First line	Short course if uncomplicated
Ampicillin (+)	2 gm IV Q4H		Use sensitivity testing to determine best regimen
Gentamicin	1 mg/kg IV Q8H × 2 weeks		
Ceftriaxone (+)	2 gm IV QD	Alternative	Short course if uncomplicated
Gentamicin	1 mg/kg IV Q8H × 2 weeks		For PCN-allergic patient
Vancomycin	1 gm IV Q12H × 4 weeks	Alternative	

Enterococcus

Ampicillin or	2 gm IV Q4H	First line	Relapse is common in the absence of gentamicin; use sensitivity testing to determine best regimen
Penicillin G (+)	2–3 million units IV Q4H		
Gentamicin	1 mg/kg IV Q8H		

***S. aureus* MSSA**

Nafcillin or Oxacillin (+)	2 gm IV Q4H	First line	Addition of gentamicin may shorten bacteremia but has no effect on final outcome
Gentamicin	1 mg/kg IV Q8H for 3–5 days		

***S. aureus* MRSA**

Vancomycin	1 gm IV Q12H	First line	

***S. aureus* (tricuspid)**

Nafcillin or Oxacillin (+)	2 gm IV Q4H	First line	Short course effective if no metastatic lesions and MSSA
Gentamicin	1 mg/kg IV Q8H × 2 weeks		
Ciprofloxacin (+)	750 mg po BID	Second line	May be effective in MSSA
Rifampin	300 mg po BID × 4 weeks		

SURGERY

- The threshold for surgery should be low and increases the likelihood of cure.
- The cardiologist and cardiac surgeon should be consulted early.
- Indications for surgery include:
  - Moderate to severe CHF
    - Delay in surgery results in irreversible left ventricular dysfunction.
    - Early surgery lowers intra- and postoperative mortality.
  - More than 1 systemic embolus
  - Uncontrolled infection
    - *S. aureus* the most common pathogen to cause persistently positive blood cultures.
    - Extravascular foci of infection should always be excluded before considering surgical intervention.
  - Resistant bacteria or a fungal pathogen
  - Perivalvular leak or myocardial abscess
    - Abscesses often continue to expand on antibiotic therapy.
- Surgery within a week of the neurologic event is not accompanied by worsening neurologic deficits.
- When possible, surgery should be delayed until blood cultures are negative.
  - Even in the setting of ongoing positive blood cultures, infection of the new valve is uncommon.
  - Reduced risk of reinfection if the surgeon thoroughly debrides the infected site.
- Intraoperative gram stains of the valve as well as cultures should always be obtained.

PROGNOSIS

- Outcome strongly correlates with the organism and valve infected.
  - *S. aureus* causes 50% mortality in patients > 50 years.
  - Fungal infections are difficult to cure.
  - Gram-negative bacilli are associated with a poor outcome.
  - Aortic valve infection has higher mortality than mitral valve infection.
- CHF or neurologic deficits = worse prognosis
- Prosthetic valve endocarditis associated with a poorer outcome
  - Early prosthetic endocarditis, cure rates only 30–50%
  - Late disease, higher cure rates, particularly with *S. epidermidis* and *S. viridans*

PREVENTION

- The efficacy of prophylaxis has not been proven; however, it is considered the standard of care.
- Two categories of patients are recommended to receive prophylaxis.
  - High risk (prosthetic valves, previous endocarditis, cyanotic heart disease, and surgical shunts)
  - Moderate risk (rheumatic and other acquired valvular dysfunction, hypertrophic cardiomyopathy, mitral valve prolapse with regurgitation)

- Prophlyaxis recommended for:
  - Dental procedures—periodontal procedures, tooth cleaning if bleeding is anticipated, initial placement of orthodontic bands, intraligamentary local anesthetic injections
  - Tonsillectomy and adenoidectomy
  - Surgical procedures that involve intestinal or respiratory mucosa
  - Sclerotherapy of esophageal varices, or esophageal dilation in high-risk patients
  - Endoscopic retrograde cholangiography with biliary obstruction
  - Gallbladder surgery in high-risk patients
  - Cystocopy, urethral dilation, or prostate surgery
- Recommended regimens for dental and ENT procedures
  - Amoxicillin, 2 g po 1 hour before the procedure, or penicillin V, 2 g po 1 hour before and 1 g 6 hr after the first dose
  - Penicillin-allergic patients: Clindamycin, 600 mg po; cephalexin or cefadroxil, 2 g po; azithromycin or clarithromycin, 500 mg po 1 hour before the procedure
  - If parenteral therapy is required, 2 g IM or IV ampicillin; in the penicillin-allergic patient, 600 mg IV clindamycin or 1 g IM or IV cefazolin 30 minutes preprocedure
- For genitourinary or gastrointestinal procedures:
  - High-risk patient—Ampicillin, 2 g IM or IV, plus gentamicin, 1.5 mg/kg ≤ 30 minutes preprocedure and 6 hour later 1 g of ampicillin IV or amoxicillin po
  - High-risk penicillin allergy—Vancomycin, 1 g IV over 1–2 hour, plus gentamicin, 1.5 mg/kg IV or IM; complete infusion within 30 minutes of start of the procedure
  - Moderate risk—Amoxicillin, 2 g po 1 hour preprocedure, or ampicillin, 2 g IM or IV 30 min before the procedure
  - Moderate risk, penicillin allergy—Vancomycin, 1 g IV over 1–2 hour; complete the infusion within 30 minutes of start of the procedure

INTRAVASCULAR CATHETER-RELATED INFECTIONS

- Potential severity: Can be life-threatening. Often prolong hospital stay and can be complicated by metastatic lesions and bacterial endocarditis.

EPIDEMIOLOGY, PATHOGENESIS, AND ETIOLOGY

- The major cause of nococomial bacteremia
- Bacteria infect catheters in 3 ways:
  1. Skin flora migrates along the catheter track
  2. Bacteria are injected into the port
  3. Hematogenous spread
- The risk of infection is greater for some devices than others:
  1. Femoral vein > internal jugular vein > subclavian catheters
  2. Nontunneled > tunneled catheters
  3. Tunneled > totally implanted devices
  4. Conventional catheter tips > silver-impregnated catheter tips
  5. Centrally inserted central venous catheters > peripherally inserted central catheters (PICC)
  6. Hemodialysis > other catheters
  7. Hyperalimentation > standard infusion ports
- Regular exchange of central venous catheters over guide wires does not reduce the incidence of infection. Not recommended; can precipitate bacteremia.

- Gram-positive cocci predominate.
  a. Coagulase-negative cocci most common; adhere to catheters by a glycocalyx
  b. *S. aureus*
  c. Enterococci
  d. Corynebacteria
- Gram-negatives account for one third.
  a. Enterobacter spp., *E. coli*, Acinetobacter spp., Pseudomonas spp., and Serratia spp.
  b. Contaminated infusate associated with Klebsiella spp., Citrobacter, or non-*aeruginosa* strains of Pseudomonas
- *Candida albicans*—also forms an adherent glycocalyx, associated with high glucose solutions

CLINICAL MANIFESTATIONS AND DIAGNOSIS

- Symptoms are nonspecific. Suggestive historical facts include:
  ○ Rigors or chills associated with infusion
  ○ Resolution of symptoms on removal of the intravenous catheter
  ○ Blood cultures positive for *S. epidermidis*, corynebacteria, or *C. albicans*
- Purulence around the catheter site provides strong evidence, but absent in many cases.
- Cytospin Gram stain or acridine orange stain of catheter sample for rapid diagnosis.
- Quantitating bacteria on catheter tip.
  ○ Roll method (the catheter is rolled across the culture plate)
    ▪ Semiquantitative (positive = > 15 cfu)
    ▪ Detects bacteria on the outer surface of the catheter
  ○ Vortex or sonication method (releases bacteria into liquid media)
    ▪ Quantitative (positive = > 100 cfu)
    ▪ Detects bacteria from the inner lumen as well as outer surface
    ▪ More sensitive than roll method
- Cultures of removed catheter tips should be performed only when a catheter-related bloodstream infection is suspected. Surveillance cultures not recommended.
- Simultaneous blood cultures should be drawn from the catheter and a peripheral vein.
  ○ Quantitative cultures:
    ▪ Catheter sample 5–10 × > peripheral sample = catheter infection
  ○ Measurement of time interval required for detection:
    ▪ Catheter positive > 2 hours earlier than peripheral sample = catheter infection

TREATMENT

- The catheter should be removed if:
  ○ The patient is severely ill.
  ○ Fever and positive blood cultures persist > 48 hours.
  ○ The patient is infected with a virulent, difficult-to-treat organism
    ▪ *S. aureus*
    ▪ Gram-negative bacilli, particularly *Pseudomonas aeruginosa*
    ▪ Fungi
  ○ Polymicrobial bacteremia
  ○ Tunnel infection, neutropenia, endocarditis, metastatic infection, septic thrombophlebitis

- Empiric therapy: Vancomycin and antipseudomonal third- or fourth-generation cephalosporin
- Duration of therapy not studied
  ○ Average duration 3 weeks
  ○ 1 week for coagulase-negative Staphylococcus, if line removed, and 2 weeks if line kept in place
  ○ 4–6 week for complicated infections
- Antibiotic lock therapy improves cure rate for tunnel catheters.
  ○ Gram-positive infection, vancomycin (25 mg in 5 ml of solution)
  ○ Gram-negative infection, gentamicin (5 mg in 5 ml)
  ○ Can improve cure rates to 60–80%
- *S. aureus*—high risk of endocarditis
  ○ Attaches to and destroys normal heart valves (70% endocardits in normal valves)
  ○ TEE helpful in determining length of therapy
    ▪ Valvular vegetations = 4–6 weeks of therapy
    ▪ Absence of vegetations = 2 weeks; without significant risk of relapse
  ○ Short-course therapy, considered only in patients who:
    ▪ Promptly defervesce on antibiotic therapy
    ▪ Do not have valvular heart disease
    ▪ Have no extravascular focus of infection
- *C. albicans*—always remove the line, treat for 2 weeks to prevent endopthalmitis
  ○ Endopthalmitis develops in 10–15% of untreated patients
  ○ Fluconazole (400 mg/day), for uncomplicated catheter-related infection
  ○ Amphotericin B (0.3–1 mg/kg/day), for severely ill, neutropenia, or infection with a resistant fungus

MYOCARDITIS

- Potential severity: Fulminant myocarditis can be fatal or lead to chronic congestive heart failure. Most cases are self-limited and are followed by full recovery.

ETIOLOGIES

- Primarily caused by viruses
  ○ Enteroviruses the primary causative agents
    ▪ Coxsackie virus most frequent
    ▪ Echoviruses less common
  ○ Adenovirus another common viral cause, particularly in adults
  ○ Other viruses implicated include cytomegalovirus and Epstein-Barr virus, varicella-zoster, and mumps
  ○ Asymptomatic HIV, incidence of mycocarditis 1.6% per year
- Other infectious agents are rare:
  ○ Legionella and Chlamydia spp.
  ○ Spirochetes: Lyme disease may present with cardiac arrhythmias (see Chap. 13)
  ○ Fungal infections due to severe disseminated Aspergillus, Candida, and Cryptococcus spp.
  ○ Parasites:
    ▪ *Trypanosoma cruzi* attacks the heart in 30% of patients with Chagas' disease.
    ▪ Trichinella can cause fatal myocarditis.
- 1–5% of systemic viral illness involves the myocardium.

RISK FACTORS FOR SYMPTOMATIC DISEASE

- Young males, pregnant women, neonates, and immunocompromised
- Forced exercise
- Steroids or nonsteroidal anti-inflammatory agents
- Ethanol
- Nutritional deficiencies
- Many patients are asymptomatic, others develop:
  - Flu-like illness, chest pain
  - Arrhythmias
  - CHF

PHYSICAL EXAM

- S_3 gallop = left-sided CHF
- Mitral regurgitation due to ring dilatation

LABORATORY FINDINGS

- Cardiac enzymes elevated in the minority of cases.
  - CK-MB levels are elevated in only 5% of cases.
  - Cardiac troponin I in 34%.
  - Usually detected within the first month of symptoms.
  - Suggest ongoing myocyte necrosis.
- EKG shows nonspecific ST and T wave changes, arrhythmias, conduction defects.
- Chest X-ray detects pulmonary edema and cardiac dilatation.
- Cardiac echo very helpful for assessing:
  - Cardiac contractility
  - Chamber size
  - Valve function
  - Wall thickness
- MRI with contrast allows assessment of extent of inflammation.
- Endomyocardial biopsy combined with PCR experimental.

TREATMENT

- Bed rest
- Drugs for CHF
- Antiarrhythmia medications
- Anticoagulation in all patients with ejection fractions < 20%
- A randomized trial of immunosuppressive agents failed to improve outcome.

OUTCOME

- Usually full recovery
- Fulminant cases may require heart transplant

PERICARDITIS

- Potential severity: Viral pericarditis usually has a self-limited benign course. However, patients with purulent pericarditis have a high mortality and require emergent care.

ETIOLOGIES

- Viral pericardidts the most frequent cause
  - ○ Enteroviruses most common (coxsackie A and B and echovirus)
- Purulent pericarditis, rare
  - ○ *S. aureus*, *S. pneumoniae*, and other streptococci are the leading etiologies
  - ○ Hematogenous spread most common
  - ○ Direct spread from:
    - Pneumonia or a subdiaphragmatic focus
    - Delayed complication of a penetrating injury
    - Following cardiac surgery
      - *S. aureus*, Gram-negative aerobic rods, and Candida spp.
- Tuberculous pericarditis
  - ○ Usually seeded during primary disease, but can spread from a pulmonary focus.
  - ○ Initially a purulent exudate, but over time the pericardium thickens, becomes fibrotic, and calcifies, causing constrictive pericarditis.

CLINICAL MANIFESTATIONS

Symptoms
- Substernal chest pain, relieved by sitting forward, most common in viral and idiopathic pericarditis.
- Fever and dyspnea in purulent pericarditis. Chest pain in one third.
- Vague, dull chest pain, weight loss, night sweats, cough, and dyspnea in tuberculous disease.

Physical Exam
- Three-component friction rub early; later disappears with increased pericardial fluid
- Pulsus paradoxicus > 10 mm abnormal
  - ○ Pericadial fluid limits the ability of the heart to expand.
  - ○ Inspiration increases right ventricular filling causing this chamber to balloon into the left ventricle and reducing left ventricular filling.
- Jugular venous distension with depressed y descent due to a rise in right ventricular filling pressure
- Rapid respiratory rate and dyspnea at rest
- Equalization of right- and left-sided cardiac pressures tends to minimize pulmonary edema and the lung fields are clear on auscultation.

DIAGNOSIS AND TREATMENT

- Echocardiography should be performed immediately.
  - Allows assessment of pericardial thickness, pericardial fluid, and tamponade
  - Can be used to guide emergency pericardiocentesis
- EKG
  - Diffuse ST and T changes
  - Depressed PR interval
  - Decreased QRS voltage and electrical alternans
- Pericardiocentesis
  - Only for those with tamponade or suspected purulent pericarditis.
  - Pericardial biopsy improves the diagnostic yield.
- Viral or ideopathic pericarditis self-limited
  - Nonsteroidals only if no myocarditis
  - Colchicine
- Purulent pericarditis (mortality 30%)
  - Emergency surgical drainage
  - Systemic antibiotics
- Tuberculous pericarditis
  - Four-drug antituberculous regimen
  - To prevent constrictive pericarditis (20–50% incidence during treatment), give prednisone simultaneously (60 mg po × 4 weeks, 30 mg × 4 weeks, 15 mg × 2 weeks, and 5 mg × 1 week).
  - Calcific form requires pericardectomy.

REFERENCES

Adler Y, Finkelstein Y, Guindo J, et al: Colchicine treatment for recurrent pericarditis: A decade of experience. *Circulation* 1998; 97:2183–85.

Aikat S, Ghaffari S: A review of pericardial diseases: Clinical, ECG and hemodynamic features and management. *Cleve Clin J Med* 2000; 67:903–14.

Andrews MM, von Reyn CF: Patient selection criteria and management guidelines for outpatient parenteral antibiotic therapy for native valve infective endocarditis. *Clin Infect Dis* 2001; 33:203–9.

Bouza E, Burillo A, Munoz P: Catheter-related infections: Diagnosis and intravascular treatment. *Clin Microbiol Infect* 2002; 8:265–74.

Dhawan VK: Infective endocarditis in elderly patients. *Clin Infect Dis* 2002; 34:806–12.

Feldman AM, McNamara D: Myocarditis. *N Engl J Med* 2000; 343:1388–98.

Haas GJ: Etiology, evaluation, and management of acute myocarditis. *Cardiol Rev* 2001; 9:88–95.

Le T, Bayer AS: Combination antibiotic therapy for infective endocarditis. *Clin Infect Dis* 2003; 36:615–21.

Lewis W: Cardiomyopathy in AIDS: A pathophysiological perspective. *Prog Cardiovasc Dis* 2000; 43:151–70.

Maisch B: Pericardial diseases, with a focus on etiology, pathogenesis, pathophysiology, new diagnostic imaging methods, and treatment. *Curr Opin Cardiol* 1994; 9:379–88.

McKay G, Bunton R, Galvin I, Shaw D, Singh H: Infective endocarditis—A twelve year surgical outcome series. *NZ Med J* 2002; 115:124–26.

Mermel LA, Farr BM, Sherertz RJ, et al: Guidelines for the management of intravascular catheter-related infections. *Clin Infect Dis* 2001; 32:1249–72.

Morris AJ, Drinkovic D, Pottumarthy S, Strickett MG, MacCulloch D, et al: Gram stain, culture, and histopathological examination findings for heart valves removed because of infective endocarditis. *Clin Infect Dis* 2003; 36:697–704.

Mylonakis E, Calderwood SB: Infective endocarditis in adults. *N Engl J Med* 2001; 345:1318–30.

Nannini EC, Singh KV, Murray BE: Relapse of type A beta-lactamase-producing *Staphylococcus aureus* native valve endocarditis during cefazolin therapy: Revisiting the issue. *Clin Infect Dis* 2003; 37:1194–98.

Olaison L, Schadewitz K: Enterococcal endocarditis in Sweden, 1995–1999: Can shorter therapy with aminoglycosides be used? *Clin Infect Dis* 2002; 34:159–66.

Piper C, Korfer R, Horstkotte D: Prosthetic valve endocarditis. *Heart* 2001; 85:590–93.

Raad, II, Hanna HA: Intravascular catheter-related infections: New horizons and recent advances. *Arch Intern Med* 2002; 162:871–78.

Ryan EW, Bolger AF: Transesophageal echocardiography (TEE) in the evaluation of infective endocarditis. *Cardiol Clin* 2000; 18:773–87.

Trautner BW, Darouiche RO: Tuberculous pericarditis: Optimal diagnosis and management. *Clin Infect Dis* 2001; 33:954–61.

CHAPTER

8

GASTROINTESTINAL AND HEPATOBILIARY INFECTIONS

INFECTIOUS DIARRHEA

HIGHLIGHTS

- One the leading causes of death worldwide (nearly 2.5 million deaths annually).
- Most commonly encountered in developing countries.
- Pathogens causing diarrhea can be transmitted in three ways:
  1. Foodborne
  2. Waterborne
  3. Person-to-person spread
- Modes of transmission reflect differences in:
  ○ Ability to survive in the environment
  ○ The inoculum size required to cause disease
- Stool smear is helpful for differentiating invasive pathogens (PMN seen) from agents that alter bowel fluid resorption.
- Antibiotics rarely required; fluid and electrolyte replacement are the mainstay of therapy.

BACTERIAL DIARRHEA

- Potential severity—Can be life-threatening in infants, young children, and the elderly. In most patients this illness can be managed on an outpatient basis.
- The three most common bacterial causes of acute infectious diarrhea:
  ○ Salmonella
  ○ Shigella
  ○ Campylobacter
- Other important bacterial pathogens include:
  ○ *E. coli*
  ○ *Yersinia enterocolitica*
  ○ *Vibrio parahaemolyticus*
- Cannot be readily distinguished clinically, and diagnosis requires isolation of the organism on stool culture.

MICROBIOLOGY, PATHOGENESIS, AND EPIDEMIOLOGY

Salmonella
- Gram-negative bacillus, does not ferment lactose, motile
- Three major species:
  1. *S. typhi*, primarily adapted to humans
  2. *S. choleraesuis*
  3. *S. enteritidis*

Pathogenesis
- Attaches to intestinal and colonic cells and injects proteins that stimulate internalization
- Spreads to mesenteric nodes
- *S. choleraesuis* and *S. typhi* often enter the bloodstream
- The organism is acid-sensitive. Large numbers of organisms required to induce infection (10^4–10^8 organisms).
- Risk factors for disease include:
  ◦ Antacid use (acid-sensitive)
  ◦ Prior antibiotics (reduces competition by normal flora)
  ◦ Depressed immune function (AIDS and transplant patients, sickle cell disease)

Epidemiology
- Contracted from contaminated foods (more common in the summer months)
  ◦ Chicken products—eggs, undercooked meat (chickens often carry Salmonella in their stool)
  ◦ Contaminated processed foods—ice cream, unpasteurized goat cheese, whitefish, as well as contaminated fruits and vegetables
  ◦ Infected pet turtles, iguanas, birds
  ◦ Contaminated water supply—*S. typhi*
    ▪ Found in developing countries with poor sanitation

Shigella
- Shigella is a gram-negative rod, does not ferment lactose, is nonmotile.
- Four major serological groups, A–D.
  ◦ Group B, *S. flexneri*, and Group D, *S. sonnei*, most common in the United States.
  ◦ Group A, *S. dysenteriae*, and Group D, *S. boydii*, rare in the United States.

Pathogenesis
- Induces ruffling of host cells; once internalized, it escapes to the cytoplasm
- Moves through the cytoplasm and spreads from cell to cell by polymerizing actin
- Accelerates cell death, forming plaques of necrotic cells
- Induces marked inflammation and rarely invades the bloodstream
- Resistance to gastric acid allows small numbers of organisms (200 bacteria) to cause disease.
- Initially grows in the small intestine and then spreads to the colon, where it causes intense inflammation, microabscesses, and mucosal ulcerations.

Epidemiology
- Person-to-person spread.
  - Day care centers
  - Toilet seats
  - Contaminated water
  - Can be spread by flies in tropical areas
  - High incidence on U.S. Indian reservations
  - Less commonly foodborne

Campylobacter
- Campylobacter is a coma-shaped Gram-negative rod, microaerophilic.
- Grows best at 42°C, requires Campy BAP selective media or other bowel flora over-grow. Only *C. fetus* can grow at 25°C.
- Two major species cause disease in man:
  - *C. jejuni* causes infectious diarrhea.
  - *C. fetus* causes prolonged bacteremia.

Pathogenesis
- Internalized by and lives in monocytes and intestinal epithelial cells, induces cell death, bowel ulceration, and intense inflammation.
- *C. fetus* is carried by monocytes to the bloodstream, resists serum bactericidal activity, and causes persistent bacteremia.
- Like Salmonella, sensitive to gastric acid and requires a high inoculum ($> 10^4$ bacteria) to cause disease

Epidemiology
Similar to epidemiology of Salmonella

- *C. jejuni* survives well in chickens because of their high body temperature (30% of carcasses culture positive as compared to 3% positive for Salmonella).
- Carried in water, raw milk, sheep, cattle, swine, and reptiles.
- Infections are more common in the summer months.

Escherichia coli
- Serotyping identifies specific O (lipopolysaccharide) and H antigens (flagellar proteins)
- There are 5 pathogenic classes.
  1. Entertoxigenic (ETEC)
     - Produce a choleralike toxin that stimulates secretion of chloride causing watery diarrhea
     - Spread by human sewage–contaminated water in developing countries
  2. Enteropathogenic (EPEC)
     - Induce pedestals that cause mild inflammation
     - Watery diarrhea primarily in children < 3 years old
     - Transmitted by contaminated food and water and by person-to-person spread in nurseries
     - Primarily found in developing countries
  3. Enterohemorrhagic (EHEC)
     - Produce verotoxins or Shiga-like cytotoxins that inhibit protein synthesis and cause cell death.
     - Toxin damages vascular endothelium in the bowel and glomeruli, causing hemorrhagic colitis and hemolytic uremic syndrome.
     - O157:H7 causes hemolytic-uremic syndrome.
     - Epidemiology

- Cattle primary reservoir; undercooked hamburger
- Less commonly:
  - Unpasteurized milk
  - Contaminated apple cider and mayonnaise
- Person-to-person spread can occur in day care centers and nursing homes.
- Primarily an infection of industrialized nations.
- Usually occurs during the summer months.

4. Enteroinvasive (EIEC)
   - Similar to Shigella
   - Requires large inoculum (10^8 organisms) to cause disease.
   - Usually associated with contaminated foods in developing countries.
5. Enteroaggregative (EaggEC)
   - Adhere as large aggregates to the colonic mucosa.
   - Enterotoxin produces watery diarrhea that is often prolonged.
   - Contracted by ingesting contaminated water or food.
   - A major cause of traveler's diarrhea.

Yersinia
- *Y. enterocolitica*, an aerobic Gram-negative bacillus, requires large inoculum (10^9).
- Infects terminal ileum; mesenteric node inflammation mimics appendicitis.
- Common in northern Europe, South America, Africa, and Asia, rare in United States.
- Found in contaminated meat products and milk; grows at $4°C$.
- Most common in children; more frequent during winter months.

Vibrio cholerae
- Vibrio is a slightly curved Gram-negative bacillus with a single flagellum. Requires special culture media (tellurite taurocholate gelatin)
- Two strains associated with diarrhea are *V. cholera* and *V. parahaemolyticus*.
- Attaches to small intestine and produces cholera toxin
  - Toxin binds to a receptor that increases cyclic AMP, which promotes chloride and water secretion.

Epidemiology
- Survives in algae, plankton, and shellfish.
- Can convert to dormant state or form aggregates surrounded by biofilm (rugose).
- Spread by contaminated water (10^3–10^6 organisms) or food (10^2–10^4 organisms).
- Noncholera toxin strains in Gulf of Mexico.
- Cholera toxin strains spread by contaminated water in India, Bangladesh, Asia, Africa, Europe, South America (Peru), and Central America.
- Occur in the hot seasons of the year.

V. parahaemolyticus
- Nonhemolytic strains are nonpathogenic.
- Produces an entertoxin causing moderate inflammation and watery diarrhea.
- Thrives in salt water; concentrates in shellfish.
- Very common in Japan, being contracted from sushi.
- Incidence may increase in the United States as sushi becomes more popular.

CLINICAL MANIFESTATIONS

Gastroenteritis
- Incubation period
  - 8–24 hours for Salmonella
  - 36–72 hours for Shigella
  - 4 days EHEC
- Diarrhea varies in volume and consistency.
  - Watery with EPEC, ETEC, EaggEC, and Vibrio
  - Mucousy with Shigella
  - Bloody with Shigella, Campylobacter, EHEC, and EIEC
- Tenesmus and pain on defecating when colon involved. Most common with Shigella.

Physical Exam
- Significant percentage of patients have fever, usually in the 38–39°C range.
- Abdominal pain and tenderness
  - Associated with hyperactive bowel sounds and diffuse tenderness
  - Can be severe, mimicking appendicitis or cholecystitis

Laboratory Findings
- Leukocyte count is often normal; some develop moderate leukocytosis.
- Fluid loss can be profound, leading to hypotension and electrolyte abnormalities.
- Blood cultures may be positive in Salmonella enterocolits, but are rare in Shigella or *C. jejuni* infections.

Enteric Fever
- Caused by *S. typhi*, *S. paratyphi*, *C. fetus*, and *Yersinia enterocolitica*
- Incubation period 8–14 days, longer with lower inocula
- Influenza-like syndrome:
  - Headache
  - Muscle aches
  - Malaise and lethargy
  - Nonproductive cough
- Initially mild abdominal discomfort
  - Worsens over time
  - Associated with constipation or minimal bloody diarrhea

Physical Exam in the Later Phases
- High fever (40°C) and slow pulse (temperature-pulse dissociation)
- Abdomen markedly distended and tender, splenomegaly
- Skin: small rose-colored macules = rose spots
  - Found in upper abdomen and chest regions
  - In 80% of patients by the second to third week
- 10% mortality in the third week due to:
  - Septic shock
  - Bowel perforation

Laboratory Findings
- Normochromic, normocytic anemia, leukopenia
- Positive blood cultures in 90% in first wk
- Stool cultures often positive for Salmonella for many weeks

Diagnosis
- Direct examination of the stool using methylene blue stain to assess PMN response
  - Abundant PMN seen in Shigella, Campylobacter, and EIEC
  - With Salmonella, moderate PMN; with *S. typhi* may see monocytes
  - PMN also seen with amebic dysentery and *C. difficile* toxin–associated diarrhea
- Gram stain showing seagull-shaped Gram-negative forms = Campylobacter
- Stool culture with standard media and Campylobacter-selective media
- *E. Coli* strains identified by slide agglutination tests using specific O antisera

Treatment and Outcome (see Table 8-1)
- Self-limiting diseases usually lasting 3–7 days, and often do not require antibiotic treatment.
- Fluid and electrolyte replacement most important.
- Avoid agents that slow peristalsis, increase the risk of bacteremia, prolong fever and carrier state.
- Antibiotic treatment of Salmonella gastroenteritis prolongs the carrier state.
  - When antibiotics required continue for 48–72 hours or until afebrile
  - An oral fluoroquinolone, amoxacillin, or trimethoprim sulfamethoxazole (see Table 8-1 for doses)
- To prevent complications associated with bacteremia, treat Salmonella gastroenteritis in:
  - Neonates
  - Persons > 50 years old
  - Immunocompromised patients or those with prosthetic valve or synthetic vascular grafts
- Treat enteric fever emergently with ciprofloxacin or ceftriaxone for 10–14 days (see Table 8-1).
- Shigella: ciprofloxacin for 3 days reduces person-to-person spread (see Table 8-1).
- *Campylobacter jejuni*: erythromycin, azithromycin, or ciprofloxacin shortens the carrier state (see Table 8-1).
- Yersinia: usually not treated; for severe cases use trimethoprim-sulfa (1DS po BID) or ciprofloxacin (500 mg po BID) for 3 days.
- *Vibrio cholerae*: treat with doxycycline, trimethoprim-sulfa, or ciprofloxacin for 3 days (see Table 8-1). *V. parahaemolyticus* usually does not require treatment.
- Traveler's diarrhea: ciprofloxacin × 3–5 days shortens the course of illness.

Prevention
- Investigation of sources of contamination is a cost-effective preventive measure.
- Salmonella fecal carriage can be prolonged.
  - Carrier state can often be eradicated by prolonged therapy (4–6 weeks) with amoxicillin (2 gm po TID + probenecid 750 mg po TID) or ciprofloxacin (500–750 mg po BID).
  - Carrier state cannot be eliminated in patients with gallstones.

TABLE 8-1

ANTIBIOTIC THERAPY FOR GASTROINTESTINAL INFECTIONS

Drug	Dose	Relative efficacy	Comments
Salmonella gastroenteritis			Antibiotics prolong the carrier state
Ciprofloxacin (or)	500 mg po BID, 2–3 days	Equivalent	Use in the neonates, those
Amoxacillin (or)	1 gm po TID, 2–3 days		> 50 years old, with prosthesis,
Trimethoprim-sulfa	1 DS po BID, 2–3 days		or immunocompromised
Salmonella enteric fever			
Ciprofloxacin (or)	500 mg po BID × 10–14 days	Equivalent	Give emergently, resistant to
Ceftriaxone	1–2 gm IV QD × 10–14 days		chloramphenicol
Shigella gastroenteritis			
Ciprofloxacin	500 mg po BID × 3 days		Prevents person-to-person spread; increased
Campylobacter jejuni			
Erythromycin (or)	250 mg po QID × 5–7 days	Equivalent	Shortens the carrier state
Azithromycin (or)	500 mg, then 250 mg po QD × 4 days		
Ciprofloxacin	500 mg po BID × 5–7 days		
Vibrio cholerae			
Doxycycline (or)	300 mg po × 1	Equivalent	
trimethoprim-sulfa (or)	1 DS po BID × 3 days		
Ciprofloxacin	500 mg po BID × 3 days		
Traveler's diarrhea			
Ciprofloxacin	500 mg po BID × 3–5 days	First line	Shortens course of illness

TABLE 8-1
ANTIBIOTIC THERAPY FOR GASTROINTESTINAL INFECTIONS (Continued)

Drug	Dose	Relative efficacy	Comments
C. difficile toxin diarrhea			
Metronidazole	500 mg po Q8H × 10 days	First line	
Vancomycin	125 mg po QID × 10–14 days	Alternative	Increases the risk of VRE
Primary peritonitis			
Ceftriaxone (or)	1 gm IV QD × 10 days	First line	Give emergently
Cefotaxime	2 gm IV Q8H × 10 days		
Secondary peritonitis, mild			
Cefoxitin (or)	1.5–2 gm IV Q6H	Equivalent	Continue until leukocyte count and
Cefotetan (or)	1.5–2 gm IV Q12H		temperature are normal;
Ticarcillin-clavulinate (or)	3 gm IV Q6H		usually 5–7 days
Piperacillin-tazobactam	3 gm IV Q6H		
Secondary peritonitis, severe			
Cefoxitin or cefotetan (+)	(doses as above)		Continue until leukocyte count and
Gentamicin (or)	2 mg/kg iv, then dose by levels		temperature are normal; some
Ceftriaxone (+)	1 gm IV Q12H		recommend imipenam-cilastin
Metronidazole (or)	750–1000 mg IV Q12H		be combined with an
Ciprofloxacin (+)	400 mg IV Q12H		aminoglycoside
Metronidazole (or)	(same as above)		
Clindamycin (+)	600–900 mg IV Q6–8H		
Aztreonam (or)	1–1.5 gm IV Q6H		
Imipenam-cilastin alone	0.5–1 gm IV Q6H		

VIRAL DIARRHEA

- Potential Severity: A self-limited disease that can cause dehydration. The most common form of infectious diarrhea.
- Caused primarily by 4 viral groups
  1. Norwalk virus—a calicivirus
     - Blunts intestinal villi, causes mild malabsorption
     - Virus is shed in the stool for 24–48 hours after the onset of illness.
     - Transmission by:
       - Contaminated water (including swimming pools)
       - Foods
         - Shellfish a leading food source
         - Virus is relatively heat-resistant, and cooking contaminated food does not completely eliminate risk of infection.
         - Infected food handlers can contaminate food, resulting in large outbreaks.
       - Person-to-person spread
     - Large outbreaks reported in closed environments
       - Ships
       - Military installations
       - Hospitals and nursing homes
       - Resistant to chlorine, making decontamination difficult
     - Primarily a disease of adults, but can infect infants and children
  2. Rotavirus
     - Causes lactase deficiency
     - Primarily infects infants
     - Resists hand washing
     - Peaks in winter
  3. Enteric adenovirus
     - Infects infants and young children
     - Peaks in summer months
  4. Astroviruses
     - Infect children in pediatric wards and the elderly in nursing homes
- Clinical spectrum: mild watery diarrhea to severe nausea, vomiting, and fever
- No PMN in the stool
- Commercial ELISA available for rotavirus
- Self-limited diseases; supportive care with hydration

PARASITIC INFECTIONS

- Amebiasis can mimic bacterial enterocolitis.
- *Giarida lamblia*, Cryptosporidium, *Isospora belli*, and Microsporidia mimic viral gastroenteritis.
- However, parasitic gastroenteritis is not self-limited and persists for prolonged periods.

AMEBIASIS

LIFE CYCLE AND EPIDEMIOLOGY

- Caused by *Entamoeba histoloytica*
  - Trophozoite contains ingested red blood cells
  - 10–60 μm in diameter

- Other amoebae do not cause disease in humans: *Entamoeba dispar*, *Entamoeba coli*, *E. hartmanni*, *E. polecki*, *Endolimax nana*, and *Iodamoeba buetschlii*
- Binds to galactose receptors and kills host cells, causes flask-like ulcers
- Able to lyse host PMN; acute inflammatory cells rarely seen in areas of infection; protection by cell-mediated immunity
- Able to invade portal vein and form abscesses in the liver
- Disease contracted by ingesting cysts
  ○ Under unfavorable environmental conditions forms dormant cysts
  ○ Has a distinctive morphology consisting of rounded structure with 3–4 distinct nuclei (see Fig. 8-1)
  ○ Dormant cysts can survive for months in moist warm environments
  ○ Contaminate food and water
  ○ Very common in developing countries
- In United States found in institutionalized patients, homosexuals, and tourists

CLINICAL MANIFESTATIONS

- Clinical presentation depends on the degree of invasion
  ○ Watery diarrhea associated with superficial infection
  ○ Bloody diarrhea, tenesmus, abdominal pain, and tenderness associated with more invasive disease
  ○ Invasive intestinal disease presents with the gradual onset (1–3 weeks) of abdominal pain, and bloody diarrhea associated with tenesmus and abdominal tenderness
  ○ Fever is noted in the minority of patients.
  ○ Misdiagnosed as ulcerative colitis; corticosteroids can lead to toxic megacolon.
  ○ Liver abscess presents with right upper quadrant, right shoulder pain and hepatomegaly in half of cases.

DIAGNOSIS

- Stool smears: PMN < shigellosis, trophozoites destroy PMN
- Stools **always** heme-positive
- Alkaline phosphatase and ESR usually elevated in hepatic abscess
- Stool examination × 3 usually reveals trophozoites or cysts
- Serum antiamebic antibody positive in most patients after 1 week of symptoms
- CT scan should be performed in patients with symptoms consistent with hepatic disease, and readily identifies abscesses
- Liver abscess aspirate brownish sterile liquid without PMN, parasite not seen

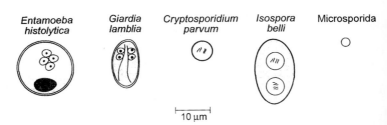

FIGURE 8-1

Parasites that cause diarrhea. Each pathogen is schematically drawn to scale and represents the form most commonly detected on stool smears.

TREATMENT

- Metronidazole (750 mg po TID × 10 days)
  - Alternatives
    - Diloxanide fuoroate (500 mg po TID × 10 days) for colitis
    - Tinidazole (2 gm po QD divided in TID doses × 3–5 days, not available in the United States) for hepatic abscess or invasive colitis
- For asymptomatic cysts excretors:
  - Idodoquinol (650 mg po TID × 20 days) or
  - Paromomycin (25–35 mg/kg/day po in TID doses × 7 days)

GIARDIA LAMBLIA

LIFE CYCLE AND EPIDEMIOLOGY

- Giardia exists as trophozoites and dormant cysts
  - Trophozoite consists of a dorsal convex surface and a flat disk-shaped ventral surface made up of microtubules and microribbons, two nuclei, and four pairs of flagella.
  - On stained preparations it has the appearance of a bearded human face (see Fig. 8-1).
- Trophozoites attach to GI endothelial cells, cause disacharidase deficiency, malabsorption, and inflammation
- Patients with X-linked agammaglobulinemia at increased risk of contracting severe prolonged disease
- Giardia cyst spread:
  - By contaminated water
  - Person to person
  - Less commonly by food
- Infection found worldwide. Common in mountainous regions of the United States
  - A disease of campers (sterilization of water critical for prevention)
  - Day care centers
  - Sexually active homosexuals

CLINICAL MANIFESTATIONS, DIAGNOSIS, AND TREATMENT

- Clinical manifestations usually mild, self-limited lasting 4–6 weeks
  - In adults, symptoms mild: abdominal cramps, anorexia, watery diarrhea, nausea, and belching
  - Children have more severe watery diarrhea.
  - Can cause a chronic malabsorption syndrome, primarily with immunoglobulin deficiency
- Diagnosis
  - Stool smear: no PMN, cysts seen in 90% after 3 stool exams
  - ELISA or immunofluorescence antigen tests have high sensitivity (up to 98%) and specificity (90–100%); tests of choice.
  - Endoscopy no longer necessary
- Treat with metronidazole (250 mg po TID × 5–7 days).

DIARRHEAL ILLNESSES PRIMARILY ASSOCIATED WITH IMMUNOCOMPROMISED HOSTS

- These intestinal protozoa survive and replicate on or in the mucosal epithelial cells of the intestine.

CRYPTOSPORIDIUM

- Protozoa survive and replicate within the intestinal microvilli.
- Generates oocysts that are excreted in the stool and are responsible for the spread of infection (see Fig. 8-1).
- Small numbers of oocysts can cause disease (130 oocysts).
- Can spread via contamination of the water supply; oocysts resist chlorination.
- Person-to-person spread has also been reported.
  - Can occur in households as well as in institutional settings such as day care centers and hospitals.
  - Animal-to-person spread can take place following exposure to infected farm animals.
- Primarily infects AIDS patients with severely depressed cell-mediated immunity.

ISOSPORA BELLI

- More frequent in tropical environments.
- Identified as a cause of watery diarrhea in AIDS patients in the United States.
- A characteristic oocyst is excreted in the stool (see Fig. 8-1).

MICROSPORIDIA

- In 1985 intestinal microsporidiosis was first described in an AIDS patient.
- Infects mucosal epithelial cells causing villous atrophy, and may ascend into the biliary tract to cause cholangitis.
- Causes significant diarrhea only in immunocompromised hosts.
- Very small as compared to the other parasites that cause diarrhea (see Fig. 8-1).
- Previously classified as a protozoa, now recognized to be related to fungi.
- All three organisms cause watery diarrhea and abdominal cramps, dehydration, and malnutrition.

DIAGNOSIS BY STOOL SMEAR

- Cryptosporidium cysts modified Kinyoun acid-fast-positive
- *Isospora belli* sporocysts transparent, fluoresce with UV light
- Microsporidium—modified trichrome and fluorescence stains sensitive and specific

TREATMENT

- Cryptosporidia: no satisfactory therapy, other than antiretroviral therapy for AIDS patients
- *Isospora belli:* trimethoprim-sulfa (1 DS QID × 10 days) and for sulfa-allergic persons, pyramethamine (75 mg/kg/day) combined with folinic acid (10–25 mg/day)
- Microsporidium: fumagillin (20 mg TID × 2 weeks)
  - Results in clearance of spores and relapse occurs in minority of patients.
  - Toxic to the bone marrow and may result in reversible neutropenia and/or thrombocytopenia.

ANTIBIOTIC-ASSOCIATED DIARRHEA

- Potential severity: Undiagnosed *C. difficile* can progress to severe colitis that may require colectomy or result in bowel perforation and death.
- *C. difficile* the only pathogen definitively proven to cause antibiotic-associated diarrhea.
  - 20–30% of patients with antibiotic-associated diarrhea caused by *C. difficile.*
  - 50–75% of those who develop antibiotic-associated colitis.
- *C. difficile* is an obligate anaerobic, spore-forming, Gram-positive rod.
  - Produces two cytotoxins, Toxin A and Toxin B, which bind to and kill host cells.
  - Bowel wall necrosis leads to acute inflammation.
- Develops in 10% of patients hospitalized for over 2 days; rarely encountered in outpatients. Risk factors for disease:
  - Broad-spectrum antibiotic administration reduces competing normal flora.
    - Clindamycin associated with highest incidence
    - Other common antibiotics:
      - Ampicillin/amoxacillin
      - Cephalosporins
  - Cancer chemotherapy
  - Bowel enemas or stimulants, enteral feedings
  - Elderly, patients with underlying disease, and after GI surgery
  - Spread from patient to patient by hospital personnel, spores carried on hands
- Symptoms do not correlate with the level of toxin production.
  - High titers of IgG directed against toxin A appear to be protective and are often high in the asymptomatic carrier.
- Mild to moderate disease
  - Diarrhea usually begins 5–10 days after the initiation of antibiotics.
    - Can develop up to 10 weeks after the completion of antibiotic therapy
  - Watery diarrhea and crampy abdominal pain
  - Low-grade fever and mild leukocytosis common
  - Patients with colitis have same symptoms plus pseudomembranes seen on colonoscopy
- Severe disease in 2–3% of patients; has a high fatality rate
  - Diarrhea or constipation
  - Diffuse abdominal pain and tenderness, signs of peritonitis = impending perforation
  - CT scan: toxic megacolon > 7 cm bowel dilatation, air fluid levels, bowel wall thickening, and thumb printing (can mimic ischemic bowel)
  - Marked leukocytosis (25–35,000/mm^3), lactic acidosis = impending perforation

DIAGNOSIS

- Stool smear—50% have PMN in stool, may be heme positive
- ELISA assays for Toxins A and B are the preferred assays. Many assays detect only Toxin A and can miss *C. difficile* which produces only Toxin B.
- The cytotoxicity assay remains the gold standard, is expensive, and takes several days.
  - Stool filtrate is overlaid onto fibroblasts, and cells round up and detach if the toxin is present.
  - Specificity is confirmed if these effects are blocked by toxin-neutralizing antibody.
- Endoscopy usually not required. Can cause perforation.

TREATMENT (SEE TABLE 8-1)

- Discontinue antibiotics whenever possible to allow the bowel to recolonize.
- Oral metronidazole is the treatment of choice.
- Oral vancomycin used only for severe illness because of the risk of VRE superinfection.
- 10–25% relapse rate because of residual spores; re-treat with metronidazole.
- Intravenous metronidazole usually effective, excreted in the bile.
- Avoid drugs that slow bowel motility.
- Severe disease may require bowel resection, mortality 30–50%.

PREVENTION

- Spread by hospital personnel; hand washing is critical.
- Limiting the use of clindamycin may reduce the attack rate.
- Avoid prolonged broad-spectrum antibiotics.

INTRA-ABDOMINAL INFECTIONS

HIGHLIGHTS

- Intra-abdominal infections often fall between the interface of internal medicine and surgery.
- Care needs to be taken to coordinate care with the infectious disease specialist, gastroenterologist, radiologist, and general surgeon.
- Broad-spectrum antibiotics are the mainstay of therapy, combined with surgical or percutaneous drainage in secondary peritonitis, cholangitis, and liver abscess.

PRIMARY OR SPONTANEOUS PERITONITIS

- Potential severity: A frequently fatal infection that requires immediate paracentesis and empiric antibiotic therapy.

Pathogenesis and Microbiology

- Most commonly associated with end-stage liver disease and portal hypertension.
- Organisms infect the ascitic fluid by hematogenous spread, lymphatic spread, and bowel leakage.

- Infecting organisms
  - Enteric Gram-negatives most common—*E. coli* and *Kleb*
  - *S. pneumoniae* and enterococci
  - Anaerobes and *S. aureus* uncommon

Clinical Manifestations
- Presentation may be subtle.
  - Low-grade fever (38°C)
  - Constant, diffuse abdominal pain and tenderness
  - Guarding not usually present
    - Ascites separates the visceral and parietal peritoneum, preventing severe inflammatory irritation of the abdominal wall muscles.
  - Worsening mental status
  - Grave prognosis if hypotension and hypothermia develop before the initiation of antibiotics

Diagnosis, Treatment, and Outcome
- Paracentesis needs to be performed when this diagnosis is considered.
  - Bleeding requiring transfusion $< 1\%$ of patients despite elevated prothrombin times
  - 10 cc of fluid in a blood culture flask for culture
  - Cell count from an anticoagulated sample $> 300 \, WBC/mm^3$ with predominance of PMN ($> 250 \, PMN/mm^3$)
  - Gram stain positive in 20–30%
  - Elevated protein, LDH, amylase, and low glucose suggest secondary peritonitis.
- Begin empiric antibiotics emergently as soon as cultures are obtained (see Table 8-1):
  - Ceftriaxone or cefotaxime, add metronidazole if suspect secondary peritonitis
  - Mortality 60–70%, reduced to 40% with early treatment
- Marker of severe end-stage liver disease. Patients should be considered for liver transplant.
- Trimethoprim-sulfa (1DS po QD 5 of 7 days) or ciprofloxacin (750 mg po once per week) prophylaxis recommended for patients at risk.

SECONDARY PERITONITIS

- Potential severity: A life-threatening illness that usually requires acute surgical intervention.

Pathogenesis and Microbiology
- Bacteriology depends on the site of perforation.
  - Gastric perforation: mouth flora including Candida and anaerobes
  - Lower bowel contains 10^{11} bacteria/ml and perforation causes massive soilage:
    - Anaerobes a major component, *Bacteroides fragilis* common
    - Aerobic Gram-negative bacteria: *E. coli* predominates; Klebsiella spp., Proteus spp., Enterobacterium spp. also common
    - Gram-positive *S. viridans*, enterococci, and *Clostridia perfringens*
- Peritoneum exudes 300–500 cc/hr of proteinacious material, masses of PMN, to lymphatics then bloodstream. Fibrinous material can wall off abscesses.
- Metabolic acidosis, hypoxia, multiorgan failure and death may follow.

nical Manifestations
- Abdominal pain is usually sharp and begins at the site of spillage.
- Pain accompanied by:
  - Loss of appetite and nausea
  - Fever and chills
  - Constipation and abdominal distension
- Any movement or deep breathing worsens the pain.
- Bowel sounds are decreased or absent, and the abdomen is tender to palpation.
- Peritoneal inflammation causes abdominal spasm (guarding) and rebound.
- Rectal tenderness may be found.
- Elderly often do not have the typical findings of peritonitis.
  - Only mild to moderate tenderness
  - Do not exhibit guarding or rebound
  - At increased risk for diverticulitis, perforated colonic carcinoma, and bowel ischemia

Diagnosis
- Serial abdominal exams should be performed and vital signs closely monitored.
- Peripheral leukocytosis should be present (17,000–25,000 WBC/mm^3 with an increased percentage of PMN and band forms).
- KUB X-ray with upright view should be performed looking for:
  - Free air, indicating bowel or gastric perforation
  - An abnormal bowel gas pattern
  - Areas of thickened edematous bowel wall
- CXR should always be performed to exclude basilar pneumonia.
- CT scan with oral and intravenous contrast is the diagnostic study of choice, allows:
  - Accurate diagnosis of appendicitis
  - Localization and needle aspiration of abscesses
  - Identification of areas of bowel obstruction

Treatment
- Empiric antibiotics should be initiated emergently (see Table 8-1).
  - Mild to moderately severe disease—single-drug therapy with cefoxitin, cefotetan, ticarcillin-clavulinate, or piperacillin-tazobactam
  - Severe disease—combination therapy with cefoxitin or cefotetan + gentamicin, metronidazole + third-generation cephalosporin, metronidazole + fluoroquinolone (ciprofloxacin, levofloxacin, or gatifloxacin), clindamycin + aztreonam, or a carbapenem alone (imipenam-cilastin)
- Surgical consultation immediately to follow the abdominal exam
  - Laparotomy often required for drainage and bowel repair.
  - Peritoneal lavage and placement of drains often required.
  - Intraoperative cultures help direct antibiotic coverage.

Secondary Peritonitis Associated with Peritoneal Dialysis
- Clinical presentation similar to primary peritonitis accompanied by cloudy dialysate.
- *S. epidermidis* and *S. aureus* most common; *Pseudomonas aeruginosa*, fungi, atypical mycobacteria also found; *M. tuberculosis* less common
- Diagnosis
  - WBC in peritoneal fluid > 100/mm^3 with a predominance of PMN
    - Predominance of lymphocytes suggests fungal or tuberculous infection.
  - Culture 10 cc peritoneal fluid into blood culture flask × 2; blood cultures rarely positive

- Empiric therapy with intraperitoneal antibiotics:
  - First-generation cephalosporin (cefazolin, 500 mg/L loading dose, followed by 125 mg/L in each bag)
  - Combined with once per day aminoglycoside (gentamicin or tobramycin, 20 mg/L, or amikacin, 60 mg/L once per day)

HEPATIC ABSCESS

- Potential severity: Usually presents subacutely. With appropriate drainage and antibiotics, prognosis is excellent.

Pathogenesis and Microbiology

- Bacteria seed the liver by multiple routes:
  - Biliary tract most common
  - Portal system in association with intra-abdominal infection
  - Direct extension from intra-abdominal infections
  - Penetrating wounds and postoperative complications
  - Hematogenous
- Bacteriology usually similar to secondary peritonitis.
  - Microaerophilic streptococci frequent, in particular *S. milleri*
  - Candida in leukemia patients following neutropenia
  - Amebic liver abscess is rare, complicates 3–9% of patients with amebic colitis.

Clinical Manifestations, Diagnosis, and Treatment

- Symptoms and signs:
  - Fever with or without chills the most common complaint
    - May present as FUO
  - Half of patients note dull right-upper-quadrant pain associated with right upper quadrant tenderness.
  - Weight loss of $\geq$ 10 pounds during $\leq$ 3 months
- Laboratory findings: leukocytosis (often > 20,000 WBC/mm^3) and elevated alkaline phosphatase
- CT scan the diagnostic study of choice
- Treatment
  - Percutaneous drainage
    - Brownish fluid without a foul odor suggests amebic abscess.
  - Broad-spectrum coverage using the same regimens as for secondary peritonitis (see Table 8-1)
  - Open drainage for patient with:
    - Biliary obstruction
    - Multiloculated abscess other than Echinococcus (see Chap. 12)
    - Viscous exudate

PANCREATIC ABSCESS

- Potential severity: A serious, but usually not fatal, complication of pancreatitis that presents subacutely.
- Necrotic tissue can become infected by contaminated bile or hematogenous spread.
- Abscesses are polymicrobial.
- CT scan and ultrasound to guide drainage.
- Open surgical drainage usually required to debride necrotic tissue.
- Same broad-spectrum coverage used for secondary peritonitis is recommended (Table 8-1).
- Fatal outcome is more likely in the elderly.
  - More often have accompanying biliary tract disease.

CHOLECYSTITIS AND CHOLANGITIS
- Potential severity: An acute potentially life-threatening infection that can be complicated by sepsis. Rapid treatment reduces morbidity and mortality.
- Caused by obstruction of the biliary tree leading to necrosis and inflammation.
- Polymicrobial infection occurs in over half of cases: *E. coli*, Klebsiella spp., enterococci, and anaerobes.
- Charcot's triad may be noted: fever, RUQ pain, and jaundice. The elderly may present with hypotension and no abdominal pain.

Diagnosis
- Leukocytosis with mature PMN and band forms
- Elevated alkaline phosphatase, GGT, and bilirubin. Transaminases can rarely reach 1,000 IU
- Blood cultures often positive
- Abdominal ultrasound the preferred diagnostic screening tool; detects:
  - Gallstones
  - Dilatation of the gallbladder
  - Dilatation of the biliary ducts including the common bile duct
- Endoscopic retrograde cholangiopancreatography (ERCP) confirmatory
  - Always perform under antibiotic coverage
  - Avoid in cases of cholangitis; risk of precipitating high-level bacteremia

Treatment
- Broad-spectrum antibiotics as in secondary peritonitis (Table 8-1)
- ERCP now the treatment of choice. Allows:
  - Biliary drainage
  - Stone removal
  - Dilation of the sphincter of Oddi
  - Placement of stints to maintain biliary flow in fibrotic constricted biliary channels
- Surgery for perforated or gangrenous gallbladder
- Mortality in severe cholangitis approaches 50%.

HELICOBACTER PYLORI–ASSOCIATED PEPTIC ULCER DISEASE
- Potential severity: A chronic disease that causes discomfort, but is not life-threatening
- A small curved microaerophilic Gram-negative rod
  - Survives and grows on the mucosal surface of the stomach
  - Synthesizes high concentrations of urease that produce ammonium ions to neutralize acid
  - Chronic inflammation produces aplastic changes in the gastric mucosa and predisposes to gastric carcinomas.
- Dyspepsia, belching, and heartburn most common symptoms

Diagnosis—Test Only Symptomatic Patients
- Endoscopic biopsy
  - Clotest used to detect urease in the specimen
  - Immunofluorescence, Giemsa, silver, and Gram stain can detect
- Culture only for refractory cases
- Urease breath test expensive, but accurate
- ELISA antibody test, false positive in those > 50 years; titer decreases with treatment

Treatment
- Triple therapy × 2 weeks 90% cure rate:
  - Proton pump inhibitor: lansoprazole, 30 mg BID, or omeprazole, 20 mg BID
  - Amoxacillin: 1 g po BID (substitute metronidazole, 500 mg BID, in penicillin-allergic patients)
  - Clarithromycin: 500 mg po BID × 2 weeks
- Alternative:
  - Proton pump inhibitor
  - Bismuth: 525 mg po QID
  - Amoxacillin
  - Clarithromycin (or metronidazole or tetracycline, 500 mg po QID)

VIRAL HEPATITIS

HIGHLIGHTS

- Hepatitis A spreads by contaminated food or person to person.
- Hepatitis B and C are primarily spread parenterally.
- Clinical presentation is similar with all forms, having incubation, preicteric, icteric, and convalescent stages.
- Hepatitis C often results in asymptomatic chronic active infection that leads to cirrhosis.
- Interferon helpful for the treatment of hepatitis B and C.

Potential severity: Fulminant hepatitis is rare, but usually fatal. Chronic active hepatitis can lead to liver failure and require liver transplantation.

- Acute viral hepatitis affects approximately 700,000 Americans per year.
- Primary causes of acute viral hepatitis:
  - Hepatitis A
  - Hepatitis B
  - Hepatitis C virus
- Rarer causes: hepatitis D or delta agent and hepatitis E
- Other viral agents affect multiple organs in addition to the liver.
  - Epstein-Barr virus and cytomegalovirus most common
  - Herpes simplex viruses, varicella-zoster virus, coxsackie B, measles, rubella, rubeola, and adenovirus can infect the liver
- Fulminant hepatitis is rare; 1% of cases with icteric hepatitis.
  - Caused primarily by hepatitis B and D
  - In pregnant woman can develop with hepatitis E

CLINICAL MANIFESTATIONS OF ACUTE HEPATITIS

- No clinical features definitively differentiate one form of viral hepatitis from another.
- Four clinical stages
  1. Incubation period—asymptomatic
  2. Preicteric stage—nonspecific symptoms
     - Malaise, fatigue, generalized weakness
     - Anorexia, nausea and vomiting, loss of taste for cigarettes
     - Minority develop a serum-sickness syndrome

    3. Icteric stage
-   Symptoms dramatically resolve with the onset of jaundice
-   Itching may develop
-   Dark urine and pale stools
-   Icterus that can be detected in the sclera or under the tongue when bilirublin levels reach 2.5–3.0 mg/dl
-   Slight hepatic enlargement with mild to moderate tenderness

    4. Convalescent stage—duration varies

- Fulminant hepatitis leads to encephalitis with asterixis (irregular flapping of the outstretched hands after forcible dorsiflexion).

LIVER TESTS

- Transaminase values 1,000–2,000, IU AST/ALT < 1 (> 1.5 with alcoholic hepatitis)
- High direct bilirubin = cholestasis; high indirect bilirubin = hemolysis
- High PT = bad prognosis; > 100 = liver transplant
- Liver biopsy generally not required to diagnose acute viral hepatitis.
  - Performed when several causes of hepatitis are possible or when therapy is being considered.
  - Histopathology: ballooning and hepatocyte necrosis, disarray of liver lobules, mononuclear cell infiltration, and cholestasis

COMPLICATIONS

- Chronic active hepatitis B or C
- Vasculitis and glomerulonephritis
  - Polyarteritis nodosa associated with persistent hepatitis B
- Cirrhosis

HEPATITIS A (SEE TABLE 8-2)

VIROLOGY, PATHOGENESIS, AND EPIDEMIOLOGY

- A single-stranded RNA picornovirus that is highly resistant to heating and drying
- Survives in protein solutions; killed by chlorine
- Enters via the gastrointestinal tract, penetrates the bowel, infects hepatocytes, and multiplies in the cytoplasm; excreted in the bile, high concentrations in the feces
- Epidemiology
  - Spread by fecal-oral route in day care centers; children < 2 years have asymptomatic infection.
  - Sexual transmission among homosexuals
  - Intravenous drug abusers; not usually spread by blood transfusions
  - Foodborne: water, milk, bivalved shellfish, contaminated fruits and vegetables, and food contaminated by food handlers
  - Decontaminate surfaces with 1:100 dilution of household bleach

CLINICAL COURSE AND DIAGNOSIS

- Incubation period 4 weeks
- Self-limited illness of 2–3 months' duration
- Relapse can occur up to 6 months after the primary attack.

- Chronic hepatitis does not develop.
- Fulminant hepatitis is rare; usually coinfected with hepatitis C or hepatitis B.
- Diagnosis
  - IgM antibody titer detected at the time of symptoms, persists 6 months
  - IgG antibody titer increases later and peaks at 4 months, persists for decades

TREATMENT AND PREVENTION

- No therapy available
- Pooled immunoglobulin (IG) protective if given within 2 weeks of exposure
  - 0.02 ml/kg IM affords 2 months of protection.
  - 0.06 ml/kg usually protects for 5 months.
- IG prophylaxis recommended
  - Household and sexual contacts
  - Day care center staff and attendees
  - Classroom contacts in school-centered outbreaks
  - Persons residing or working in institutions with crowded living conditions
  - Hospital personnel with direct contact with feces or body fluids from an infected patient
  - Travelers to endemic areas
  - Not recommended for casual contacts or in common-source outbreaks
- Formalin-killed vaccine is safe and effective; indications are evolving
  - Homosexual men and illicit drug users
  - Heterosexuals with multiple sexual partners
  - Persons requiring repeated administration of concentrated coagulation factors
  - Occupational risk of exposure
  - Patients with preexisting chronic liver disease
  - Travelers to endemic areas > 3 times over 10 years
  - Children over age of 2 years where high incidence of hepatitis A (> 20/1,000)
  - Duration of protection has been estimated to be 20–30 years.

HEPATITIS E (SEE TABLE 8-2)

- A single-stranded RNA virus related to the caliciviruses
- Incubation period 1 month
- Transmitted by the fecal-oral route
- Reported in developing countries with poor sanitation, not in the United States, except for travelers
- A self-limited disease
- Causes fulminant hepatitis in women in their 3rd trimester of pregnancy
- No blood test available
- Pooled immunglobulins are not helpful for prevention.

HEPATITIS B (SEE TABLE 8-2)

VIROLOGY AND PATHOGENESIS

- An enveloped, partially double-stranded DNA hepadnavirus
  - Outer core contains lipid and a surface hepatitis B antigen (HbsAg)
  - Inner core is released by nonionic detergent and is called core antigen (HbcAg)

TABLE 8-2
CLINICAL CHARACTERISTICS OF THE DIFFERENT FORMS OF VIRAL HEPATITIS

Virus type	Incubation period	Epidemiology	Sequelae
Hepatitis A	4 weeks	Fecal-oral route Foodborne Water Sexually transmitted	Self-limited disease Can relapse up 6 months post primary attack Fulminant hepatitis rare
Hepatitis B	12 weeks	Person to person Blood and blood products Other body fluids iv drug abuse Sexually transmitted	Chronic infection common 90% neonates, 20–50% children, 5–10% adults Hepatocellular carcinoma
Hepatitis C	6–10 weeks	Person to person Blood and blood products iv drug abuse Sexual transmission rare Higher risk with HIV infection	Usually a chronic infection Cirrhosis in 25% Require liver transplant Hepatocellular carcinoma
Hepatitis D + B	12 weeks	Person to person Blood and blood products Other body fluids iv drug abuse Sexual transmission Household contacts	Same as Hepatitis B Hepatic failure more common among IV drug abusers
Hepatitis E	4 weeks	Fecal-oral route Only in developing countries	Self-limited disease Fulminant hepatitis in pregnancy

210

- ○ E antigen (HbeAg) remains when the core is treated with the ionic detergent SDS
- ○ Presence of HbeAg = active viral replication
  - ▪ Except for a mutant Eastern European strain that does not release HbeAg during replication
- Enters and replicates in hepatocytes, but cannot be grown in tissue culture
  - ○ Survives in serum at 4 °C for months, but is killed by heating to 98 °C
    - ▪ Integrates into host DNA, which may explain increased risk of hepatocellular carcinoma

EPIDEMIOLOGY

- Spread from person to person primarily by blood and blood products
  - ○ Screening of donors has reduced the risk to 1/63,000 transfusions.
- Contaminated needles:
  - ○ Intravenous drug abusers who share needles
  - ○ Reuse of needles for tattoos and ear piercing
- In other body fluids (urine, bile, saliva, semen, breast milk, and vaginal secretions); not found in feces
- Mucosal contact with infected body fluid can transmit infection to:
  - ○ Homosexual or heterosexual sexual partners of infected individuals
  - ○ Neonate following vaginal delivery from an infected mother
  - ○ Crowded environments such as institutions for the mentally handicapped
- Hepatitis B–infected organ transplant
- 280,000 new cases per year in the United States; estimated to have infected 5% worldwide

CLINICAL COURSE AND DIAGNOSIS

- Incubation period 12 weeks
- Acute disease similar clinically to hepatitis A except not always self-limited
  - ○ Symptoms usually resolve over 1–3 months.
  - ○ Transaminase values usually return to normal within 1–4 months.
  - ○ Persistent infection develops in:
    - ▪ 90% of infants
    - ▪ 20–50% of children 1–5 years old
    - ▪ 5–10% of adults
- Diagnosis is made by serologic testing (see Fig. 8-2).
  - ○ HbsAg appears within 10 weeks of exposure, persists for 4–6 months; > 6 months = chronic disease.
  - ○ HbsAb often develops after HbsAg disappears; HbsAb usually persists for life. HbsAb and HbsAg may be negative during this "window" transition period.
  - ○ HbcAb IgM positive early, a marker for acute disease, but can persist for 2 years and can increase during exacerbations of chronic active hepatitis. Used for blood screening.
  - ○ HbeAg indicates active viral replication. Disappearance of HbeAg and appearance of HbeAb = clearance of virus.
  - ○ HBV-DNA—quantitation of DNA used to assess responses to therapy of chronic disease.

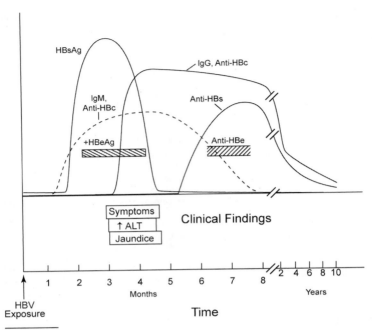

FIGURE 8-2
Clinical course of hepatitis B. (Adapted from *Hoeprich Infectious Diseases*, 1994.)

TREATMENT AND PREVENTION

- Treatment is the same as for hepatitis A; supportive measures
- Hepatitis B immune globulin (HBIG) (0.05–0.07 ml/kg IM) provides maximal protection when given within 48 hours and is recommended within 7days for:
  - Needle stick or mucosal exposure to blood or fluids from HbsAg-positive person
  - Intimate contact with someone who has acute or chronic hepatitis B
  - Neonates born to a hepatitis B–infected mother
- Recombinant vaccine is safe and efficacious and should be given intramuscularly in three doses at months 0, 1–2, and 6–12 to:
  - Health care workers, laboratory workers who handle blood and blood products
  - Patients requiring repeated blood transfusions or clotting factors
  - Hemodialysis patients
  - Morticians
  - Persons with multiple sexual partners
  - Intravenous drug users
  - Residents and staff of closed institutions
  - Household and sexual contacts of carriers.
  - Neonates born to mothers with unknown or positive HBsAg
    - First dose of vaccine given within 12 hours of delivery
    - Booster doses at 1 and 6 months

TREATMENT AND PROGNOSIS OF CHRONIC HEPATITIS B

- Chronic hepatitis B defined as positive HbsAg $\geq$ 20 weeks
- Three stages:
  - Replicative stage with immune tolerance
    - LFTs WNL
    - Viral load high
    - This stage may last 20–30 years after neonatal infection
  - Replicative stage with immune clearance
    - LFTs are abnormal
    - Associated with a rise in anti-HBc IgM levels
    - HBeAg and viral DNA may clear from the serum.
    - In others the viral replication continues = episode of abortive immune clearance
  - Nonreplicative stage
    - HbeAg disappears and anti-HBe appears.
    - HbsAg may persist.
- Chronic carriers can:
  - Progress to cirrhosis and hepatic failure
  - 1.6% incidence of hepatocellular carcinoma per year
- Treatment
  - Goal of therapy is to achieve seroconversion from HBeAg positive to negative
  - Reserved for patients who have persistent HBe-Ag and elevated transaminase values
  - Three potential treatment regimens:
    - Lamivudine (100 mg po QD × 1 year) doubles the seroconversion rate from HbeAg positive to negative.
    - Adefovir dipivoxil (10 mg po QD) improves hepatic histopathology and is not associated with the development of resistance over 48 weeks.
    - Interferon alpha (5–10 million units QD 3×/week for 12–24 weeks) triples seroconversion rate.

HEPATITIS D (SEE TABLE 8-2)

- A single-stranded RNA virus that is surrounded by hepatitis B envelope
- Only replicates in the presence of hepatitis B virus
- Replicates rapidly in the host cell nucleus
- Clinically indistinguishable from other forms of acute hepatitis
- Endemic in the Mediterranean basin; first discovered in Italy. Also high prevalence in the eastern Asia (Pacific Islands, Taiwan, Japan)
- Person-to-person spread by body fluids and blood or blood products
  - Sexual transmission
  - Intravenous drug abusers
  - In United States primarily contracted by multiple blood transfusions
- Diagnosis is made by measuring anti–hepatitis D IgM and IgG serum titers.
  - Tests for hepatitis D not commercially available

HEPATITIS C (SEE TABLE 8-2)

VIROLOGY, PATHOGENESIS, AND EPIDEMIOLOGY

- Single-stranded RNA virus.
- Viral replication is associated with inaccurate proof reading and multiple mutations yielding multiple quasispecies. Mechanism for evading the immune system.
- Primarily infects hepatocytes; may also infect hematopoietic cells. Infects only humans and chimpanzees.
- Chronic active hepatitis is characterized by periportal infiltration with lymphocytes and piecemeal necrosis; often followed by fibrosis leading to cirrhosis.
- 2.4 million chronically infected people in the United States.
- Spread by:
  - Blood and blood products
  - iv drug abuse
  - Mother-to-neonate spread less common than for hepatitis B
  - Sexual transmission rare
  - Higher risk of infection in HIV-infected persons

CLINICAL MANIFESTATIONS AND DIAGNOSIS

- Incubation period 6–10 weeks
- Only 25% of patients develop symptoms of acute hepatitis.
- 50–75% progress to chronic infection.
- Serum transaminase values fluctuate during chronic illness.
  - Normal in some periods
  - At other times increase to 7–10 times normal values
- Diagnosis
  - ELISA that detects antibodies directed against specific hepatitis C antigens, 95% sensitivity
  - In low-risk populations confirm with recombinant immunoblot assay (RIBA)
  - PCR methods able to detect viral load (can detect 100 copies/ml)

TREATMENT AND PROGNOSIS

- Spontaneous clearance is rare in hepatitis C
- 20–25% of patients with chronic hepatitis C progress to cirrhosis over 20–30 years
- One of the leading diseases requiring liver transplantation
- Increases the risk of hepatocellular carcinoma
- Combined therapy has the highest cure rate
  - Pegylated interferon (Pegintron, 1.5 µg/kg sq, Q1week or Pegasys, 180 mg SQ, Q1week)
  - Combined with ribovirin (1–1.2 gm po QD)
- Duration of therapy depends on initial viral load.
  - >2 million copies/ml, 48 weeks
  - Lower viral loads 24 weeks

REFERENCES

Infectious Diarrhea

Ashkenazi S, Levy I, Kazaronovski V, Samra Z: Growing antimicrobial resistance of Shigella isolates. *J Antimicrob Chemother* 2003; 51:427–29.

Glass RI, Noel J, Ando T, et al: The epidemiology of enteric caliciviruses from humans: A reassessment using new diagnostics. *J Infect Dis* 2000; 181 (Suppl 2):S254–61.

Gonvers JJ, Bochud M, Burnand B, Froehlich F, Dubois RW, Vader JP: 10. Appropriateness of colonoscopy: Diarrhea. *Endoscopy* 1999; 31:641–46.

Goodgame RW: Viral causes of diarrhea. *Gastroenterol Clin North Am* 2001; 30:779–95.

Gumbo T, Hobbs RE, Carlyn C, Hall G, Isada CM: Microsporidia infection in transplant patients. *Transplantation* 1999; 67:482–84.

Ilnyckyj A: Clinical evaluation and management of acute infectious diarrhea in adults. *Gastroenterol Clin North Am* 2001; 30:599–609.

Okeke IN, Nataro JP: Enteroaggregative *Escherichia coli. Lancet Infect Dis* 2001; 1:304–13.

Oldfield EC III, Wallace MR: The role of antibiotics in the treatment of infectious diarrhea. *Gastroenterol Clin North Am* 2001; 30:817–36.

Sirinavin S, Garner P: Antibiotics for treating Salmonella gut infections. *Cochrane Database Syst Rev* 2000; CD001167.

Stanley SL, Jr: Amoebiasis. *Lancet* 2003; 361:1025–34.

Antibiotic-Associated Diarrhea

Bartlett JG: Clinical practice: Antibiotic-associated diarrhea. *N Engl J Med* 2002; 346:334–39.

Yassin SF, Young-Fadok TM, Zein NN, Pardi DS: Clostridium difficile-associated diarrhea and colitis. *Mayo Clin Proc* 2001; 76:725–30.

Primary Peritonitis

Navasa M, Rodes J: Management of ascites in the patient with portal hypertension with emphasis on spontaneous bacterial peritonitis. *Semin Gastrointest Dis* 1997; 8:200–9.

Soares-Weiser K, Paul M, Brezis M, Leibovici L: Evidence based case report: Antibiotic treatment for spontaneous bacterial peritonitis. *Br Med J* 2002; 324:100–2.

Secondary Peritonitis

Alapati SV, Mihas AA: When to suspect ischemic colitis: Why is this condition so often missed or misdiagnosed? *Postgrad Med* 1999; 105:177–80, 183–84, 187.

Gupta H, Dupuy DE: Advances in imaging of the acute abdomen. *Surg Clin North Am* 1997; 77:1245–63.

Liver Abscess

Bornstein JD, Byrd DE, Trotter JF: Relapsing hepatitis A: A case report and review of the literature. *J Clin Gastroenterol* 1999; 28:355–56.

Ch Yu S, Hg Lo R, Kan PS, Metreweli C: Pyogenic liver abscess: Treatment with needle aspiration. *Clin Radiol* 1997; 52:912–16.

Acute Hepatic Failure

Schiodt FV, Davern TJ, Shakil AO, McGuire B, Samuel G, et al: Viral hepatitis–related acute liver failure. *Am J Gastroenterol* 2003; 98:448–53.

Hepatitis A

Levy MJ, Herrera JL, DiPalma JA: Immune globulin and vaccine therapy to prevent hepatitis A infection. *Am J Med* 1998; 105:416–23.

Hepatitis B

Gitlin N: Hepatitis B: Diagnosis, prevention, and treatment. *Clin Chem* 1997; 43:1500–6.

Lee WM: Hepatitis B virus infection. *N Engl J Med* 1997; 337:1733–45.

Marcellin P, Chang TT, Lim SG, Tong MJ, Sievert W, et al: Adefovir dipivoxil for the treatment of hepatitis B antigen-positive chronic hepatitis B. *N Engl J Med* 2003; 348:808–16.

Nakhoul F, Gelman R, Green J, Khankin E, Baruch Y: Lamivudine therapy for severe acute hepatitis B virus infection after renal transplantation: Case report and literature review. *Transplant Proc* 2001; 33:2948–49.

Hepatitis C

Fried MW, Shiffman ML, Reddy KR, Smith C, Marinos G, et al: Peginterferon alfa-2a plus ribavirin for chronic hepatitis C virus infection. *N Engl J Med* 2002; 347:975–82.

Moradpour D, Wolk B, Cerny A, Heim MH, Blum HE: Hepatitis C: A concise review. *Minerva Med* 2001; 92:329–39.

Shamoun DK, Anania FA: Which patients with hepatitis C virus should be treated? *Semin Gastrointest Dis* 2000; 11:84–95.

9

GENITOURINARY TRACT INFECTIONS AND SEXUALLY TRANSMITTED DISEASES (STDs)

URINARY TRACT INFECTION (UTI)

HIGHLIGHTS

- One of the most common infections encountered by practitioners
- Predominantly occurs in sexually active females
- Helpful to attempt to differentiate upper tract disease (fever, flank pain, chills) from lower tract disease
- Short-course therapy, 3 days, for lower tract disease and 2-week therapy for upper tract disease
- Urinalysis is ordered for all patients, initial urine Gram stain and culture for upper tract disease
- Initial therapy for lower tract disease trimethoprim-sulfa in some areas of the country, but resistance is increasing
- Fluoroquinolones, third-generation cephalosporins, aminoglycosides for upper tract disease
- Potential severity: Often outpatient infections; however, the development of pyelonephritis can lead to sepsis and death. These infections need to be promptly treated.

PATHOGENESIS

- Bacterial characteristics that predispose to UTI:
  - Adherence via fimbria that attach to mannose-sensitive and mannose-insensitive host cell receptors
  - Hemolysin production
  - Resistance to serum cidal activity
  - Ability to synthesize the essential amino acids arginine and glutamine
  - Urease production (*Proteus mirabilis*)

- Host characteristics that predispose to UTI:
    - ○ Urine—usually inhibits bacterial growth; exceptions pregnant women and diabetics (glucose)
    - ○ Mechanical properties
        1. Obstruction, importance of flushing, conditions that cause obstruction:
            - Prostatic hypertrophy
            - Urethral strictures
            - Defective bladder contraction (paraplegia)
            - Renal stones
            - Vesicoureteral reflux
        2. Short urethral length and colonization of the vaginal area
            - Higher risk in women, 1–3% incidence/year; 10–20% develop symptomatic urinary tract during their lifetime
            - < 0.1% in men
        3. Bladder catheterization—bypasses the urethra
            - All patients with a bladder catheter in place will eventually develop a urinary tract infection.
    - ○ Renal medulla—high ammonia concentration blocks complement, high osmolality inhibits PMN migration

ETIOLOGY (SEE TABLE 9-1)

- The majority of organisms causing community-acquired UTI come from the fecal and vaginal flora
    - ○ *E.coli* the most frequent pathogen
    - ○ Klebsiella and Proteus next most frequent
    - ○ *S. saprophyticus* causes 5–15% of cystitis in young, sexually active women
- Nosocomial infections
    - ○ Enterobacter spp.
    - ○ Pseudomonas spp.
    - ○ Enterococci
    - ○ Candida
    - ○ *S. epidermidis* and Corynebacterium

TABLE 9-1
COMMON URINARY PATHOGENS

	Outpatient	Inpatient
E. coli	75%	Common
Klebsiella	15%	Common
Proteus	5%	Common
Enterococci	2%	Common
S. epidermidis	< 2%	Common
Group B streptococci	< 2%	Common
Pseudomonas	Rare	Common

CLINICAL MANIFESTATIONS

- Overlap between the symptoms of cystitis and pyelonephritis
  - Cystitis
    - Dysuria (pain, tingling, or burning in the perineal area during or just after urination) and urinary frequency
    - Hematuria
    - Suprapubic discomfort
  - Pyelonephritis
    - In addition to cystitis symptoms:
      - Fever and chills
      - Costovertebral angle pain and tenderness
      - Nausea and vomiting
    - Pyelonephritis more likely in:
      - Diabetics—often have only symptoms of cystitis
      - Elderly—may present with confusion or somnolence
      - Cystitis symptoms for > 7 days
- Asymptomatic bacteriuria
  - Positive urine culture
  - No symptoms
  - No pyuria
  - Usually do not treat except:
    - Pregnant women to prevent low-birth-weight neonates
    - Adolescent children to prevent renal scarring
    - Treatment not required for diabetics
- Urethritis can be mistaken for cystitis
  - No suprapubic tenderness unless associated with pelvic inflammatory disease
  - Usually < 10^5 bacteria
  - More PMN in the early-voided sample as compared to a mid-void or late-void sample
- Vaginitis can mimic cystitis
  - Pelvic exam recommended in women with UTI symptoms
  - Particularly if symptoms are associated with vaginal discharge
- Physical findings associated with urinary tract infection
  - Usually minimal
  - Cystitis may have suprapubic tenderness
  - Pyelonephritis
    - Patients often are acutely ill, appearing toxic
    - High fever
    - Hypotensive and elevated heart rate may indicate early septic shock
    - Costovertebral angle or flank tenderness due to inflammation and swelling of the infected kidney
    - Elderly patient can present with confusion and somnolence

DIAGNOSIS (SEE FIG. 9-1)

- Urinalysis should be performed in all patients with possible UTI
  - > 5–10 WBC/hpf = pyuria
  - WBC casts are strong evidence for pyelonephritis (a rare finding)
  - Leukocyte esterase dip stick usually sensitive
- Unspun urine Gram stain helpful: 1 bacterium/hpf = $\geq 10^5$ organisms
- Urine culture requires quantitation in order to differentiate contamination from true infection

- ○ Not required in sexually active adult women with early symptoms of cystitis
- ○ Women $\geq 10^5$/ml organisms = infection. Symptomatic women can have 10^3 organisms
- ○ Men $\geq 10^3$/ml organisms = infection
- ○ Cultures must be processed immediately
- ○ After therapy all patients should have a follow-up culture
- • Imaging studies
  - ○ Ultrasound, the imaging study of choice
    - ▪ Perform in patients with upper tract disease
    - ▪ Preschool girls with 2nd UTI, boys, or men with UTI
  - ○ IVP may be required to further delineate anatomic defects; avoid with multiple myeloma or renal failure
  - ○ CT scan with contrast in patients who fail to respond to antibiotics within 48 hours to exclude perinephric abscess formation

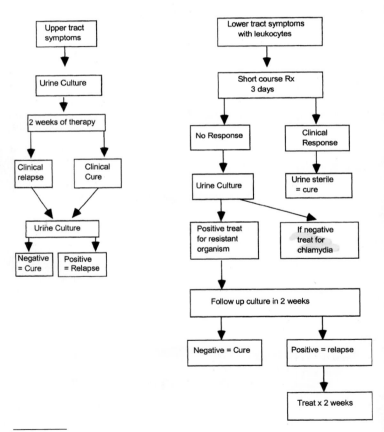

FIGURE 9-1
Schematic diagram of how to manage urinary tract infections.

TREATMENT (SEE TABLE 9-2)

- Cystitis: short course × 3 days
  - Do not use for men, diabetics, women × 7 days of symptoms, elderly
  - Multiple possible regimens
    - Trimethoprim-sulfamethoxazole (least expensive, but increasing percentages of *E. coli* becoming resistant)
    - Ofloxacin (preferred by many physicians); other fluoroquinolones also efficacious   *FLOXIN ; OCUFLOX*
    - Trimethoprim alone also effective *PRIMSOL ; PROLOPRIM*
    - Cephalexin, poorer response rates
- Pyelonephritis: treat for 2 weeks
  - Nontoxic, not vomiting can use oral antibiotics; use urine Gram stain as guidance:
    - Gram-positive cocci in chains (streptococci), amoxacillin
    - Gram-positive cocci in clusters (*S. aureus*), oral amoxacillin-clavulinate or cephalexin
    - Gram-negative rods, fluoroquinolones preferred
  - Suspected bacteremia with chills, toxic, hypotensive, vomiting, hospitalize and give IV antibiotics:
    - IV ciprofloxacin superior to IV trimethoprim-sulfamethoxazole
    - Aztreonam (no Gram-positive coverage, confirm Gram-negative pathogen by unspun Gram stain)
    - Third- or fourth-generation cephalosporin (ceftazidime or cefepime, ceftriaxone)
    - Extremely ill patients usually treated with two antibiotics: aminoglyoside, such as gentamicin, and a second antibiotic
  - If a patient relapses:
    - A 2-week course of therapy should be repeated.
    - If relapse follows a second treatment, a 4–6-week course should then be given.
    - All patients with relapse should be studied for anatomic defects or stones.

PREVENTION

- Voiding and/or single-dose trimethoprim-sulfa after intercourse reduces UTIs in women.
- Anatomic defects that predispose to UTI, can prevent recurrence by daily low dose of:
  - Trimethoprim-sulfa (1/2 tablet po QD) or
  - Nitrofurantoin (50 mg po QD)
- Antibiotic prophylaxis for bladder catheters not recommended; remove bladder catheters as soon as possible.

PROSTATITIS

- Potential severity: Acute prostatitis can lead to sepsis and requires acute empiric antibiotic therapy.
- Primarily caused by Gram-negative enteric organisms
  - *E. coli* most frequent
  - Klebsiella, Proteus, Pseudomonas, Enterobacter spp. and Serratia also cultured
  - Gram-positives rare, except enterococcus

TABLE 9-2
TREATMENT OF URINARY TRACT INFECTIONS

Drug	Dose	Relative efficacy	Comments
Lower Tract			
Trimethoprim-sulfa (TMP-SMX)	1 DS po BID × 3 days	First line	Least expensive; *E. coli* increasing resistance
Ofloxacin	400 mg BID × 3 days	First line	More expensive
Trimethoprim (TMP)	100 mg BID × 3 days	First line	
Cephalexin	500 mg po QID × 3 days	Second line	Inferior outcome as compared to TMP-SMX, fluoroquinolone or TMP
Upper Tract (oral)			
Ciprofloxacin	500 mg po BID × 14 days	First line	Preferred empiric regimen
Trimethoprim-sulfa	1 DS po BID × 14 days	Alternative	Preferred if organism known to be sensitive
Gram positive pathogen			
Amoxacillin or	500 mg po TID × 14 days	First Line	
Amoxacillin-clavulinate	500 mg po TID × 14 days		
Upper Tract (iv)	Total antibiotic duration 14 days		
Ciprofloxacin	400 mg IV Q12H	First line	Better outcomes than TMP-SMX
Trimethoprim-sulfa	10–15 mg/kg/day (TMP) divided into 3–4 doses	Alternative	Inexpensive, but more side effects, poorer outcome
Aztreonam	1–2 gm IV Q6–8H	Alternative	No Gram-positive coverage
Cefapime ± gentamicin	1–2 gm IV Q12H 5–6 mg/kg load, adjust by levels	Alternative for very ill patient	Broader coverage
Gram-positive pathogen ampicillin-sulbactam ± gentamicin	1–2 gm IV Q6H (amp) (as above)	First line	Ticarcillin-clavulinate or piperacillin-tazobactam alternatives

- Pathogenesis unclear
  - Reflux from urethra, often associated with UTI
  - Prostatic antibacterial factor (PAF) becomes depleted
- Clinical manifestations
- Acute prostatitis
  - Fever and chills
  - Dysuria, and urinary frequency
  - Bladder outlet obstruction
  - Prostate tender, do **not** message; can precipitate bacteremia
- Chronic prostatitis
  - Low-grade fever
  - Myalgias and arthralgias
  - Recurrent UTIs
- Diagnosis by urine or blood cultures
- Treatment
  - Acute disease
    - Ticarcillin-clavulinate (3 gm IV Q4–6H) or piperacillin-tazobactam (3 gm IV Q4–6H)
    - Ampicillin (1–2 gm Q4–6H) + gentamicin (5–6 mg/kg, then dose by levels)
  - Chronic disease—prolonged therapy with:
    - Trimethoprim-sulfa (1 DS po BID) × 4–16 weeks
    - Ciprofloxacin (500 mg po BID) or ofloxacin (400 mg po BID × 4–6 weeks)
    - May require prostatectomy for cure

SEXUALLY TRANSMITTED DISEASES (STDs)

HIGHLIGHTS

- STDs are increasing in frequency; highest incidence in teenagers and early 20s.
- PID a leading cause of infertility.
- GU ulcers caused by syphilis, herpes simplex, chancroid, and lymphogranuloma venerium.
- Syphilis is increasing in frequency and associated with a higher risk of HIV infection.
- Important to diagnose and treat latent syphilis to prevent tertiary CNS and cardiovascular disease.
- Warrant continued public health measures, including education and tracking of secondary cases.
- The importance of aggressive case finding and early treatment cannot be overemphasized.

Potential severity: Usually outpatient infections that can cause significant discomfort, but are rarely life-threatening.

URETHRITIS

- Etiologies
  - *Chlamydia trachomatous* and *Neisseria gonorrhoeae* associated with a purulent discharge
  - *Ureaplasma urealyticum* and noninfectious causes of nonpurulent urethritis

- Symptoms and signs
  - Burning on urination, worse with concentrated urine and after drinking EtOH
  - Staining of underwear, mucous in the urine
  - Meatus erythematous, milk discharge from penis
- Diagnosis
  - Primarily by DNA probes
  - Gram stain—In gonorrhea almost always find intracellular Gram-negative diplcocci; a negative Gram stain = nongonococcal urethritis (NGU)
  - Culture of *N. gonorrhoeae* using 5% CO_2, have to plant culture immediately
- Treatment (see Table 9-3)
  - A third-generation cephalosporin or fluoroquinolone for gonorrhea
  - Macrolide, tetracycline, fluoroquinolone, or sparfloxacin for NGU

PELVIC INFLAMMATORY DISEASE (PID)

- PID is the most common gynecologic disease managed in emergency rooms.
- Estimated that 1 million cases are diagnosed annually in the United States.

Etiology and Pathogenesis

- Primarily caused by *N. gonorrhoeae* and *Chlamydia trachomatis*. Other less common pathogens:
  - *S. pyogenes* and *Haemophilus influenzae* most frequently accompany gonorrhea and chlamydia.
  - Group B streptococci, *E. coli*, Klebsiella spp., *Proteus mirabilis*, and anaerobes less common.
- Cervical canal usually prevents vaginal flora from invading the endometrium.
  - Caused by spread of cervical microbes to the endometrium, fallopian tubes, ovaries, and surrounding pelvic structures.
  - Menstruation allows bacteria to bypass the cervix; PID usually begins 7 days after menstruation.
  - Delayed treatment of urethritis leads to PID. 15% of patients with urethritis develop PID.
- Risk factors for PID
  - Young age (sexually active teenagers at highest risk)
  - Multiple sexual partners
  - Past history of PID
- Risk reduced by:
  - The use of condoms and spermicidal agents
  - The placement of an IUD does not increase the risk for pelvic inflammatory disease in women with a stable monogamous relationship

Symptoms and Clinical Findings

- Lower abdominal pain during or immediately following menses
  - Made worse by jarring motions
  - In one third accompanied by vaginal bleeding
  - Vaginal discharge common
- On physical exam:
  - Only half the patients have fever.
  - Bilateral lower quadrant tenderness, cervical, uterine, and bilateral adnexal tenderness. Absence of tenderness makes PID unlikely.
  - Right upper quadrant tenderness = Fitz-Hugh-Curtis syndrome.
  - Localized tenderness to one adnexa suggests tubo-ovarian abscess.

TABLE 9-3
TREATMENT REGIMENS FOR STDS (CDC 2002)

Drug	Dose	Relative efficacy	Comments
Gonococcal Urethritis			
Cefixime	400 mg po × 1	First line	Some discomfort with the IM injection
Ceftriaxone	125 mg IM × 1	First line	Increased resistance to fluoroquinolones in
Ciprofloxacin	500 mg po × 1	First line	Honolulu, Hawaii
Ofloxacin	400 mg po × 1		
Levofloxacin	250 mg po × 1 (500 mg QD for disseminated disease)		
Combine with azithromycin (or) Doxycycline	1 g po × 1 100 mg po BID × 7 days		
Spectinomycin	2 gm IM × 1	Alternative	
Ceftizoxime	500 mg IM × 1	Alternative	
Cefoxitin	2 gm IM with probenecid 1 gm po × 1	Alternative	
Disseminated Gonococcal Disease			
Ceftriaxone	1 gm IV or IM QD	First line	Continue for 24–48 hours after clinical improvement, switch to an oral regimen above, to complete 7 days, minimum
Cefotaxime (or)	1 gm IV Q8H	Alternative	Same duration and po regimen as for ceftriaxone
Ceftizoxime	1 gm IV Q8H		
Ciprofloxacin (or)	400 mg IV BID	Alternatives	Same duration and po regimen as for ceftriaxone
Ofloxacin (or)	400 mg IV BID		
Levofloxacin	250 mg IV QD		
Spectinomycin	2 gm IM QD	Alternative	Same duration and po regimen as for ceftriaxone

TABLE 9-3
TREATMENT REGIMENS FOR STDS (CDC 2002) *(Continued)*

Drug	Dose	Relative efficacy	Comments
Nongonococcal urethritis			
Axithromycin	1 g po × 1	First line	
Doxycycline	100 mg po BID × 7 days	First line	
Erythromycin base	500 mg po QID × y days	Alternative	
Ofloxacin	300 mg po BID × 7 days	Alternative	
Levofloxacin	500 mg po QD × 7 days	Alternative	
Amoxicillin	500 mg po TID × 7 days	Alternative	In pregnancy only
Metronidazole	2 gm po × 1		Use if recurrent urethritis to treat *T. vaginalis*
Pelvic inflammatory dis.	**IV regimens**		
A) Cefotetan (or	2 g IV Q12H	First line	Continue IV for 24 hours after improvement
Ceftriaxone (+)	2 g IV Q6H		
Doxycycline	100 mg po BID × 14 days		
B) Clindamycin (+)	500 mg IV Q8H	First line	Continue IV × 24 hours after improvement, then switch to clindamycin 450 mg po QID to complete 14 days
Gentamicin	1.5 mg/kg IV Q8H or 7 mg/kg IV QD		Metronidazole adds anaerobic coverage
Ofloxacin (or	400 mg IV Q12H	Alternative	
Levofloxacin (+/−)	500 mg IV QD		
Metronidazole	500 mg IV Q8H		
Amp/sulbactam (+)	3 g IV Q6H	Alternative	
Doxycycline	100 mg IV or po Q12H		

PID "Oral" regimens

A) Ofloxacin (or)   400 mg po BID   First line
Levofloxacin (+/−)   500 mg po QD
Metronidazole   500 mg po BID × 14 days   Metronidazole adds anaerobic coverage

B) Ceftriaxone (or)   250 mg IM × 1   First line
Cefoxitin (+)   2 gm IM + probenecid 1 gm
Doxycycline (+/−)   100 mg po BID × 14 days
Metronidazole   500 mg po BID × 14 days   Metronidazole adds anaerobic coverage

Genital Ulcers

Herpes Simplex 1st episode

Drug	Dose	Line	Cost
Acyclovir	400 mg po TID × 7–10 days	First line	
Acyclovir	200 mg po 5x/day 7–10 days	First line	
Famciclovir	250 mg po TID × 7–10 days	First line	
Valacyclovir	1 g po BID × 7–10 days	First line	

Episodic therapy, HIV neg

Drug	Dose	Line	Cost
Acyclovir	Same as 1st episode × 5 days	First line	
Acyclovir	800 mg BID × 5 days	First line	Less expensive
Famciclovir	125 mg BID × 5 days	First line	Less expensive
Valacyclovir	500 mg po BID × 5 days	First line	
Valacyclovir	1 g QD × 5 days	First line	

Episodic therapy, HIV pos

Drug	Dose	Line	Cost
Acyclovir	Same as 1st episode × 5–10 days	First line	
Famciclovir	500 mg po BID × 5–10 days	First line	Less expensive
Valacyclovir	1 gm po BID × 5–10 days	First line	

Daily suppressive therapy
HIV negative

Drug	Dose	Line	Cost
Acyclovir	400 mg po BID	First line	Less expensive

TABLE 9-3
TREATMENT REGIMENS FOR STDS (CDC 2002) (Continued)

Drug	Dose	Relative efficacy	Comments
Famciclovir	250 mg po BID	First line	
Valacyclovir	500 mg po QD	First line	
Valacyclovir	1 g po QD	First line	
Daily suppressive therapy			
HIV positive			
Acyclovir	400-800 mg BID or TID	First line	Less expensive
Famciclovir	500 mg BID	First line	
Valacyclovir	500 mg BID	First line	
Chancroid			
Azithromycin	1 g po × 1	First line	Most convenient
Ceftriaxone	250 mg IM × 1	First line	IM injection painful
Ciprofloxacin	500 mg po BID × 3 days	First line	
Erythromycin base	500 mg QID × 7 days	First line	Least convenient
Lymphogranuloma venereum (LGV)			
Doxycycline	100 mg po BID × 21 days	First line	
Erythromycin base	500 mg po QID × 21 days	First line	No data on azythromycin
Donovanosis			
Trimethoprim-sulfa	1 DS po BID × 21days	First line	
Doxycycline	100 mg po BID × 21 days	First line	
Ciprofloxacin	750 mg BID × 21 days	Alternative	

228

Erythromycin base	500 mg QID × 21 days	Alternative	
Azithromycin	1 g po Q 1 week × 3	Alternative	
Syphilis Primary and Secondary			
Benzathine penicillin	2.4 million units IM × 1	First line	
Doxycycline	100 mg po BID × 14 days	Alternative for PCN allergic	Retreatment Q1 week × 3
Tetracycline	500 mg po QID × 14 days	Alternative for PCN allergic	
Erythromycin	500 mg po QID × 28 days	Alternative for PCN allergic	Less effective requires close follow-up
Latent Syphilis Early, < 1 y			
Benzathine penicillin	2.4 million units IM × 1	First line	
Late or Tertiary (except Neurosyphilis)			
Benzathine penicillin	2.4 million units IM Q 1 week × 3	First line	
Neurosyphilis			
Aqueous penicillin G	3–4 million units IV Q4H × 10–14 days	First line	
Procaine penicillin + Probenecid	2.4 million units IM QD + 500 mg po QID × 10–14 days	First line	A painful regimen
Ceftriaxone	2 g IV QD × 10–14 days	Alternative	

- Other diseases that may present with similar clinical findings:
  - Appendicitis
  - Ectopic pregnancy
  - Diverticulitis
  - Adnexal torsion
  - Ruptured or hemorrhage of an ovarian cyst
  - Nephrolithiasis
  - Pancreatitis
  - Perforated bowel.

Diagnosis and Treatment

- There is no specific test for PID, usually a clinical diagnosis.
  - A pregnancy test should be performed during the initial evaluation to exclude tubo-ovarian pregnancy.
  - Peripheral WBC is elevated in half of cases.
  - ESR and C-reactive protein are elevated; normal values make this diagnosis unlikely.
  - ≥ 3 WBC/hpf of the vaginal exudate, 80% sensitivity, 40% specificity.
  - Urinalysis is recommended in all cases to exclude cystitis or pyelonephritis.
- Definitive diagnosis can be made by:
  - Laparoscopy, high specificity, but low sensitivity; should be reserved for the seriously ill patient
  - Histologic evidence of endometritis on biopsy
  - Ultrasound to exclude tubo-ovarian abscess. Will also reveal:
    - Thickened, fluid-filled oviducts with or without free pelvic fluid
    - Tubo-ovarian swelling
- Low threshold for treatment to prevent infertility and chronic pain (see Table 9-3)
  - Outpatient
    - Ofloxacin or levofloxacin plus metronidazole × 14 days or
    - Ceftriaxone × 1 day, plus doxycycline with or without metronidazole × 14 days
  - Inpatient treatment
    - IV cefoxitin or cefotetan plus doxycycline or
    - IV clindamycin plus gentamicin
  - Laparoscopy for tubo-ovarian abscess or persistent fever and pain × 72 hours
  - Laparotomy for ruptured abscess
- The sequelae following PID can include:
  - Infertility
  - Chronic pelvic pain
  - Increased risk of ectopic pregnancy

GENITAL ULCERS

- The most commonly diagnosed and treated venereal diseases of skin and mucous membranes

Etiology

- 5 major etiologies in the United States
  - Herpes simplex type II most common
  - Syphilis—*Treponema pallidum*
  - Chancroid—*Haemophilus ducreyi*
  - Lymphogranuloma venerium (LGV)—*Chlamydia trachomatis*
  - Behçet's syndrome

- Donovanosis or granuloma inguinale—*Calymmatobacterium granulomatosis*
  - Not found in the United States
  - Common in India, Papua New Guinea, the West Indies, and parts of Africa and South America
- All sexually transmitted except for Behçet's syndrome
  - A complete sexual history and a past history of STDs important
- Diagnosis usually made by clinical characteristics of the ulcer (not always reliable) (see Table 9-4)
  - Size and location
  - Pain and tenderness
  - Appearance of base and edges
  - Lymphadenopathy
- Laboratory studies—VDRL, HIV antibody, Gram stain if suspect chancroid, viral culture for HSV, LGV serum titers, dark field for syphilis
- Treatment (see Table 9-3)
  - HSV—acyclovir, valacyclovir, or famciclovir
  - Syphilis—penicillin
  - Chancroid—azithromycin or ceftriaxone
  - Donovanosis—trimethoprim-sulfa or doxycycline
  - LGV—doxycycline or erythromycin

SYPHILIS (*TREPONEMA PALLIDUM*)

- Potential severity: Not life-threatening, but untreated primary infection can lead to debilitating complications 20–30 years later.

Epidemiology
- Transmitted person to person by sexual intercourse.
- Can cross the placenta and cause congenital disease.
- Direct contact with an infected lesion can rarely spread the disease.
- Blood transfusion drawn from a patient with early disseminated disease can transmit disease.
- Incidence in the United States is 28,000 cases a year.
- Incidence waxes and wanes depending on changes in sexual practices and public health funding.

Pathogenesis and Clinical Manifestations
- *Treponema pallidum* is a very thin (0.1–$0.2\,\mu$m) and long (5–$20\,\mu$m) spirochete.
  - Moves by flexing
  - Doubling time is very slow (30 hours)
  - Cannot be grown by conventional methods
- Able to penetrate skin and initially multiplies subcutaneously
- Stimulates acute inflammation followed by cell-mediated and humoral immunity
- The natural history of syphilis can be broken down into three stages.
- Stage 1: Primary syphilis, caused by:
  - Inflammation that leads to tissue destruction and formation of a painless skin ulcer or chancre (see above) approximately 3 weeks after exposure
  - Ulcer teaming with spirochetes that can be readily seen by darkfield or phase microscopy
- Stage 2: Secondary syphilis
  - After skin penetration *T. pallidum* enters the lymphatics and bloodstream.
  - Disseminates throughout the body causing symptomatic disease in 30%.
  - Manifestations usually begin 2–8 weeks after exposure.

TABLE 9-4
CLINICAL CHARACTERISTICS OF GENITAL ULCERS

Diseases	Number and location	Tenderness	Ulcer appearance	Adenopathy
HSV	Clusters of ulcers Labia and penis	Tender	Uniform size Clean based Erythematous border	Very tender inguinal nodes
Syphilis	One or two Vagina and penis	1/3 Tender	Clean base Indurated border	Rubbery, mildly tender
Chancroid	Labia and penis	Tender	Can be large Ragged and necrotic base Undermined edge	Very tender, fluctuant inguinal nodes
LGV	Ulcer lasts 2–3 weeks Labia and penis	Painless	Ulcer spontaneously heals at time of fluctuant adenopathy	Fluctuant inguinal nodes groove sign
Donovanosis	Kissing lesions Labia and penis	Painless	Clean, beefy red base Stark white heaped-up ulcer edges	Nodes usually firm, can mimic LGV
Behçet's syndrome	Mouth and scrotum or vulva	Painful	Yellow necrotic base	Adenopathy minimal

- ○ 90% develop a pink to red, macular, macular-papular, or pustular rash, begins on trunk, then spreads to extremities, palms, and soles.
- ○ Less commonly see:
    - Condyloma lata: painless gray-white, erythematous, highly infectious plaques; can develop in the moist groin area.
    - Areas of alopecia in eyebrows and beard.
    - Generalized lymphadenopathy; enlarged epitrochlear nodes suggest this diagnosis.
    - Basilar meningitis can cause ocular motor, pupillary, facial nerve, and hearing deficits.
    - Also causes anterior uveitis, glomerulonephritis, hepatitis, synovitis, and periostitis.
    - Called "The Great Imitator."
- 3rd stage: Tertiary or late syphilis: Patients who remain untreated for syphilis have a 40% risk of developing late syphilis. This disease causes three major syndromes:
    - ○ Late neurosyphilis
        - Meningovascular syphilis causes arteritis and cerebral infarction. A rare cause of stroke in younger patients. Occurs within 5–10 years of primary disease.
        - General paresis is due to direct damage of the cerebral cortex by spirochetes, 15–20 years after primary disease.
            - Emotional lability, paranoia, delusions, hallucinations, megalomania
            - Tremors, hyperreflexia, seizures, slurred speech, Argyll Robertson pupils, optic atrophy
        - Tabes dorsalis is caused by demyelination of the posterior column, 15–20 years after primary disease.
            - Ataxic gait, loss of position sense, lightening pains, absent DTRs, loss of bladder function
            - Charcot's joints, skin ulcers
    - ○ Late cardiovascular syphilis
        - Arteritis of the vasa vasorum causes damage to the aortic vessel wall, 15–30 years after primary disease, and leads to:
            - Dilatation of the proximal aorta leading to aortic regurgitation and CHF
            - Saccular aneurysms primarily of the ascending and transverse aorta
            - CXR may demonstrate linear calcifications of the aorta
    - ○ Gummas are granulomatous-like lesions, rare except for AIDS patients
        - Skin gummas can break down and form a chronic ulcer
        - Lytic bone lesions can cause tenderness, and draining sinuses
        - Mass lesions of cerebral cortex, liver, and gastric antrum
- *Latent syphilis*
    - ○ After dissemination the organism is controlled by the immune system.
    - ○ Can persist in the body without causing symptoms.
    - ○ During this period the sphirochetes slow their metabolism and doubling time.
    - ○ Defined as the asymptomatic period of greater than 1 year after primary infection; often lasts 20–30 years.

Diagnosis

- Serologic testing remains the primary method of making a diagnosis in most cases.
- Nontreponemal tests—VDRL and RPR test the ability of serum to flocculate a cardiolipin-cholesterol-lecithin antigen.
    - ○ Few false positives with modern tests, usually associated with connective tissue disease.

- ○ Prozone phenomenon observed in 2% of cases.
  - ▪ When the antibody titer is high, a flocculate is not observed in the undiluted sample.
  - ▪ Sample needs to be diluted.
- ○ Use as a marker for response to therapy.
  - ▪ Highest in secondary or early latent disease; following appropriate treatment usually decreases to < 1:4.
  - ▪ In one quarter of patients the VDRL or RPR becomes negative.
  - ▪ With treatment of primary or secondary syphilis, usually a 4-fold decline by 6 months and an 8-fold decline by 12 months.
  - ▪ Treatment of late syphilis usually causes a slower decline of 4-fold over 12 months. A 4-fold or greater decline is considered significant.
  - ▪ The rate of titer decline is slower in patients with:
    - • Prolonged infection
    - • History of recurrent infection, and a high pretreatment titer
  - ▪ In a small number of patients the test remains persistently positive and the patients are called chronic persistors.
  - ▪ A persistent elevation, particularly when the titer remains elevated above 1:4, represents:
    - • A false positive
    - • Persistent active infection
    - • Reinfection
- • Treponemal tests—Measure antibody directed against the treponeme
  - ○ Specific and sensitive, antibody titers may persist for life
  - ○ Not useful for assessing disease activity; used to verify a positive VDRL or RPR
- • CSF tests
  - ○ VDRL positive in the CSF in 1/2 of cases of neurosyphilis
  - ○ Peripheral VDRL positive in 3/4
  - ○ Specific treponemal test positive in all cases; order when considering neurosyphilis

Treatment (see Table 9-3 for doses and complete regimens)

- • Penicillin is the drug of choice.
  - ○ Therapy needs to be prolonged (2 weeks) because of the slow rate of growth of the treponeme.
  - ○ Jarisch-Herxheimer reaction is common: 10–25% most stages, 70–90% in secondary disease.
- • Primary, or secondary syphilis—im benzathine penicillin × 1 or PCN-allergic doxycycline × 2 weeks
- • Early late syphilis (< 1 y)—im benzathine penicillin × 1 or in PCN-allergic doxycycline × 4 weeks
- • Late latent syphilis—im benzathine penicillin × 3 or in the PNC-allergic doxycycline × 4 weeks
- • Neurosyphilis—iv aqueous penicillin G × 2 weeks or IM procaine penicillin + probenecid × 2 weeks
- • Late syphilis (other than neuro)—im benzathine penicillin × 3 or doxycycline × 4 weeks

PAPULAR GU LESIONS

- Condyloma acuminata or anogenital warts are caused by the human papilloma virus.
- Vary in size and can be visualized by treatment with 3–5% acetic acid.
- Predispose to epithelial cell cancers by altering the function of p53 protein.
- Palliative treatment available:
  - Cryotherapy with liquid nitrogen
  - Laser surgery
  - Topical therapy with 10% pododphylin, 0.5% podophyllotoxin (podofilox), or 5% 5-fluorouracil crème
  - Intralesional interferon
- Molluscum contagiosum is a rarer form of venereal warts due to a poxvirus seen in AIDS.

REFERENCES

UTI

Bent S, Nallamothu BK, Simel DL, Fihn SD, Saint S: Does this woman have an acute uncomplicated urinary tract infection? *JAMA* 2002; 287:2701–10.

Gupta K, Hooton TM, Roberts PL, Stamm WE: Patient-initiated treatment of uncomplicated recurrent urinary tract infections in young women. *Ann Intern Med* 2001; 135:9–16.

Gupta K, Scholes D, Stamm WE: Increasing prevalence of antimicrobial resistance among uropathogens causing acute uncomplicated cystitis in women. *JAMA* 1999; 281:736–38.

Harding GK, Zhanel GG, Nicolle LE, Cheang M: Antimicrobial treatment in diabetic women with asymptomatic bacteriuria. *N Engl J Med* 2002; 347:1576–83.

McIsaac WJ, Low DE, Biringer A, Pimlott N, Evans M, Glazier R: The impact of empirical management of acute cystitis on unnecessary antibiotic use. *Arch Intern Med* 2002; 162:600–5.

Raz R, Chazan B, Kennes Y, Colodner R, Rottensterich E, et al: Empiric use of trimethoprim-sulfamethoxazole (TMP-SMX) in the treatment of women with uncomplicated urinary tract infections, in a geographical area with a high prevalence of TMP-SMX-resistant uropathogens. *Clin Infect Dis* 2002; 34:1165–69.

Scholes D, Hooton TM, Roberts PL, Stapleton AE, Gupta K, Stamm WE: Risk factors for recurrent urinary tract infection in young women. *J Infect Dis* 2000; 182:1177–82.

Prostatitis

Collins MM, Meigs JB, Barry MJ, Walker Corkery E, Giovannucci E, Kawachi I: Prevalence and correlates of prostatitis in the health professionals follow-up study cohort. *J Urol* 2002; 167:1363–66.

Collins MM, Stafford RS, O'Leary MP, Barry MJ: How common is prostatitis? A national survey of physician visits. *J Urol* 1998; 159:1224–28.

Naber KG, Sorgel F, Kinzig M, Weigel DM. Penetration of ciprofloxacin into prostatic fluid, ejaculate and seminal fluid in volunteers after an oral dose of 750 mg. *J Urol* 1993; 150:1718–21.

PID

McNeeley SG, Hendrix SL, Mazzoni MM, Kmak DC, Ransom SB: Medically sound, cost-effective treatment for pelvic inflammatory disease and tuboovarian abscess. *Am J Obstet Gynecol* 1998; 178:1272–78.

Ness RB, Soper DE, Holley RL, et al: Effectiveness of inpatient and outpatient treat-
    ment strategies for women with pelvic inflammatory disease: Results from the
    Pelvic Inflammatory Disease Evaluation and Clinical Health (PEACH) Ran-
    domized Trial. *Am J Obstet Gynecol* 2002; 186:929–37.
Scholes D, Stergachis A, Heidrich FE, Andrilla H, Holmes KK, Stamm WE: Pre-
    vention of pelvic inflammatory disease by screening for cervical chlamydial in-
    fection. *N Engl J Med* 1996; 334:1362–66.

STDs
CDC. Sexually transmitted diseases guidelines 2002. *MMWR* 2001; 51:1–77.

10

SKIN AND SOFT TISSUE INFECTIONS

HIGHLIGHTS

- Soft tissue infections vary in severity depending on the depth of infection, as well as the offending organism.
- It is important to differentiate soft tissue infections that can be treated with antibiotics alone (erysipelas and cellulitis) from those that require emergent surgical debridement (necrotizing fasciitis and myositis).
- *Staphylococcus aureus* and *Streptococcus pyogenes* are the most common pathogens.
- Clostridia myonecrosis is a fulminant disease that is often fatal and requires very aggressive debridement to healthy tissue.

Potential severity: Can progress rapidly to shock and death. For deeper soft tissue infections, immediate antibiotic therapy is required, often accompanied by surgical debridement.

CLASSIFICATION OF SKIN AND SOFT TISSUE INFECTIONS (SEE FIG. 10-1)

- Superficial infections usually can be treated on an outpatient basis
  - Most superficial—impetigo, erysipelas, and folliculitis
  - Deeper localized infections—furunculosis, hidroadenitis, and skin abscesses
- Deeper infections require hospitalization, parenteral antibiotics, and surgical debridement
  - Cellulitis is the most superficial and usually is not life-threatening.
  - Necrotizing fasciitis involves the fascia and can result in severe illness.
  - Myonecrosis is often fatal.

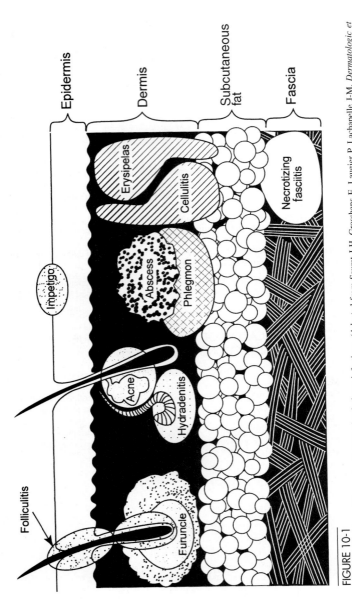

FIGURE 10-1

Schematic drawing of the anatomic sites of soft tissue infections. (Adapted from Saurat J-H, Grosshans E, Laugier P, Lachapelle J-M, *Dermatologic et Vénéréologie*, 2nd ed. Editions Masson, 1990, p. 109.)

238

SEVERE SKIN AND SOFT TISSUE INFECTIONS

CELLULITIS

- An infection of the skin with some extension to the subcutaneous tissues
- Predisposing factors:
  - Venous or lymphatic insufficiency
  - Diabetes mellitus
  - Alcoholism
  - 50% have no clear predisposing factor
- Erythema, edema, diffuse tenderness, indistinct border, lymphadenopathy
  - Systemic toxicity with fever, chills, and myalgias seen in patients presenting with severe cellulitis
- Usually caused by:
  - Group A Streptococci (GAS)
  - Other strains of Streptococci (groups B, C, and G)
  - *S. aureus*
  - *H. influenzae* in children
- Subclasses of cellulitis include:
  - Erysipelas
    - Superficial, very sharp raised border
    - Almost always due to group A streptococci (uncommonly group C, G, or B)
  - Clostridia cellulitis—associated with crepitance, no muscle involvement
  - Anaerobic cellulitis—foul smelling, more common in diabetics
- Diseases confused with cellulitis
  - Deep venous thrombosis
  - Radiation damage

Treatment (see Table 10-1)
- Antibiotics the mainstay of therapy
  - Penicillinase-resistant penicillin (oxacillin, nafcillin) or
  - First-generation cephalosporin (cefazolin)
  - Vancomycin for the penicillin-allergic patient
- Other measures:
  - Immobilization and elevation reduce swelling
  - Cool sterile saline dressings to remove a purulent exudate
- Despite antibiotic treatment, resolution of local findings is typically slow.
  - Can require 1–2 weeks of therapy.
  - Local desquamation can be seen during the early convalescence.

NECROTIZING FACIITIS

- Deep subcutaneous infection that causes necrosis of the fascia and subcutaneous fat
- Often fatal; requires rapid institution of appropriate therapy
- Inciting factors:
  - Usually begins with trauma.
  - Inciting event may be a simple contusion, minor burn, or insect bite.
  - Can result from bacterial superinfection of varicella.
  - Use of nonsteroidal anti-inflammatory drugs (NSAIDs) may increase the risk.

TABLE 10-1
ANTIBIOTIC TREATMENT OF SKIN AND SOFT TISSUE INFECTIONS

Drug	Dose	Relative efficacy	Comments
Cellulitis			
Nafcillin or oxacillin	See Text for duration	First line	
Cefazolin	1–1.5 gm IV Q4H	First line	Inexpensive, less frequent dosing
Vancomycin	1–1.5 gm IV Q8H	Alternative	For PCN-allergic patient
	1 gm IV Q12H		
Necrotizing fasciitis	See text for duration		
Penicillin G (+)	4 million units IV Q4H	First line	PCN dose for adults > 60 kg and
Clindamycin	600–900 mg IV Q8H		normal renal function
Piperacillin-tazobactam (or)	3/0.375 gm IV Q6H	Alternatives	Useful forms of monotherapy
Ticarcillin-clavulinate (or)	3.1 gm IV Q4-6H		
Imipenam	500 mg IV Q6H		
Myonecrosis	See text for duration		
Penicillin G (+)	4 million units IV Q4H	First line	PCN dose for adults > 60 kg and
Clindamycin	600–900 mg IV Q8H		normal renal function
Impetigo	Treat × 10 days		Treatment prevents poststreptococcal
			complications
Erythromycin	250 mg po QID	First line	May cause GI toxicity
Dicloxacillin	250 mg po QID	First line	
Cephalexin	250 mg po QID or 500 mg po BID	Alternative	
Mupirocine	Polyethylene glycol ointment apply BID	Alternative	
Skin abscesses			
Clindamycin	150 mg po QID	First line	
Dicloxacillin	250 mg po QID	First line	

240

Etiologies
- Group A streptococci
- Mixed infection with Gram-positive and Gram-negative aerobes (*S. aureus*, group A streptococci, and *E. coli*) and anaerobes (Peptostreptococcus, Clostridia, Provotella, Porphyromonas, and Bacteroides spp.)
- Certain underlying conditions affect the bacteriology
  - *Diabetes mellitus*
    - Mixed flora occur more often in diabetic patients.
    - Usually begins on the feet, rapidly extending up the fascia of the leg
      - Also can develop in the head and neck region and the perineum
    - In diabetic patients with cellulitis consider necrotizing fasciitis when:
      - Tachycardia and leukocytosis
      - Marked hyperglycemia and acidosis
  - *Cervical necrotizing fasciitis*
    - Breach of the integrity of mucous membranes after surgery or instrumentation or due to an odontogenic infection
    - Can reult in necrotizing fasciitis and/or "Ludwig's angina," a rapidly expanding inflammation in the submandibular and sublingual spaces
  - *Fournier's gangrene*
    - Penetration of the gastrointestinal or urethral mucosa
    - Abrupt onset of severe pain
    - May spread rapidly onto the anterior abdominal wall, into the gluteal muscles and, in men, onto the scrotum and penis

Symptoms and Signs
- Toxic appearance, tachycardia, and hypotension
- Excruciating pain in the absence of any cutaneous findings
- Within 24–48 hours, erythema may develop or darken to a reddish-purple color.
- Bullae can also develop in normal-appearing skin, often associated with extensive deep soft tissue destruction
- Fever, malaise, myalgias, diarrhea, and anorexia in the first 24 hours
- Infection typically spreads rapidly and causes multiple-organ failure, adult respiratory distress syndrome, and death.

Diagnosis (early diagnosis is critical for survival)
- Surgical exploration or punch biopsy is required for rapid diagnosis.
- Imaging studies, such as soft tissue X-rays, CT scan, and MRI, are helpful if there is gas in the tissue, but may delay definitive diagnosis and treatment.

Treatment must include:
- Early, aggressive, and often repeated surgical debridement
  - All necrotic tissue has to be removed to prevent progression.
- Systemic antibiotics (see Table 10-1)
  - Group A Streptococcus (GAS)
    - High doses of intravenous penicillin
    - Clindamycin usually, because this antibiotic:
      - Is not affected by inoculum size or the stage of growth
      - Suppresses exotoxin production by GAS
      - Facilitates phagocytosis of *S. pyogenes*
      - Has a long postantibiotic effect
  - Mixed infection
    - Ticarcillin-clavulinate, piperacillin-tazobactam, or imipenam

- Additional measures
  - Volume replacement: 10–20 L/day of IV fluid often necessary to maintain tissue perfusion.
  - Combined with vasopressors such as dopamine or epinephrine.
  - High-dose immunoglobulins may be beneficial.

MYONECROSIS

- Clostridial gas gangrene due to *C. perfringens* occurs after:
  - Trauma, deep, penetrating injury (e.g., knife or gunshot wound, or crush injury classically occurring in war wounds)
  - Bowel surgery
  - Postabortion and with retained placenta
  - Spontaneous and nontraumatic disease due to hematogenous spread usually due to *C. septicum* with gastrointestinal portals of entry such as adenocarcinoma
  - Spontaneous gangrenous myositis can also be caused by group A Streptococcus.
- Other infectious diseases that involve muscle need to be considered
  - Tropical myositis
    - Primarily due to *S. aureus* and, less often, other organisms
    - Causes a primary muscle abscess (pyomyositis)
    - More common in tropical areas
  - Necrotizing infections due to *Vibrio vulnificus*
    - Most common among patients with cirrhosis, consumers of raw seafood, or inhabitants of coastal regions

Pathophysiology

- Clostridia inoculated into damaged tissue
  - An anaerobic environment with low oxidation-reduction potential and acid pH is optimal for growth of clostridial organisms.
- Tissue and systemic effects are the result of toxin production.
  - Clostridial theta toxin destroys host tissues and inflammatory cells and systemic diffusion results in vascular leukostasis, endothelial cell injury, and regional tissue hypoxia.
  - Alpha toxin, a phospholipase C, directly suppresses myocardial contractility and lyses cell membranes, causing hemolysis and the destruction of leukocytes.

Clinical Presentation

- Mean incubation period less than 24 hours.
- First symptom in traumatic or bacteremic gas gangrene is usually the sudden onset of severe pain at the site of infection.
- Skin initially appears pale, quickly changes to bronze and then purplish red, and becomes tense and exquisitely tender, with overlying blisters.
- Crepitus is readily palpated in most cases.
- Systemic toxicity, tachycardia, and hypotension are common.
- Clostridial bacteremia may be associated with extensive hemolysis.

Diagnosis

- Gas within the soft tissue shown by soft tissue X-rays, computerized tomographic (CT) scan, or magnetic resonance imaging (MRI)
- Definitive diagnosis made by Gram stain showing large, Gram-variable rods at the site of injury; PMN not usually seen

Treatment must be rapid and outcome is often fatal
- High-dose intravenous penicillin and clindamycin the treatment of choice (see Table 10-1). Clindamycin used to reduce clostridia toxin production
  - Other antibiotics also have excellent activity against *C. perfringens* and other strains.
    - Metronidazole
    - Cefotetan and cefoxitin
- Emergent surgical debridement may be lifesaving
  - All necrotic tissue must be removed
    - Dead muscle can be identified by its brown color and lack of contraction on electrical stimulation
    - Amputation of the infected limb almost always required
- Hyperbaric oxygen likely to be helpful

BURN INFECTIONS

- Burned skin provides a fertile environment for bacterial growth.
- Organisms associated with invasive infection include:
  - Gram-positive aerobic bacteria—*S. aureus* and *epidermidis*, enterococcus
  - Gram-negative aerobic bacteria—Enterobacter, *E. Coli*, Klebsiella, Pseudomonas spp., and Acinetobacter
- When burn wound infections become invasive:
  - Concentration of microorganisms rises to greater than one million per gram of tissue.
  - Developing granulation tissue becomes edematous and pale, associated with occlusion and thrombosis of new blood vessels.
  - Lack of bleeding is evident on surgical exploration of the wound.
  - Infection advances, the surface becomes frankly necrotic, and the infection spreads rapidly.
- Aggressive wound care and extreme vigilance are required to control the concentration of organisms in the burn wound.
  - Frequent debridement
  - Topical antimicrobial therapy
  - After 2–3 weeks a layer of granulation tissue forms where the eschar separates, and the improved blood supply and wound hypermetabolism limit the proliferation of microbes
- Clinical manifestions
  - The burn patient's "normal" hyperdynamic state mimics some of the typical signs of sepsis.
  - Changes in status, rather than the presence or absence of specific abnormalities, are most helpful in deciding whether or not patient has developed an invasive infection.

Treatment
- Broad-spectrum antibiotics are given when sepsis is suspected based on previous surgical wound cultures.
- Operations performed in patients with a deteriorating cardiovascular status and pulmonary function are extremely hazardous.

LESS SEVERE, MORE COMMON, AND LOCALIZED SKIN INFECTIONS

- Impetigo causes superficial vesicular lesions that crust over
  - Caused by group A streptococci and *S. aureus*
  - Treatment (see Table 10-1) with amoxacillin-clavulinate, dicloxacillin, cephalexin, or erythromycin
  - For localized disease, may use topical mupirocine
- Folliculitis—infection localized to the hair follicles
  - *S. aureus* most common, often associated with nasal carriage
  - *P. aeruginosa* associated with "whirlpool" folliculitis
  - Candida usually follows the use of broad-spectrum antibiotics
  - Treated with topical antibiotics or antifungals; systemic antibiotics not recommended

FURUNCULOSIS AND CARBUNCLES

- Furuncles are nodular lesions that are result of progression from folliculitis.
- Carbuncles are larger subcutaneous abscesses that represent a progression from furuncles.
- Both infections are caused by *S. aureus*.
- Can be dangerous
  - On the face, can lead to cavernous sinus infection
  - Bacteremia can occur if the lesions are manipulated.
- Treatment may include (see Table 10-1):
  - Hot compresses to promote spontaneous drainage
  - Oral antibiotics if fever develops—dicloxacillin, cephalexin, clindamycin
  - Surgical drainage if spontaneous drainage fails to occur
- Prevention—chlorhexidine solutions, mupirocin in the nose to prevent carriage, prophylactic antibiotics

SKIN ABSCESSES

- Localized infection of the dermis and subcutaneous tissue, usually deeper than carbuncles
- Can arise from local trauma, IV drug abuse, and bacteremic seeding
- *S. aureus* most common etiology
- Therapy should include (see Table 10-1):
  - Oral clindamycin (adds anaerobic coverage) or dicloxacillin
  - If cellulitis—iv clindamycin, nafcillin, oxacillin, or cefazolin
  - In perirectal, oral, or vaginal area—amoxacillin-clavulinate
- Preventive measures
  - If recurrent furunculosis, carbuncles, or abscesses, exclude diabetes mellitus, neutrophil dysfunction, and hyper-IgE syndrome
  - Prophylactic antibiotics prior to incision and drainage, if high risk for endocarditis

TETANUS

- Rare in the United States (most cases in age > 60 due to waning immunity), but common in developing countries
- Most cases develop following punctures or lacerations.
- *C. tetani* produces tetanospasmin, blocks normal inhibition of motor neurons.

Clinical presentation
- Masseter muscle trismus or "lockjaw."
- Generalized muscle spasm leading to arching of the back (opisthotonus), flexion of the arms, and extension of the legs.
- Spasms may be triggered by any sensory stimulus and are very painful.
- Spasm of the diaphragm and throat can lead to respiratory arrest and sudden death.
- Autonomic dysfunction can lead to hyper- or hypotension, bradycardia or tachycardia.
- Neonatal tetanus develops following infection of the umbilical stump.
  - Most commonly reported in developing countries.
  - Present with generalized weakness followed by increased rigidity; mortality exceeds 90%.

Treatment
- Human tetanus immunoglobulin (HITIG) 500 IU im
- Diphtheria-pertussis-tetanus vaccine (DPT, 0.5 ml)
- Metronidazole (500 mg Q8H iv) × 7–10 days
- iv Diazepam, short-acting β-blockers, vaspopressors, fluids
- Intubation and tracheostomy
- Two additional doses of DPT vaccine are recommended.
  - One dose at discharge
  - A third dose 4 weeks later
- Mortality ranges from 6% in milder cases to 60% in severe disease.

Prevention
- DPT Q10 years
- If a potentially contaminated wound, DPT booster after 5 years
- If high-risk wound or immunocompromised patient, also give HITIG

ANIMAL AND HUMAN BITES
- A leading cause of visits to the E.R. (approximately 1% of visits)
- More common in children, dog bites > in boys, cat bites > in girls
- Teeth of cats very sharp
  - Commonly penetrate the skin
  - Puncture the underlying bone, increasing the risk of osteomyelitis

Microbiology
- Pasteurella species found in 50% of dog bites and 70% of cat bites
- *S. aureus*, streptococcal spp., *Capnocytophaga canimoris*, and anaerobic bacteria also frequently cultured from these wounds
- Infections are usually polymicrobial.
- Prophylactic antibiotics recommended because of the high risk of infection:
  - iv ampicillin-sulbactam (3 gm iv × 1) followed by amoxacillin-clavulinate (875 mg po BID) × 3–5 days
  - In penicillin-allergic patients: clindamycin (900 mg IV followed by 300 mg po Q6H) plus ciprofloxacin (400 mg IV followed by 500 mg po BID) × 3–5 days; in place of ciprofloxacin use trimethoprim-sulfamethoxazole in children

Treatment
- Same antibiotic regimens as prophylaxis, but more prolonged, 10–28 days
- First-generation cephalosporins, dicloxacillin, and erythromycin should be avoided; do not cover Pasteurella spp.
- Rabies prophylaxis
- Tetanus prophylaxis

HUMAN BITES
- Often associated with alcohol or other drugs; clenched fist injuries most common
- Polymicrobial infections, often includes *Eikenella corrodens*
  - Other organisms: *S. viridans* and *S. aureus*, Bacteroides spp., Fusobacterium spp., and peptostreptococci

Prophylaxis and Treatment
- Ampicillin-sulbactam IV followed by amoxicillin-clavulinate (see above) or cefoxitin (2 gm IV Q6H)
- Avoid oxacillin, nafcillin, clindamycin, metronidazole, and many cephalosporins because *Eikenella corrodens* is resistant
- Duration depends on response, tissue damage, and bony involvement

REFERENCES

Bonnetblanc JM, Bedane C: Erysipelas: Recognition and management. *Am J Clin Dermatol* 2003; 4:157–63.
Duvanel T, Auckenthaler R, Rohner P, Harms M, Saurat JH: Related articles: Quantitative cultures of biopsy specimens from cutaneous cellulitis. *Arch Intern Med* 1989; 149(2):293–96.
Stamenkovic I, Lew PD: Early recognition of potentially fatal necrotizing fasciitis: The use of frozen-section biopsy. *N Engl J Med* 1984; 310(26):1689–93.
Wong CH, Chang HC, Pasupathy S, Khin LW, Tan JL, Low CO: Necrotizing fasciitis: clinical presentation, microbiology, and determinants of mortality. *J Bone Joint Surg Am* 2003; 85-A:1454–60.

11

BONE AND JOINT INFECTIONS

OSTEOMYELITIS

HIGHLIGHTS

- Often presents as localized pain associated with low-grade fever.
- Three forms are managed differently: hematogenous, contiguous spread following trauma, and contiguous spread associated with ischemic skin ulcers.
- With the exception of pediatric cases, bone biopsy and culture are required to guide antibiotic therapy, and amputation is usually necessary for ischemic disease.
- Prolonged high-dose antibiotic therapy (4–8 weeks) is required for cure.
- Necrotic bone (sequestrum) must be surgically removed.
- Relapse is common, and cure as defined as > 1 year without symptoms after the completion of therapy.

Potential severity: A subacute to chronic infection that can cause severe disability if improperly managed.

- A progressive infectious process that can involve one or multiple components of bone, including:
  - Periosteum
  - Medullary cavity
  - Cortical bone
- Characterized by progressive:
  - Inflammatory destruction of bone
  - Necrosis
  - New bone formation

CLASSIFICATION

- Acute osteomyelitis develops over days to weeks.
- Chronic osteomyelitis develops over weeks to months and can persist for years.
- Hematogenous osteomyelitis occurs in the children and the elderly.
- Infections at contiguous sites spread to bone after:
  - Traumatic injury
  - Penetrating injuries
  - Postoperative orthopedic surgery infections
- Diabetic as well as other forms of ischemic ulcer can spread infection to bone.

HEMATOGENOUS OSTEOMYELITIS
OF LONG BONES AND VERTEBRAL BODIES

- Bacteria are trapped in small end vessels.
  - At the metaphysis of long bone in children
    - Lodge in small end vessels that form sharp loops near the epiphyses
    - Tibia and femur most common locations
  - In vertebral bodies in the elderly
    - Can seed via small bifurcating arteries
    - Also can spread via a plexus of veins lacking valves, called Batson's plexus. May allow bladder and pelvic infections to spread to vertebral bodies.
    - The lumbar segments > thoracic regions > the cervical region (rare)

TABLE 11-1
THE MICROBIOLOGY OF OSTEOMYELITIS

Type of Osteomyelitis	Common Pathogens
Hematogenous (usually 1 organism)	
Infant (< 1 year)	*S. aureus* Group B Streptococci *E. coli*
Children (1–16 years)	*S. aureus* *S. pyogenes* *H. influenzae*
Adults (> 16 years)	*S. aureus* Coagulase-negative staphylococci Gram-negatives—*E. coli,* Pseudomonas, Serratia
Contiguous spread (polymicrobial)	
Microbiology depends on the primary site of infection.	*S. aureus* *S. pyogenes* Enterococcus Coagulase-negative staphylococci Gram-negatives Anaerobes
Diabetic foot (polymicrobial)	*S. aureus* Streptococcus spp. including Enterococcus Gram-negatives—*Proteus mirabilis,* Pseudomonas Anaerobes

- Microbiology reflects the causes of bacteremia in the different age groups (see Table 11-1)
  - Infants: *S. aureus* and group B streptococci most frequent
  - Children: *S. aureus*, other streptococci, and coagulase-negative staphylococci
  - Elderly: *S. aureus* most common, followed by Gram-negatives
  - Immunocompromised: fungi
  - iv drug abusers—*Pseudomonas aeruginosa* predilection for cervical vertebra and clavicles

CLINICAL MANIFESTATIONS

- Long bones: fever, chills, and malaise associated with soft tissue swelling and pain, usually develops in children
- Vertebral osteomyelitis: back pain and localized tenderness accompanied by a high ESR

DIAGNOSIS (SEE FIGS. 11-1 THROUGH 11-3)

- Plain films require 2–3 weeks to become positive (require a 50% loss of bone calcium); in vertebral osteomyelitis can take 6–8 weeks. (see Fig. 11-1). They may show:
  - Periosteal elevation
  - Areas of demineralization and loss of a sharp bony margin, "moth-eaten" appearance
  - Soft tissue swelling
  - Late stages areas of increased calcification or sclerosis
- CT scan more sensitive (see Fig. 11-2). Allows more accurate:
  - Detection of disruption of the bony margins
  - Detection of collapse of the disc space in vertebral osteomyelitis
- MRI increasingly being used; may prove to be the most sensitive tool for assessing early osteomyelitis (see Fig. 11-3) as well as detecting dead bone.
  - More sensitive than CT scan for detecting early osteomyelitis
    - Early edema of the bone marrow and decreased signal intensity of the disc and infected vertebral bodies are observed on T2-weighted images.
    - Loss of end plate definition seen on T-1 images.
    - Contrast enhancement of the infected regions is also observed.
  - Helpful for guiding surgical debridement
    - Able to detect areas of dead bone, also termed sequestrum.
    - Necrosis of long bones results in bone marrow death, which produces a unique MRI signal.
    - Allows a more complete surgical debridement of sequestrum.
    - Also helpful in detecting the spread of vertebral infection to the epidural space (see Chap. 6).
- Bone scan: can detect early disease, but not as accurate as MRI.
  - False positives common, particularly when soft tissue infection is overlying bone
  - Gallium preferred for vertebral osteomyelitis
- Vertebral osteomyelitis needs to be differentiated from metastatic bone lesions, which can also cause erosions of the vertebral margin.
  - Osteomyelitis almost always involves two adjacent vertebral bodies and the disc space.
  - Neoplastic processes usually involve a single vertebral body and do not extend across the disc space.

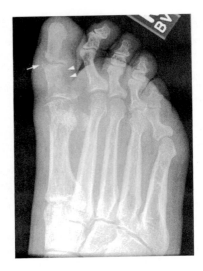

FIGURE 11-1
Plane X-ray showing changes of osteomyelitis of the great toe. Arrow points to fragmentation of the distal interphalangeal joint. Arrowheads outline the expected location of the medial margin of the proximal phalangeal bone. Multifocal areas of cortical destruction and ill-defined lytic areas are found throughout the distal first metatarsal and both first toe phalanges. (Courtesy of Maria T. Calimano, M.D., and Andres R. Acosta, M.D., University of Florida.)

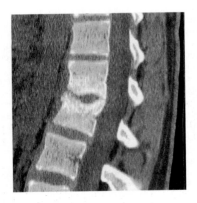

FIGURE 11-2
Sagittal CT scan showing typical changes of vertebral osteomyelitis. Obliteration of the disc space is seen with marked irregularity and sclerosis of the cortical endplates. (Courtesy of Maria T. Calimano, M.D., and Andres R. Acosta, M.D., University of Florida.)

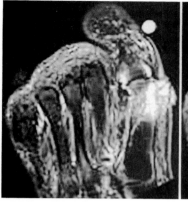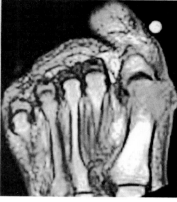

FIGURE 11-3

MRI changes of early osteomyelitis. *Left*: T2 image shows increased signal in the bone marrow of the metatarsal and the surrounding soft tissue. *Right*: T1 post contrast image showing loss of the bone marrow fat signal and cortical margins in the metatarsal. (Courtesy of Maria T. Calimano, M.D., and Andres R. Acosta, M.D., University of Florida.)

- 2–3 blood cultures should be drawn, but are positive in only a small percentage of cases.
- For patients who traveled to endemic areas, Brucella serology is useful (see Chap. 13).
- Tissue sample for culture and histopathology should be obtained except when blood cultures are positive.
  - Long bone infection in children may be treated empirically because operative intervention may damage the epiphyseal plate.
  - Long bone infection in adults usually requires operative culture.
  - In vertebral osteomyelitis use CT guided-needle biopsy.
    - The number of potential pathogens is large in vertebral osteomyelitis, and effective antimicrobial therapy requires guidance by culture results.
    - Needle aspirates should be submitted in parallel for bacteriologic and pathologic evaluation.
    - Pathology helpful in patients who previously received antibiotic therapy, and in patients with suspected mycobacterial disease.
    - If the first biopsy is culture negative, a second biopsy guided by CT scan should be obtained.
    - If the second sample fails to establish a diagnosis, an open surgical biopsy should be considered.

TREATMENT

- Antibiotic therapy (see Table 11-2)
  - Empiric antibiotic therapy is usually avoided.
  - In vitro susceptibility testing should be performed to guide treatment.
  - Therapy must be prolonged.

TABLE 11-2
ANTIBIOTIC TREATMENT OF HEMATOGENOUS
OSTEOMYELITIS IN ADULTS

Microorganisms Isolated	Treatment of Choice (iv unless specified)	Alternatives
S. aureus		
Penicillin-sensitive	Penicillin G (4 million units, every 6 hours)	A cephalosporin II,[a] clindamycin (600 mg, every 6 hour) or Vancomycin
Penicillin-resistant	Nafcillin[b] (2 gm, every 6 hour)	A cephalosporin II, clindamycin (600 mg, every 6 hour), or Vancomycin
Methicillin-resistant	Vancomycin (1 gm, every 12 hour)	Teicoplanin[c] (400 mg every 24 hour, first day every 12 hour)
Various streptococci (group A or B β-hemolytic; *S. pneumoniae*)	Penicillin G (3 million units every 4–6 hour)	Clindamycin (600 mg, every 6 hour), Erythromycin (500 mg, every 6 hour), or Vancomycin
Enteric Gram-negative rods	Quinolone (Ciprofloxacin, 500–750 mg every 12 hour, IV or oral)	A cephalosporin III[d]
Serratia spp. (or) *P. aeruginosa*	Piperacillin[e] (2–4 gm, every 4 hour) and Gentamicin (1.5 mg/kg/day)	A cephalosporin III[e] or a quinolone (with aminoglycosides)
Anaerobes	Clindamycin (600 mg, every 6 hour)	Ampicillin-sulbactam (2.2 gm every 8 hour) or Metronidazole for Gram-negative anaerobes (500 mg every 8 hour)
Mixed infection (aerobic and anaerobic microorganisms)	Ampicillin-sulbactam (2.2 gm every 8 hour)	Imipenem[f] (500 mg every 6 hour)

[a]II, second generation; [b]Flucloxacillin in Europe; [c]Teicoplanin is at present only available in Europe; [d]III, third generation; [e]depends on sensitivities; piperacillin/tazobactam and imipenem are useful alternatives; [f]in cases of aerobic Gram-negative microorganisms resistant to amoxicillin–clavulanic acid.

- Treat a minimum of 4–6 weeks, often followed by prolonged oral antibiotic treatment (months).
- Therapy must be dated from the day on which effective antimicrobial therapy was begun.
  - Recommended antibiotics for specific pathogens:
    - *S. aureus*: methicillin-sensitive, nafcillin or oxacillin; MRSA—vancomycin
    - Streptococci: penicillin G
    - Enteric Gram-negatives: ciprofloxacin
    - Serratia or *Ps. aeruginosa*: piperacillin-tazobactam combined with gentamicin
    - Anaerobes: clindamycin or metronidazole
- Surgical debridement not necessary if early treatment.
  - Required to remove necrotic long bone
  - Rarely required in vertebral osteomyelitis; surgery if:
    - Infection is unresponsive to antibiotic therapy
    - Vertebral instability
    - Cord compression
    - Development of a soft tissue abscess

OSTEOMYELITIS SECONDARY TO A CONTIGUOUS INFECTION

- Clinical presentation of osteomyelitis associated with a comminuted fracture is subtle.
  - Following corrective surgery, pain initially improves.
  - As the patient begins to bear weight, pain reappears.
  - Mild fever develops.
  - The wound becomes more erythematous accompanied by a slight discharge.
- Other forms of osteomyelitis due to contiguous spread include:
  - Acute purulent frontal sinusitis spreading to the frontal bone and causing edema of the forehead (Pott's puffy tumor)
  - Dental root infection leading to local bony destruction
  - Deep-seated pressure sores spreading to underlying bone, usually the sacrum

DIAGNOSIS

- Imaging procedures often difficult to interpret
- Based on clinical findings and surgical exploration
- Microbiology may reveal multiple organisms (see Table 11-1).
  - *S. aureus* most common
  - Streptococci
  - Enterobacteriaceae, *Ps. aeruginosa*
  - Anaerobes

DIABETIC FOOT INFECTION: OSTEOMYELITIS SECONDARY TO VASCULAR INSUFFICIENCY

- Located almost exclusively on the lower extremities
- Most common clinical presentation is a painless ulcer that extends to bone.

PHYSICAL EXAM

- Mild cellulitis.
- Often there is no tenderness at ulcer site (secondary to neuropathy). If acute bone necrosis, can be tender.
- Crepitance with anaerobes or enterobacteriaceae.
- Important to carefully examine the vascular supply to the affected limb and evaluate the concomitant neuropathy.

DIAGNOSIS

- Plain X-rays of the bone should be part of the initial evaluation.
- The ulcer should be gently probed; if the probe reaches bone, the patient is treated for osteomyelitis.
- If bone cannot be detected by probing and the plain radiography does not suggest osteomyelitis, treat for soft tissue infection.
- Because occult osteomyelitis may be present, radiography should be repeated in 2 weeks.
- MRI is recommended in doubtful cases.
- Microbiology—mixed Gram-positive, Gram-negatives and anaerobes (see Table 11-1)

TREATMENT (SEE TABLE 11-2)

- Prognosis for cure is poor because of:
  - Impaired host defenses in the ischemic region
  - Inability of systemic antibiotics to gain entry into the site of infection
- Must determine the amount of vascular compromise by:
  - Transcutaneous oximetry (once inflammation has been controlled)
  - Pulse pressure measurements by Doppler ultrasonography
  - Arteriography of the lower extremity including the foot vessels should be considered if serious ischemia is suspected.
- Revascularization may be considered prior to amputation.
- Therapy depends on the extent of vascular perfusion in the area.
  - If good oxygen tension at the infected site:
    - Debridement and a 4–6-week course of antimicrobial therapy sometimes followed by oral antibiotics can lead to a high cure rate.
  - If poor oxygen tension at the site of infection:
    - The wound often fails to heal.
    - Amputation of infected bone is ultimately required.
    - Treat with antimicrobial agents for 4 weeks when infected bone is transected surgically.
    - Treat 2 weeks if the infected bone is completely removed in order to clear residual soft tissue infection.
- Hyperbaric oxygen is of no proven benefit for these patients.

GENERAL PRINCIPLES FOR THE MANAGEMENT OF OSTEOMYELITIS

- Three critical elements to good care:
  1. Adequate tissue must be obtained for culture and histopathology.
     ○ Obtain deep infected tissue (specimens obtained superficially from ulcers or from fistulas are often misleading).
     ○ A bone biopsy should be performed, and the sample obtained should be submitted for:
       - Aerobic and anaerobic cultures
       - Histopathologic evaluation, including Gram stain
       - Ideally should be fully analyzed before therapy is begun
  2. A specific antibiotic regimen should be designed based on antibiotic sensitivity tests.
     ○ Empiric antimicrobial therapy is often required to reduce the risk of bacteremia or spread of infection.
     ○ The antimicrobial regimen should subsequently be modified on the basis of culture and susceptibility results.
     ○ Maximal doses of antibiotics should be used because of the poor penetration of most antibiotics into bone.
     ○ Therapy must be prolonged because revascularization of bone after debridement takes 3–4 weeks.
       - Parenteral therapy recommended for 4–6 weeks.
       - If severe bone necrosis, therapy may be prolonged to 12 weeks.
       - The start of this therapy is usually dated from the last major debridement.
     ○ Early antibiotic treatment, given before extensive bone destruction has occurred, produces the best results.
     ○ Single-agent chemotherapy is usually adequate for the treatment of osteomyelitis due to hematogenous spread (see Table 11-2).
     ○ Outpatient parenteral therapy (OPAT) has become increasingly popular, but requires a team of dedicated nurses and physicians.
     ○ For chronic osteomyelitis, oral therapy extending over months, and more rarely years, will reduce acute flare-ups.
     ○ The efficacy of local administration of antibiotics, either by instillation or by gentamicin-laden beads, has not been proven by controlled studies.
       - Antibiotic diffusion is limited in time and space.
       - May be of some additional benefit in osteomyelitis secondary to a contiguous focus of infection.
     ○ Fluoroquinolones have been shown to be highly effective in experimental infections, and in several randomized and nonrandomized studies in adults.
       - Excellent bone levels achievable.
       - The drug of choice for most Enterobacteriaceae (which are very sensitive to fluoroquinolones).
       - Their advantage over conventional therapy in osteomyelitis due to Pseudomonas or Serratia species, as well as Gram-positive organisms (in particular *S. aureus*), remains to be demonstrated.
  3. Proper surgical management requires:
     ○ Proper drainage
     ○ Thorough debridement
       - Including removal of all orthopedic appliances except those deemed absolutely necessary for stability
       - Often must be repeated at least once for the removal of all nonviable tissue

- ○ Obliteration of dead space
- ○ Open wounds must be covered to prevent bacteria from reinfecting the bone.
- Assessment of response and cure is difficult.
  - ○ ESR and symptomatic improvement best parameters
  - ○ Serial radiologic or MRI studies are not recommended during therapy.
    - ▪ Radiologic and MRI changes of osteomyelitis can worsen for several weeks on appropriate antibiotic therapy.
  - ○ Cure is defined as resolution of all signs and symptoms for > 1 year after completion of therapy.
  - ○ Failure is defined as a lack of apparent response to therapy, as evidenced by one or more of the following:
    - ▪ Persistence of drainage
    - ▪ Recurrence of a sinus tract or failure of a sinus tract to close
    - ▪ Persistence of systemic signs of infection (chills, fever, weight loss, bone pain)
    - ▪ Progression of bone infection shown by imaging methods

INFECTIONS IN PROSTHETIC JOINTS

HIGHLIGHTS

- A feared postoperative complication that necessitates removal of the prosthetic material in almost all cases.
- Biofilm provides a protective environment that usually prevents cure by antibiotics alone.

CLASSIFICATION

- Can be divided into three categories based on time course and pathogenesis:
  - ○ Acute contiguous infection (≤ 6 months after surgery)
    - ▪ Contracted from infected skin, subcutaneous tissue, muscle, and/or operative hematoma
  - ○ Chronic contiguous infection (6–24 months after surgery)
    - ▪ Contamination at the time of surgery with microorganisms of lower pathogenicity
    - ▪ The infection progresses slowly to a chronic form before it is recognized
  - ○ Hematogenous spread (> 2 years after surgery)
    - ▪ Caused by transient bacteremia
    - ▪ Can be caused by a wide variety of organisms

MICROBIOLOGY

- 3/4 due to Staphylococcus
- Coagulase-negative Staphylococcus most common
- *S. aureus*

CLINICAL MANIFESTATIONS

- Difficult to differentiate from mechanical loosening
  - ○ Joint pain
  - ○ Fever often not present

DIAGNOSIS

- Joint aspiration, with quantitative culture and Gram stain to differentiate from skin contamination of the culture

TREATMENT

- Removal of the prosthesis is usually required
  - One-step procedure
    - Infected components are excised
    - Surgical debridement is performed
    - A new prosthesis is immediately placed
    - Many surgeons use antibiotic-impregnated cement
  - Two-step approach (Mayo Clinic approach)
    - Removal of all foreign bodies
    - Debridement of the bone and soft tissues
    - A minimum of 4 weeks of parenteral antimicrobial therapy
    - With less virulent pathogens, replacement ≥ 3 months
    - With more virulent pathogens, replacement > 1 year
- A stable joint with early infection may occasionally be cured with antibiotics alone
- A difficult infection to cure. Relapse is:
  - 10% at 3 years
  - 26% after 10 years

SEPTIC ARTHRITIS (EXCLUDING REACTIVE ARTHRITIS)

HIGHLIGHTS

- Monoarticular arthritis is septic arthritis until proven otherwise.
- Diagnosis requires arthrocentesis and yields high numbers of neutrophils.
- High-dose antibiotics should be accompanied by joint drainage to remove damaging proteases released by neutrophils.
- The most common cause is *S. aureus*.

Potential severity: Delays in appropriate therapy can lead to irreversible joint damage.

PATHOGENESIS

- Usually hematogenous
  - Bacteria enter synovial membrane lining the joint, resulting in an acute inflammatory reaction.
  - Bacteria and inflammatory cells quickly spread to the synovial fluid, leading to joint swelling and erythema.
  - Cytokines and proteases are released into the synovial fluid and, if not quickly treated, cause cartilage damage and eventually joint space narrowing.
  - Causes of bacteremia leading to septic arthritis include urinary tract infection, intravenous drug abuse, intravenous catheters, soft tissue infections, and bacterial endocarditis, particularly due to *S. aureus* or enterococcus.

- Patients at higher risk:
  - ○ Those with underlying joint disease due to rheumatoid arthritis and os- teoarthritis. Damage to the synovial membrane increases the likelihood of bacterial invasion.
  - ○ HIV infected are at higher risk of septic arthritis due to fungus or mycobac- teria.
  - ○ Patients with minor trauma or an upper respiratory infection.
  - ○ Intra-articular injection of corticosteroids can lead to bacterial superinfection.

ETIOLOGY

- *S. aureus* is the most common cause of infectious arthritis.
- In young adults, *Neisseria gonorrhoeae* (presenting sometimes as disseminated gonococcal infection, see below).
- Elderly are at higher risk for Gram-negative bacilli (often secondary to urinary tract infection).
- Viruses such as parvovirus B19, hepatitis B, rubella, mumps, and HIV can be causes of acute arthritis.
- Mycobacterial and fungal infections can cause chronic monoarticular arthritis.
- Lyme arthritis caused by *Borrelia burgdorferi* is a diagnosis to be considered in the appropriate epidemiologic setting:
  - ○ May occur as an acute transient arthritis
  - ○ Less commonly presents as late chronic arthritis (see Chap. 13).

CLINICAL MANIFESTATIONS

- Classic findings: swelling and pain in a single joint accompanied by fever
  - ○ Connective tissue diseases present with bilateral joint involvement.
  - ○ Any patient with monoarticular arthritis should be considered to have septic arthritis until proven otherwise.
- Elderly patients may be afebrile at the time of presentation.
- On exam:
  - ○ Swollen and warm to touch
  - ○ Any movement of the joint is accompanied by exquisite pain.
  - ○ Knee most commonly involved (40–50%), hip (15–20%), followed by shoul- der, wrist, ankle, and elbow.
  - ○ In children the hip joint is most commonly affected (60%) followed by the knee joint (35%). Nearly half of patients who develop septic arthritis have un- derlying chronic joint disease, such as rheumatoid arthritis and osteoarthritis. It is likely that damage to the synovial membrane increases the likelihood of bacterial invasion.

DIAGNOSIS PRIMARILY MADE BY JOINT ASPIRATION

- Synovial fluid leukocyte count is normally < 180 cells/mm^3; a count that exceeds 200 is generally considered inflammatory.
- In acute infections, the count is often > 50,000, with predominance of polymor- phonuclear leukocytes.
- Gram stain smears are positive in 75–80% of patients with Gram-positive mi- croorganisms, but lower in the presence of Gram-negative or *N. gonorrhoeae* infection.
- Blood cultures are positive in a significant proportion of cases.

- Selected gonococcal media may be useful to plate from pharyngeal, rectal, cervical, or urethral specimens when *N. gonorrhoeae* infection is suspected.
- PCR has been used with success to detect *B. burgdorferi* DNA and gonococcal arthritis.
- Crystals should be sought, because crystal arthropathy may be inflammatory in the absence of infection.

THERAPY SHOULD INCLUDE

- Complete drainage and washing of the purulent joint
  - By arthroscopy (example: the knee joint)
  - Or by surgery (example: the hip joint)
  - Particularly important for *S. aureus* or Gram-negative infection
  - If activated polymorphonuclear leukocytes are allowed to remain in the joint space, this condition can result in irreversible cartilaginous damage.
- Systemic antibiotics × 3–4 weeks
  - Nafcillin or oxacillin (10–12 gm QD IV divided Q4H) for *S. aureus*
  - Third- or fourth-generation cephalosporin (Ceftriaxone 1–2 gm IV QD, Cefepime 2 gm IV Q8–12H) or fluoroquinolone (ciprofloxacin 500 mg po or 400 mg IV Q12H) for Gram negatives

OUTCOME

- One third of patients suffer significant residual joint damage.
- Adverse outcome is more likely in the elderly and in patients with preexisting joint disease.

DISSEMINATED GONOCOCCAL INFECTION

- 1–3% of patients infected with *N. gonorrhoeae* develop disseminated disease.
- Most commonly occurs in patients with asymptomatic mucosal infections
  - More common in women, 3 × more likely than in men
  - Higher incidence following menstruation or postpartum
    - During endometrial bleeding bacteria can more readily invade the bloodstream.
  - Patients with congenital or acquired deficiencies (including patients with systemic lupus erythematosus) of the terminal complement components (C5–C8) have a higher risk of developing disseminated gonococcal as well as meningococcal infection.
  - As compared to strains that cause urethritis, most strains associated with disseminated disease are penicillin-sensitive.
- Two clinical syndromes associated with dissemination:
  - Tenosynovitis, dermatitis, polyarthritis
    - The first manifestations of disease are fever, malaise, and arthralgias.
    - Subsequently inflammation of the tendons in the wrist, fingers, and, less commonly, the ankles and toes is noted.
    - On exam tenderness is noted over the tendon sheaths, and pain is exacerbated by movement.
    - The development of tenosynovitis in a young person is virtually pathopneumonic for disseminated gonococcemia.

- Pustular, pustular-vesicular, and, less commonly, hemorrhagic or papular skin lesions accompany the onset of tenosynovitis.
  - Lesions are often periarticular, relatively few in number (usually 4–10, rarely > 40 lesions)
  - Transient, spontaneously resolving over 3–4 days
- If untreated, patients with this syndrome may progress to purulent arthritis.
- Purulent arthritis without skin lesions
  - Similar to other forms of septic arthritis (see above)
  - High numbers of PMNs are found in the synovial fluid.

DIAGNOSIS

- Blood cultures are positive in about half of cases. More frequently positive in patients with the tenosynovitis-dermatitis-polyarthritis syndrome.
- Cultures and Gram stains of joint aspirates should also be performed, but are frequently unrevealing.
- Cultures and Gram stains of cervical and urtheral exudate, as well as skin lesions, should also be obtained.

TREATMENT (SEE TABLE 9-3)

- Parenteral ceftriaxone (1 g IV or im/day) continue for 24–48 hours after clinical improvement.
- Can then be switched to an oral regimen such a cefixime, ciprofloxacin, ofloxacin, or levofloxacin to complete 7–10 days of therapy.
- Alternative regimens including parenteral administration of other third-generation cephalosporins; a fluoroquinolone, or spectinomycin.
- Management of purulent joint effusions is identical to that of other forms of septic arthritis. As compared to *S. aureus*, and Gram-negative bacilli, residual joint damage is unusual following *N. gonorrhoeae*.

REFERENCES

Caputo GM, Cavanagh PR, Ulbrecht JS, Gibbons GW, Karchmer AW: Assessment and management of foot disease in patients with diabetes. *Engl J Med* 1994; 331(13):854–60.

Gentry LO: Approach to the patient with chronic osteomyelitis. In: *Current Clinical Topics in Infectious Diseases 8*. New York: McGraw-Hill Book Co., 1987, pp. 62–83.

Lew DP, Waldvogel FA: Use of quinolones in osteomyelitis and infected septic arthritis. *Drugs* 1999; 58 (Suppl 2):85–91.

Lew DP, Waldvogel FA: Osteomyelitis. *N Engl J Med* 1997; 336:999–1007.

Mader JT, Norden C, Nelson JD, Calandra GB: Evaluation of new anti-infective drugs for the treatment of osteomyelitis in adults. Infectious Diseases Society of America and the Food and Drug Administration. *Clin Infect Dis* 1992; 15 (Suppl 1):S155–S161.

McHenry MC, Easley KA, Locker GA: Vertebral osteomyelitis: Long-term outcome for 253 patients from 7 Cleveland-area hospitals. *Clin Infect Dis* 2002; 34: 1342–50.

Obrien JP, Goldenberg DL, Rice PA: Disseminated gonococcal infection: A prospective of 49 patients, and a review of the pathophysiology and immune mechanisms. *Medicine* 1983; 62:395.

12

PARASITIC INFECTIONS

- With the marked rise in international travel, parasitic infections are now increasingly being diagnosed in the United States, Europe, and other developed countries.
- Immunosuppressants and HIV allow dormant parasites to reactivate and cause disease.
- Thorough travel and exposure histories are critical steps in accurately diagnosing parasitic infections.
- An awareness of geography and environmental conditions and a familiarity with the life cycles of parasites are all required for proper diagnosis and treatment.

BLOOD PROTOZOA

Malaria

HIGHLIGHTS

- Beware of the international traveler who returns with a flu-like illness. Malaria should always be excluded.
- The clinician must differentiate *P. falciparum*, which is life-threatening, from other forms of malaria.
- In *P. falciparum* levels of > 5%, parasitemia greatly increase the risk of cerebral and renal complications, and constitute a medical emergency.
- Hospitalize all patients with *P. falciparum* who do not have prior immunity.
- Oral quinine or IV quinidine recommended for chloroquine-resistant *P. falciparum*, and oral chloroquine for other forms of malaria, combined with primaquine for *P. vivax* and *P. ovale* to treat hepatic hypnozoites.

Potential severity: Hours can make the difference between life and death. Rapid diagnosis and treatment are critical.

PREVALENCE

- The worldwide annual incidence of malaria is between 300 and 500 million cases, causing 2–3 million deaths.
- Areas with significant numbers of malaria cases include: Africa, the Middle East, India, Southeast Asia, South America, Central America, and parts of the Carribean.
- Chloroquine resistance is now the rule.

261

- *P. falciparum* in Southeast Asia is frequently resistant not only to chloroquine, but also to pyrimethamine-sulfadoxine, mefloquine, and halofantrine.
- Chloroquine-sensitive areas include Central America and the Caribbean, in particular Haiti.
- Updated patterns of resistance can be the CDC website (Internet address: www.cdc.gov/travel).

EPIDEMIOLOGY

- Humans contract malaria after being bitten by the anophiline female mosquito.
  - Certain strains appear to be more efficient transmitters
    - *Anopheles gambiae* and *Anopheles finestus* in Sub-Saharan Africa.
  - Preventive measures in addition to chemoprophylaxis include mosquito netting, long-sleeved shirts, long pants, insect repellant, and staying in a protected environment when the mosquito population is highest.

LIFE CYCLE (SEE FIG. 12-1)

- The female anopheline mosquito introduces sporozoites into the human bloodstream that quickly travel to the liver and invade hepatocytes.
- Within hepatocytes sporozoites mature to tissue schizonts.
- In *P. vivax* and *P. ovale* some sporozoites become dormant forming hypnozoites that can remain dormant for 6–11 months.
- Schizonts in hepatocytes then produce merozoites that are released into the bloodstream.
- Merozoites in turn can invade a single red blood cell and replicate.
  - Bind to a specific red blood cell membrane receptor (glycophorin A in *P. falciparum* and Duffy factor in *P. vivax*)
- The production of merozoites is followed by red blood cell lysis and release of merozoites that infect additional red blood cells.
- Merozoites in the red blood cell mature to a trophozoites forming signet rings that can be readily seen on RBC smears following Giemsa or Wright staining (see Fig. 12-2).
- As the trophozoites mature to red blood cell schizonts they split into multiple merozoites.
- Some merozoites mature in RBC into sexual forms called gametocytes.
- Mosquitoes bite humans, and gametocytes enter the mosquito where they sexually mate forming zygotes that develop into oocysts.
- Oocysts then form thousands of infectious sporozoites that move to the mosquito salivary gland where they are transmitted to the human host.

HUMAN | MOSQUITO

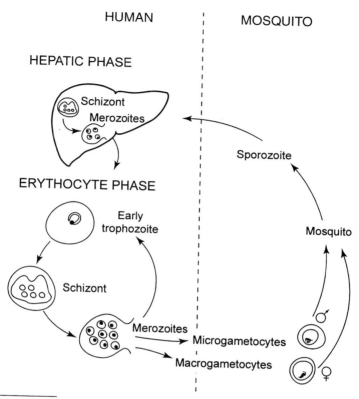

FIGURE 12-1
Life cycle of plasmodium.

DIFFERENCES IN THE LIFE CYCLE AMONG THE DIFFERENT *PLASMODIUM* SPECIES

- *Plasmodium falciparum* is the most dangerous form.
  - Has no dormant phase in the liver.
  - Merozoites can infect red blood cells of all ages allowing very high levels of parasitized red blood cells.
  - Multiple merozoites can infect and mature within a single red blood cell, and usually lyse the RBC within 48 hours.
  - Rapid asexual reproduction results in a rapid rise in the percentage of infected host red blood cells.
  - The risk of death or serious complications directly correlates with the level of parasitemia.

○ Adherence of *P. falciparum*–infected RBCs to blood vessel walls explains damage to humans.
  ■ Invasion is uniquely associated with the formation of red blood cell membrane knobs that tightly adhere to the vascular endothelium.
  ■ Causes vascular occlusion and severe hypoxic damage particularly to the brain and kidneys.
  ■ Increased red blood cell adherence develops as the merozoite matures beyond the early trophozoite stage, and explains the absence of more mature forms on peripheral blood (see Table 12-1 and Fig. 12-2).
○ Other strains of malaria
  ■ *P. vivax* > *P. malaria* > *P. ovale* in frequency of human infection.
  ■ *P. vivax* and *P. ovale* can form hypnozoites that can remain dormant within the liver for months.
    • These strains can relapse 6–11 months after initial treatment.

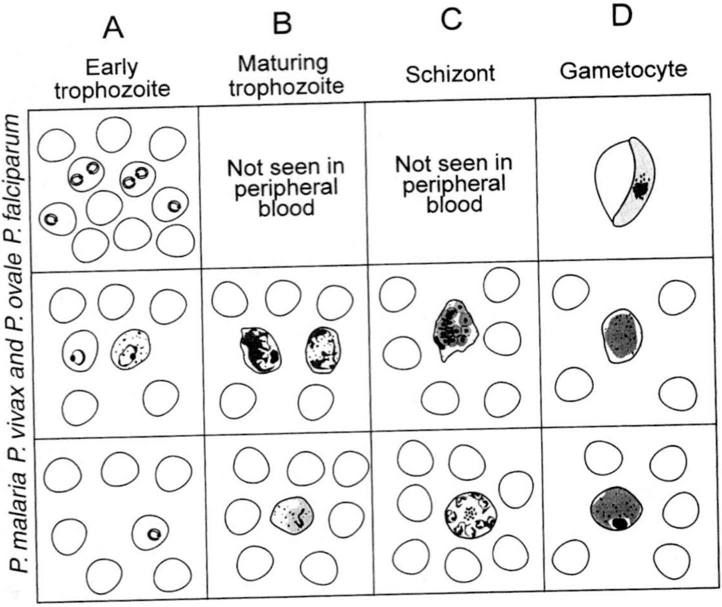

FIGURE 12-2

Typical blood smear findings of the different strains of malaria. (Adapted from Schaechter M, Engleberg NC, Eisenstein BI, Medoff G. (Eds.), *Mechanisms of Microbial Disease.* Baltimore: Lippincott Williams & Wilkins, 1999.)

TABLE 12-1
DIFFERENCES IN MALARIA STRAINS

P. falciparum	No dormant phase in the liver Multiple signet ring trophozoites per cell High percentage (> 5%) of parasitized RBCs Development stages other than the early ring trophozoite and mature gametocyte not seen
P. vivax and *P. ovale*	Dormant liver phase Single signet ring trophozoites per cell Schuffner's dots in the cytoplasm Low percentage (< 5%) of parasitized RBCs All developmental stages seen RBCs often appear enlarged in the later stages
P. malariae	No dormant phase Single signet ring trophozoites per cell Very low level of parasitemia All developmental stages seen RBCs normal size

- *P. malariae* has no dormant liver phase but can persist as a low-level infection for up to 30 years.
- Cause milder disease because that can infect only a small percentage of RBC.
  - *P. vivax* and *P. ovale* merozoites bind only young red blood cells, having the highest affinity for reticulocytes.
  - *P. malaria* tends to infect older red blood cells.

GENETIC DETERMINANTS OF SUSCEPTIBILITY TO MALARIA

- Sickle cell disease and trait are resistant to *P. falciparum*.
  - When parasitized red blood cells containing sickle cell hemoglobin become trapped in small vessels, low oxygen tension leads to sickle cell formation.
  - The polymerization of hemoglobin S kills the *P. falciparum* parasite.
- Negative Duffy blood group antigen prevents invasion by *P. vivax*, which requires this receptor for RBC entry.

CLINICAL PRESENTATION

- Presents as influenza-like syndrome
- Exposure history is critical for raising the possibility of malaria
- Incubation period:
  - 9–40 days for *P. falciparum*
  - 6–12 months for *P. vivax*
  - Years for *P. malariae* and *P. ovale*

- Fever is the primary manifestation.
  - Occurs at regular 2–3-day intervals in *P. vivax* and *P. malariae*, but has a more irregular pattern in *P. falciparum*.
  - Fever generally occurs soon after the lysis of the red blood cells and release of merozoites.
  - Three classic stages of the febrile paroxysms:
    - The "cold stage," which occurs 15–60 minutes prior to the onset of fever. The patient feels cold and has shaking chills.
    - The "hot stage," during which the body temperature rises to 39–41°C, associated with lassitude, loss of appetite as well as vague pains in the bones and joints. Commonly mistaken for influenza.
    - The "sweating" stage follows within 2–6 hours, consisting of marked diaphoresis followed by resolution of fever, profound fatigue, and a desire to sleep.
- Other symptoms primarily seen in *P. falciparum* as a consequence of severe hemolysis and small vessel occlusion particularly in tourists lacking immunity:
  - Jaundice can occur due to hemolysis and release of hemoglobin that exceeds the metabolic capacity of the liver, causing a rise in unconjugated bilirubin.
  - Dark urine as consequence of hemoglobin also may be excreted into the urine.
  - Black water fever refers to the combination of jaundice and hemoglobinuria.
  - Renal failure due to occlusion of vessels in the kidney and hemoglobinuria.
  - Pulmonary edema is a less common complication, resulting from fluid leakage from pulmonary capillaries into the alveoli.
  - CNS dysfunction results from vascular obstruction of small arteries in the central nervous system leading to hypoxia and is also due to hypoglycemia, which can develop during high-level infection.
    - Confusion and obtundation can rapidly progress to coma.
    - Grand mal seizures.

DIAGNOSIS

- The clinician must focus on differentiating *P. falciparum* from other forms of malaria (see Table 12-1).
- Blood smear remains the preferred method. The highest number of organisms is seen immediately following a fever spike.
  - The diagnosis of *P. falciparum* is favored by finding:
    - A high percentage of RBCs with ring forms
    - More that one signet ring in an RBC
    - The absence of other developmental stages
  - Smear should be repeated for 3–4 days to exclude the diagnosis.
  - Thick smears are more reliable than thin smears.
- In addition to smears, three assays are available to differentiate *P. falciparum* from other forms:
  - Enzyme-linked immunoabsorbance assay for histidine-rich *P. falciparum* antigen
  - An immunoassay for species-specific parasite lactic dehydrogenase isoenzymes
  - Polymerase chain reaction amplification of parasite DNA or mRNA

- Other laboratory tests
  - Hemolysis results in:
    - Anemia
    - Elevated lactic dehydrogenase (LDH) levels
    - Increased reticulocytes
    - Elevated unconjugated bilirubin level without a significant increase in hepatic enzymes
  - Thrombocytopenia is common.
  - Elevated serum creatinine, proteinuria, and hemoglobinuria are found in severe cases of *P. falciparum*.
  - Hypoglycemia may complicate severe cases of *P. falciparum*, requiring close monitoring of blood sugars during the acute illness.

PROPHYLAXIS

- Chemoprophylaxis should be given 2 weeks before departure to an endemic area and be continued 4 weeks after return.
- Up-to-date prophylactic and treatment regimens should be reviewed on the Center for Disease Control (CDC) web page (www.cdc.gov/travel).
- For areas with chloroquine-susceptible *P. falciparum*:
  - Chloroquine is the drug of choice. Dose 300-mg base (500 mg of chloroquine phosphate) po/week.
- For areas of chloroquine resistance:
  - Mefloquine, 250 mg (228 mg of base) po/week, or
  - Doxycyline, 100 mg po/day, or
  - Primaquine, 0.5 mg base/kg/day, or
  - Atovaquone, 250 mg combined with 100 mg proguanil (combination tablet called Malarone) po/day, or
  - The standard dose of chloroquine with proguanil, 200 mg/day.
- A vaccine is not available. The immune response required to protect the host against malaria is poorly understood, making the development of an effective vaccine a formidable task.

TREATMENT

- Hospitalize all individuals with *P. falciparum* without previous immunity.
- Patients with *P. vivax*, *P. ovale*, and *P. malariae* can usually be treated as outpatients if there is reliable follow-up.
- Antimalaria medication:
  - Chloroquine-sensitive *P. falciparum* and all other strains
    - Chloroquine, 600 mg base (1,000 mg of the phosphate) po initially followed 6 hours later by 300 mg of base (500 mg of phosphate) and again on days 2 and 3.
    - To prevent relapse of *P. vivax* or *P. ovale*, also treat with primaquine phosphate, 15.3 mg base (26.5 mg phosphate salt) po for 14 days or 45 mg base (79 mg salt) per week for 8 weeks (kills dormant hepatic hypnozoites).
    - Prior to receiving primaquine, all patients should be tested for glucose-6-phosphate dehydrogenase (G6PD) deficiency, because those with deficiency are at risk of severe hemolysis during primaquine treatment.

- ○ For chloroquine-resistant areas:
  - ▪ Quinine, 650 mg every 8 hours for 3–7 days, plus doxycycline, 100 mg bid for 7 days.
  - ▪ Alternative regimens have been recommended, including:
    - • Quinine plus pyramethamine sulfadoxine
    - • Quinine plus clindamycin (900 mg TID × 5 days)
    - • Mefloquine (1250 mg × 1). Frequently causes intolerable side effects including vertigo (10–20%), gastrointestinal disturbances, seizures, and less commonly psychosis
    - • Halofantrine (500 mg every 6 hours × 3 doses repeated in 1 week)
    - • Atovaquone (1,000 mg daily) plus proquanil (400 mg daily) (4 Malarone tablets) × 3 days
    - • Artesunate (4 mg kg/day × 3) plus mefloquine (750 mg followed in 12 hours by 500 mg)
    - • In the extremely ill patient unable to take oral medications, quinidine gluconate 10 mg salt/kg loading dose (maximum 600 mg) in normal saline should be infused slowly over 1–2 hour followed by a continuous infusion of 0.02 mg/kg/min until the patient is able to take oral medications (requires cardiac monitoring)
- • Other supportive measures:
  - ○ Severity of disease correlates with the level of parasitemia. Levels above 5% constitute a medical emergency and require intensive treatment.
  - ○ 10–15% levels of *P. falciparum* parasitemia in patients with no immunity should be considered for exchange transfusion.
  - ○ Volume status, renal function as well as serum glucose must be carefully monitored.
  - ○ Respiratory support may be required in cases of severe pulmonary edema.
  - ○ Intravenous steroids have been shown to be harmful in cases of cerebral malaria and, therefore, should not be used.
  - ○ Cardiac monitoring because of the risk of arrhythmias associated with quinine, quinidine, mefloquine, and halofantine.

Babesiosis

HIGHLIGHTS

- • A rare tick-borne infection that presents as a "summer flu."
- • More severe in the splenectomized patient and the elderly.
- • Blood smear reveals only ring forms; a tetrad ring form is pathopneumonic.
- • Treat with clindamycin and quinine.

Potential severity: Usually causes mild disease, but in splenectomized patients can be fatal.

PREVALENCE AND LIFE CYCLE

- • A rare human disease first found in Massachusetts on the islands of Nantucket and Martha's Vineyard. Subsequently found throughout New England, New York, Maryland, Virginia, Georgia, Wisconsin, Minnesota, Washington State, and California.

- Life cycle similar to that of malaria, except Babesia uses the small nymph form (2 mm in diameter) of the deer tick, *Ixodes scapularis*, to carry it from the white deer mice to humans.
- In human red blood cells the mature signet ring trophozoite multiplies by binary fission forming characteristic tetrads.
- Multiplication is asynchronous; therefore, RBC lysis is never massive.
- Babesiosis has no hepatic phase.

EPIDEMIOLOGY

- Endemic in areas where the deer population is abundant.
- Requires the presence of the white deer mouse, which harbors the infectious deer tick (*Ixodes scapularis*) nymphs.
- Human infections occur during the period of nymph feeding (May–September).

CLINICAL PRESENTATION

- Presents as the "summer flu" 1–3 weeks after exposure
- History of hiking in tick-infested areas
- Often no history of tick bite, because the *Ixodes scapularus* nymph is mistaken for a small freckle
- More serious disease occurs in splenectomized patients and can be more fulminant, being associated with severe hemolysis and death.
- More severe in the elderly. Adult respiratory distress syndrome and hypotension have been reported.
- Patients with babesiosis may also have Lyme disease because *Ixodes scapularis* transmits both infections. In one series 54% of patients with babesiosis possessed antibodies against the Lyme spirochete.

DIAGNOSIS AND TREATMENT

- Giemsa stains of the peripheral blood remain the best way to make the diagnosis.
- Only ring forms are seen, frequently mistaken for *P. falciparum*.
- Tetrad ring forms strongly support the diagnosis of babesiosis.
- Many malaria regimens, including chloroquine and primaquine, are not effective in babesiosis.
- Clindamycin, 300–600 mg every 6 hours IV or im, combined with oral quinine, 650 mg every 6–8 hours, for 7–10 days recommended.

TISSUE PROTOZOA

Leishmaniasis

HIGHLIGHTS

- Spread by the sandfly.
- Increased incidence in HIV patients and transplant patients.
- Visceral form (kala azar) often mistaken for lymphoma, usually causing hepatosplenomegaly, abdominal swelling, and weight loss.
- Cutaneous form results in large ulcerations that are "pizza-like."

- Treatment with liposomal amphotericin B for visceral form and topical paromycin and methylbenzethomium chloride for cutaneous disease.

Potential severity: Visceral disease is a chronic disease that can cause severe morbidity and death in debilitated and immunocompromised hosts.

PREVALENCE, EPIDEMIOLOGY, AND LIFE CYCLE

- Contracted in tropical areas where the Phlebotomus sandfly is common, rare in the United States. Found South America, India, Bangladesh, Middle East, and East Africa.
- Flagellated promastigote introduced by the sandfly is ingested by macrophages.
- In the macrophage develops into nonflagellated amastigote that lives happily within the macrophage phagolysosome.
- This intracellular parasite is controlled by activation of the Th-1 cell-mediated immune response that increases interferon-γ.
- Progression of infection is associated with Th-2 type response with production of interleukin-4, a cytokine that inhibits the production of Th-1 cells and the activation of interferon-γ production.
- Leishmaniasis can be an opportunistic infection in HIV and transplant patients.

CLINICAL PRESENTATION

There are three clinical forms: visceral, cutaneous, and mucosal.

Visceral Leishmaniasis (Kala-Azar)
- Caused by *L. donovani* (in India), *L. infantum* (Middle East), *L. chagasi* (Latin America), and *L. amazonensis* (Brazil).
- Incubation period is 3–8 months.
- Subacute onset: increased abdominal swelling due to massive splenomegaly and hepatomegaly, intermittent fever, and weight loss. Can be mistaken for lymphoma or infectious mononucleosis.
- Acute onset: persistent high fever mimicking bacteremia or malaria.
- Skin tends to be dry and thin, and takes on a grayish tint. This characteristic accounts for the Indian name "kala-azar," which means black fever.
- Anemia, leukopenia, and hypergammablobulinemia are common.
- Diagnosis is made by biopsy and Giemsa stain showing amastigotes.
- Enzyme-linked immunoabsorbent assays usually demonstrate high antileishmanial antibody titers. However, frequently cross-reacts with antibodies to other pathogens.
- HIV patients may have disseminated disease without a rise in antibody titer or splenomegaly. In HIV, amastigotes may be identified in macrophages from bronchoalveolar lavage, pleural effusion, bone marrow aspiration, or buffy coat samples of the peripheral blood.

Cutaneous and Mucosal Leishmaniasis
- Caused by *L. major* and *L. tropica* found in the Middle East, India, Pakistan, and Asia; and *L. mexicana*, *L. brazilensis*, *L. amazonensis*, and *L. panamensis* in Central and South America. *L. mexicana* has been reported in Texas.
- A problem for farmers, settlers, troops, and tourists.
- Found throughout the world, cases reported in Texas.
- Lesions occur primarily on exposed areas where infected sandflies bite. Incubation period 2 weeks–2 months.

- Organisms multiply within macrophages and produce a granulomatous inflammatory reaction.
- Skin lesions have a dry or moist appearance; ulcers have sharp raised borders; "pizza-like" lesions are common.
- Mucosal disease rarer, usually involves the nose, is caused by *L. braziliensis*.
- Diagnosis by biopsy; always biopsy the raised border of skin lesions.
  - Amastigotes are seen on Giemsa stain.

TREATMENT

- Visceral disease:
  - Liposomal amphotericin B in immunocompetent patients, 3 mg/kg body weight/day (in immunocompromised, 4 mg/kg) on days 1–5, 14, and 21
- Cutaneous: May spontaneously heal but if mucosa involved or in a cosmetically sensitive area treat with:
  - Topical with 15% paromycin and 12% methylbenzethomium chloride or
  - Pentavalent antimony (20 mg/kg/day × 20 days) (has many side effects) not approved in the United States or
  - Ketonconazole (400–600 mg/day × 4 weeks)

Trypanosomiasis (Trypanosome cruzi)

HIGHLIGHTS

- Transmitted by the reduviid bug found in native huts.
- Causes Chagas' disease, resulting in cardiomyopathy, megaesophagus, and megacolon.
- Treated with nifurtimax or benzidazole.

Potential severity: A chronic disorder that can lead to fatal cardiomyopathy.

PREVALENCE, EPIDEMIOLOGY, AND LIFE CYCLE

- *Trypanosome cruzi* causes Chagas' disease.
- Found throughout Central and South America. 16–18 million people worldwide; nearly one half million die from Chagas' disease annually.
- Transmitted by the reduviid bug, which carries the trypomastigote in its feces. This bug lives in the cracks of substandard housing.
- The host allows the parasite to enter the bloodstream by scratching and rubbing the infected feces into the skin.
- A disease of poor rural people, not tourists.

CLINICAL PRESENTATION

- Acute disease is associated with localized areas of swelling called chagomas.
  - Associated with local lymph node swelling.
  - Entry via the conjunctiva causes periorbital edema (the Romaña sign).
  - Local edema is quickly followed by fever, malaise, anorexia, and edema of the face and legs.

- Chronic disease develops decades after initial infection in 10–30% of cases.
- Immunocompromised hosts, such as organ transplant patients and AIDS patients, can reactivate, developing chronic disease; also at risk for brain abscess.
- Chronic diseases affects:
  ◦ The heart, causing a cardiomyopathy associated with CHF, emboli, and arrhythmias
  ◦ The GI tract, causing:
    ▪ Megaesophagus associated with dysphagia, regurgitation, and aspiration pneumonia
    ▪ Megacolon, causing constipation and bowel obstruction that can lead to perforation and bacterial sepsis

DIAGNOSIS

- Acute disease is diagnosed by Giemsa stain of a peripheral blood smear.
- Chronic disease can be diagnosed by ELISA assay that detects IgG antibody to *T. cruzi*.

TREATMENT

- Both acute and chronic disease should be treated.
  ◦ Nifurtimax, 8–10 mg/kg body weight per day divided into four oral doses for 90–120 days, cures about 70% of acute cases. Has gastrointestinal and neurologic side effects in many patients.
  ◦ Benzidazole, 5 mg/kg/day for 60 days, has a similar cure rate. Causes peripheral neuropathy, granulocytopenia, and rash.
- Treatment slows the progression of heart disease in chronic Chagas' disease.

INTESTINAL HELMINTHS

HIGHLIGHTS

- Helminths include roundworms (nematodes), flukes (trematodes), and tapeworms (cestodes).
- Large parasites, ranging in size from 1 cm to 10 meters.
- Often live in the human gastrointestinal tract without causing symptoms.
- Symptoms develop when the infection is very heavy or the worm migrates to extraintestinal sites.
- Transmission to humans in most cases results from contact with human waste.
- Diagnosis is generally made by examining the stool for eggs, larvae, or adult worms. (see Fig. 12-3).
- Treatment with mebendazole, except Strongyloides, which requires thiobendazole
- Stongyloides usually does not release eggs into the stool. Eggs hatch in the bowel, and filariform larvae reinfect the host.

Potential severity: Infections are often asymptomatic. In the immunocompromised host strongyloides can progress to a fatal hyperinfection syndrome.

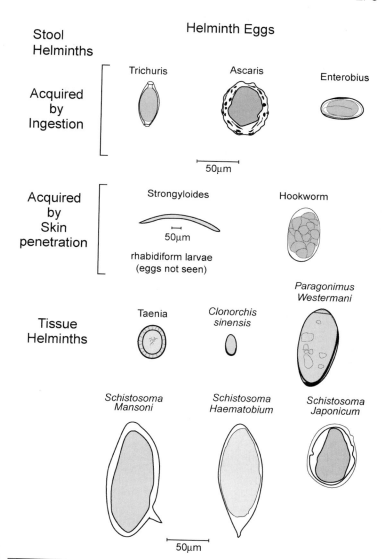

FIGURE 12-3

Helminth eggs. All eggs are drawn to scale. In Strongyloides only the rhabidiform larvae are usually seen.

INTESTINAL NEMATODES (ROUNDWORMS)

- Life cycles of the roundworm can also be classified into two groups (see Fig. 12-4), and life cycle differences account for some of the unique clinical characteristics of different species of nematodes.
    1. Trichuris and Enterobius attach and grow in the intestine soon after ingestion.
    2. Ascaris, Strongyloides, and hookworm first penetrate the venous system, enter the lungs, migrate up the trachea, are swallowed, and then take up residence in the gastrointestinal tract.

NEMATODES ACQUIRED BY INGESTION

- Tend to cause minimal symptoms and are not life-threatening
- Contracted by contact with fecal material
- *Trichuris tricura* (whipworm)
    ○ Causes iron deficiency anemia
    ○ Excretes lemon-shaped ova

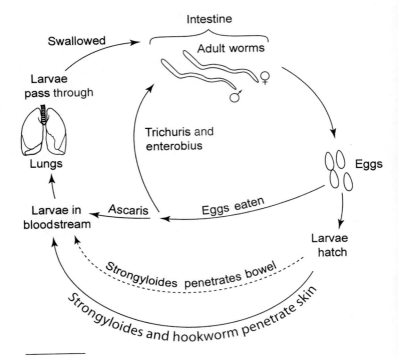

FIGURE 12-4
Comparative life cycles of intestinal nematodes. (Adapted from Schaechter M, Engleberg NC, Eisenstein BI, Medoff G. (Eds.), *Mechanisms of Microbial Disease.* Baltimore: Lippincott Williams & Wilkins, 1999.)

- Ascaris
  - After being ingested, larvae penetrate the small intestinal wall and enter the venous system.
  - Passes through the lung and can initially cause respiratory symptoms
  - Can cause biliary obstruction
  - Excretes round thick-walled ova
- Enterobius (pinworm) is common in children.
  - Readily spreads by dust and contaminated linen
  - Causes nocturnal perianal itching
  - Diagnosed by the scotch tape test demonstrates worms in the anal area
- Mebendazole 100mg po BID for 3 days is highly effective treatment and is rarely associated with side effects. A single 100 mg dose, repeated once at 2 weeks effective for enterobius.

NEMATODES ACQUIRED BY SKIN PENETRATION

Strongyloides

Prevalence, Epidemiology, and Life Cycle
- Less common than the other roundworms.
- Endemic in warm areas including the southeast United States.
- Because it can cause a fatal hyperinfection syndrome in the immunocompromised host, clinicians need to be familiar with this parasite.
- The filariform larvae excreted in the feces are capable of penetrating the skin and barefoot individuals can contract this parasite from fecal contaminated soil.
- Larvae enter the bloodstream, invade the lung, crawl up the trachea, are swallowed and mature in the small intestine (see Fig. 12-4).
- Adult worms deposit eggs in the bowel wall, where they hatch.
- Larvae in the bowel can enter the bloodstream, causing autoinfection.
- Infection can persist for 35–40 years.

Clinical Manifestations
- Many patients are asymptomatic.
- Skin penetration can cause an itchy erythematous rash.
- Lung invasion can produce a Löffler's syndrome (cough, wheezing, pneumonia, and eosinophilia).
- Heavy infection can cause abdominal pain and eosinophilia.
- When larvae penetrate the perianal area, a localized snakelike urticarial rash or a generalized urticarial rash may develop associated with eosinophilia.
- Hyperinfection syndrome
  - Treatment with high-dose steroids, severe malnutrition, or AIDS can precipitate a fatal hyperinfection syndrome (accelerated autoinfection).
  - Hyperinfection causes diffuse pneumonia, meningitis, abdominal pain, and Gram-negative sepsis. Eosinophilia is absent.
  - This clinical constellation, combined with childhood in the rural south or previous residence in a tropical region, should always raise the possibility of hyperinfection with Strongyloides.

Diagnosis and Treatment
- Diagnosis is difficult; eggs usually hatch in the gastrointestinal tract; therefore, Strongyloides eggs are rarely seen on stool smear.
- Larvae are found in the stool; duodenal aspiration may be required.

- Peripheral eosinophilia may the only finding, may increase to 10–20% of the peripheral white blood cells.
- Absence of eosinophilia, particularly in the hyperinfection syndrome, does not exclude the diagnosis.
- Serology may be helpful in immigrants, but is insensitive in travelers.
- Treat asymptomatic as well as symptomatic infections because of the danger of autoinfection. Treatment should be completed before use of immunosuppressive agents.
- Thiobendazole is the drug of choice: 25 mg/kg twice a day for 2 days (maximum dose 3 g/day).

Hookworm (*Acylostoma duodenale* and *Necator americanus*)

Prevalence, Epidemiology, and Life Cycle
- Infects nearly one quarter of the world's population.
- Found throughout the tropical and subtropical zones.
- Infection is prevalent in areas where untreated human feces are allowed to contaminate the soil and people walk barefooted.
- Larvae from the soil penetrate the skin (see Fig. 12-4).
- Larvae pass through the lung and then are ingested, taking up residence in the intestine.
- Adult worms attach to bowel wall and suck blood.
  - A single *Necator americanus* worm can remove 0.03 ml/day.
  - A single *Ancylostoma duodenale* worm can remove 0.2 ml of blood per day.
- Eggs hatch outside of the host in warm, moist soil; as a consequence, there is no autoinfection.

Clinical Manifestations, Diagnosis, and Treatment
- When hookworm larvae penetrate the skin, they can cause intense pruritis, sometimes called "ground itch."
- Like Strongyloides and Ascaris, hookworm can cause Löffler's syndrome.
- Iron-deficiency anemia is the most common manifestation.
- Other complaints may include abdominal pain, diarrhea, and weight loss.
- Individuals ≥ 50 years old have higher levels of worm infestation.
- Diagnosis made readily by seeing ova in the stool.
  - Female worms release 10,000–20,000 eggs per day.
  - The eggs are readily seen using a low-power (100×) microscope (see Fig. 12-3).
- Mebendazole, 100 mg twice a day for 3 days, is usually curative.

TISSUE AND BLOOD HELMINTHS
Trichinella

HIGHLIGHTS

- A disease contracted by eating poorly cooked pork.
- Causes eosinophilia, myositis, and periorbital edema.
- Treat with thiobendazole within 1 week of ingestion.

Potential severity: Usually asymptomatic, but heavy infections can lead to severe myocarditis, pneumonia, and encephalitis that can be fatal.

- Caused by ingesting larvae cysts, primarily from pork
- Uncommon in countries that do not feed pigs uncooked garbage
- Larvae infect skeletal and cardiac muscle
- Light infections are often asymptomatic
- Heavy infection causes:
  - Diarrhea and abdominal pain
  - Followed by:
    - Fever
    - Periorbital edema, subconjunctival hemorrhages, and chemosis
    - Muscle pain and weakness beginning in eye muscles, then involving neck and back, arms and legs
    - Occasionally a macular or petechial diffuse body rash may be seen.
    - Myocarditis
    - Symptoms usually peak within 2–3 weeks
  - Associated with marked eosinophilia and increased CPK

DIAGNOSIS

- Muscle biopsy demonstrating Trichinella larvae
- ELISA
- Often diagnosis is made clinically.
- If exposure to tainted meat is verified within 1 week of ingestion, thiabendazole, 25 mg/kg/day, can be given for 1 week. Active only against the intestinal phase
- Corticosteroids may be helpful in severe myocarditis.
- Cooking meat above 55°C until all pink flesh is browned kills encysted larvae and prevents trichinosis.

Echinococcus (Echinococcosis)

HIGHLIGHTS

- Spread primarily by sheepdogs that live around livestock.
- Forms large cysts primarily in the liver.
- Develop symptoms when lesions reach 8–10 cm in diameter.
- Treatment includes surgical resection, instillation of hypertonic saline or alcohol, and albendazole.

Potential severity: Rarely fatal. Clinical symptoms are often delayed by many years and result from the mass effect of the hydatid cyst.

PREVALENCE, EPIDEMIOLOGY, AND LIFE CYCLE

- Infections with *E. granulosus* are found worldwide, including Africa, the Middle East, southern Europe, Latin America, and the southwestern United States, and *E. multilocularis* in northern Europe, Asia, northern United States, and Arctic regions.
- Carried in the feces of sheep, goats, camels, horses, and domestic dogs that live around livestock.
- Spread primarily by sheepdogs that excrete eggs in their feces. Eggs survive in dust and contaminate food.

- Eggs hatch in the intestine and onchospheres enter the bloodstream, the liver, the lung, and less commonly the brain, forming hydatid cysts.
- Hydatid cysts consist of a germinal membrane that produces multiple tapeworm heads and also undergoes budding to form multiple septated daughter cysts within the primary cyst.

CLINICAL MANIFESTATIONS

- Most patients with echinococcosis are asymptomatic, infection being detected incidentally on an imaging study.
- Cysts can survive and grow in the host over decades, causing symptoms when they reach 8–10 cm.
- Begin compressing vital structures or erode into the biliary tract or a pulmonary bronchus.
- The cysts can also become superinfected, resulting in a bacterial abscess.
- Cyst leakage or rupture can result in an anaphylactic reaction causing fever and hypotension.

DIAGNOSIS

- CT scan, MRI, or ultrasound; often tapeworm heads can also be visualized.
- Confirmed by enzyme-linked immunsabsorbent assay (ELISA), which is highly sensitive for liver cysts, but less sensitive for cysts in other organs.

TREATMENT

- Surgical resection of the hydatid cyst is the treatment of choice.
  - Should be removed intact taking great care that the cyst not rupture, spreading the infection by daughter cysts.
  - To reduce the risk of spread, aspiration of the cyst is recommended with removal of a fraction of the contents and instillation of hypertonic saline (30% NaCl solution), iodophore, or 95% ethanol to kill the germinal layer and daughter cysts.
- Albendazole, 400 mg twice a day for 4 weeks, followed by a 2-week rest period with 3–4 cycles is recommended in the perioperative period to limit the risk of intraoperative dissemination.
- For inoperable lesions:
  - Same medical therapy as above.
  - Computed tomography–guided needle aspiration and instillation of cidal agents to sterilize inoperable lesions may be helpful, but experience is limited.

Taenia Solium (Cysticercosis)

HIGHLIGHTS

- Contracted by ingesting eggs or poorly cooked pork containing encysted larvae.
- Primarily infects the CNS, causing localized cysts.
- May cause grand mal seizures.
- Diagnosed by CT scan and serology.
- Treatment with albendazole or praziquantel reduces the incidence of seizures.

Potential severity: Causes neurologic complications in a significant number of infected patients many years after the initial infection.

PREVALENCE, EPIDEMIOLOGY, AND LIFE CYCLE

- Infections are common in Central and South America, Mexico, the Phillipines, southeast Asia, India, Africa, and southern Europe.
- Contracted by ingesting viable eggs, or infection is contracted by eating raw or undercooked pork containing encysted larvae.
- Eggs hatch or encysted larvae are released in the stomach and develop in the intestine into adult worms that can reach 8 m in length.
- Autoinfection can occur due to regurgitation of eggs into the stomach.

CLINICAL MANIFESTATIONS

- Adult intestinal worms rarely cause symptoms.
- Larvae can penetrate the intestine, enter the bloodstream, and eventually encyst in the brain causing, neurocysticercosis. Cysts may lodge in the:
  ○ Cerebral ventricles, causing hydrocephalus
  ○ Spinal cord, resulting in cord compression and paraplegia
  ○ Subarachnoid space, causing chronic meningitis
  ○ Cerebral cortex, causing seizures—the most common manifestation
  ○ Cysts may remain asymptomatic for many years until the larvae die
    ▪ Results in cyst swelling and increased inflammation

DIAGNOSIS

- Computed tomography or nuclear magnetic resonance scan is the preferred method.
  ○ Discrete cysts may enhance with contrast media depending on the degree of surrounding inflammation.
  ○ Multiple CNS lesions are usually detected.
  ○ Older lesions are often calcified.
  ○ In the absence of cerebral edema, lumbar puncture can be performed.
    ▪ CSF analysis reveals lymphocytes or eosinophils, accompanied by a low glucose level and an elevated protein level.
- Serologic tests detecting antibody directed against *T. solium* may be positive, particularly in patients with multiple cysts.

TREATMENT

- Complex and controversial.
- Praziquantel (50 mg/kg/day × 15–30 days) or albendazole (10–15 mg/kg/day × 8 days) is recommended. May temporarily increase inflammation and edema, but reduces the incidence of seizures.
- Symptomatic cysts may be surgically resected.
- Corticosteroids may be helpful for reducing edema and inflammation, and antiepileptic medications should be utilized to control seizures.

Schistosomiasis

HIGHLIGHTS

- Requires a freshwater snail as the intermediate host.
- Contracted by wading in stagnant freshwater pools where cercariae penetrate the skin.
- Migrate to the venous system of the small intestine (*S. japonicum*), large intestine (*S. mansoni*), and bladder (*S. haematobium*).
- Cause venous obstruction resulting in local symptoms involving the portal system and bladder.
- Diagnosed by biopsy or identification of eggs in the stool or urine.
- Treated with praziquantel.

Potential severity: Usually a chronic disorder resulting in debilitating complications. Occassionally fatal during the early stage of infection as a result of a severe serum sickness syndrome.

PREVALENCE, EPIDEMIOLOGY, AND LIFE CYCLE

- *S. mansoni*, *S. haematobium*, and *S. japanicum* infect 200–300 million people worldwide.
- *S. mansoni* is found primarily in South America, the Carribean, Africa, and Arab countries; *S. haematobium* in Africa and the Middle East; *S. japonicum* is found primarily in China and the Phillipines.
- Primary infection does not occur in the United States because the critical intermediate host, a specific type of freshwater snail, is absent. However, approximately 400,000 imported cases in immigrants from Puerto Rico, South America (particulary Brazil), the Middle East, and the Phillipines.
- Freshwater snails are infected by miracidia and are necessary for the production of cercariae that infect humans.
- Humans contract the disease by swimming or wading in stagnant freshwater pools or rice paddies contaminated by cercariae, which penetrate human skin.
- In the host cercariae mature to schistosomulae that enter the bloodstream and settle in the liver and lung where they mature.
- Mature worms migrate to the venous system of the small (*S. japonicum*) or large intestines (*S. mansoni*) or bladder venous plexus (*S. haematobium*).
- Release eggs for many years into stool or urine resulting in contamination of freshwater.

CLINICAL PRESENTATION

- Skin penetration causes "swimmers' itch."
- A serum sickness syndrome with eosinophilia and high IgE may follow and is called Katayama fever.
- Granulomatous reaction to egg deposition leads to chronic diarrhea, portal hypertension and hepatosplenomegaly, and pulmonary hypertension in *S. mansoni* and *S. japonicum*.
- Eggs deposited in the bladder can lead to hematuria, bladder obstruction, hydronephrosis, recurrent UTIs, and bladder cancer in cases of *S. haematobium*.

DIAGNOSIS AND TREATMENT

- Identification of eggs in stool and urine most common way to diagnose (see Fig. 12-3).
  - ○ Urine is best collected between 12 and 2 P.M. and passed through a 10-μ filter to concentrate the eggs.
  - ○ Eggs can be identified on tissue biopsies. Rectal biopsy is particularly helpful in diagnosing *S. mansoni.*
  - ○ Eggs may not be seen in chronic disease.
- Antischistosome antibody may be helpful in diagnosing chronic infection; however, the specificity and sensitivity are limited.
- Praziquantel is the treatment of choice.
  - ○ For *S. mansoni* and *S. haematobium*, 20 mg/kg given twice over 1 day.
  - ○ For *S. japonicum*, 20 mg/kg given three times in 1 day.
  - ○ Side effects of treatment are mild and include fever, abdominal discomfort, and headache.

OTHER, LESS COMMON TISSUE FLUKES

Clinorchis sinensis *(or Chinese Liver Fluke)*

- Infections result from the ingestion of raw or undercooked freshwater fish, occur in China, Hong Kong, and Vietnam.
- Worms gain entry into biliary tract via the ampulla of Vater.
- Infection can be complicated by cholangitis and later cholangiocarcinoma.
- Infections are effectively treated with praziquantel.

Fasciola hepatica

- A liver fluke found in sheep-raising areas of the world, including South America, Australia, China, Africa, and Europe.
- Ingestion of vegetables contaminated with encysted cercarae is the most common route of infection. This fluke is treated with bithionol.

Paragonimus westermani *(lung fluke)*

- Contracted by eating raw or pickled crawfish or freshwater crabs.
- Found in Central and South America, West Africa, India, and the Far East.
- Enters the gastrointestinal tract and subsequently penetrates through the diaphram, entering the pleural cavity and lungs and causing respiratory symptoms.
- Praziquantel is the treatment of choice.

Filariasis (Wuchereria bancrofti *and* Brugia malayi)

HIGHLIGHTS

- Transmitted by mosquitoes.
- Larvae enter the lymphatic system and then enter the bloodstream.
- Results in periodic fever and lymphangitis mimicking cellulitis, accompanied by peripheral eosinophilia.
- Chronic infection leads to elephantiasis.
- Diagnosis by blood smear.
- Treated with ivermectin combined with albendazole.

Potential severity: A chronic debilitating infection that can cause severe disfiguring complications by blocking lymphatic drainage.

PREVALENCE, EPIDEMIOLOGY, AND LIFE CYCLE

- Infects approximately 120 million individuals.
- *Wuchereria bancrofti* is found throughout the tropics.
- *Brugia malayi* is restricted to the southern regions of Asia.
- *Brugia timori* is found only in Indonesia.
- Infectious larvae are transmitted by the bite of a mosquito.
- Larvae pass from the skin into the lymphatic system where over several months they mature in the lymph nodes.
- Adult worms (40–100 mm in length) are then released into the bloodstream.
  - *W. bancrofti*, the highest concentration of worms in the blood around midnight.
  - Only 1% of mosquitoes are infected; therefore, large numbers of bites are required to contract the disease.

CLINICAL MANIFESTATIONS

- Many people, particularly children, are asymptomatic.
- Inflammatory filariasis:
  - Associated with periodic fever, chills, vomiting, headache, and malaise
  - Accompanied by lymphangitis of an extremity, orchitis, epididymitis, or scrotal swelling
  - Erythema, warmth, pain, and swelling mimic cellulitis; however, fails to respond to antibiotics
  - Associated with peripheral eosinophilia (6–25%)
- Chronic obstructive disease
  - Results in chronic limb swelling due to lymphatic fibrosis causing elephantiasis.
  - Can lead to recurrent bacterial cellulitis.
  - Rupture of lymphatics can cause chyluria or chylous ascites.

DIAGNOSIS AND TREATMENT

- Midnight blood smear demonstrating worms allows definitive diagnosis (except for cases from the South Pacific).
- In early and late disease worms may not be seen.

- Ultrasound of dilated lymphatics may demonstrate worms.
- Peripheral eosinophilia is common.
- Antibody titers may be helpful, but do not prove active disease.
- Diethylcarbamazine, 6 mg/kg daily by mouth for 2 weeks, kills some adult worms, but killing is not complete. Treatment may increase inflammation and may not halt progression to fibrosis and lymphatic obstruction.
- Ivermectin, 200–400 μg/kg combined with albendazole 400 mg as a single dose, is a more recent treatment regimen that may more effectively kill the adult worms.
- Anti-inflammatory agents may be used to reduce the extent of inflammation and elastic support stockings can be helpful in reducing moderate lymphedema.

PREVENTION

- Mass treatment over 5 years of individuals in areas with a moderate incidence of *W. bancrofti* have successfully controlled this infection.
- Areas with a high incidence may require more prolonged periods of mass treatment.

Dirofilariasis (Dog Heartworm)

- Humans are an accidental host.
- Most commonly found in the southeastern United States and is transmitted by mosquitoes.
- In humans the young forms migrate to the lung, but fail to develop and die, producing local granulomatous inflammation.
- Present as an asymptomatic pulmonary coin lesion mimicking an early neoplasm. Lung biopsy reveals a dead worm.
- Treatment of human cases is not necessary.

Onchocerciasis (Onchocerca volvulus)

- Found primarily in Africa, where it infects approximately 20 million people.
- Rare cases are seen in Central and South America.
- Transmitted by a black fly that swarms around the face, often biting around the eyes and depositing onchocerca larvae onto the skin.
- Larvae penetrate and crawl through the skin and connective tissue. The worms initially cause an itchy erythematous rash. Later fibrous skin nodules develop.
- Worms often migrate into the anterior chamber of the eye, causing inflammation and blindness. Because the black fly is commonly found near streams, this disease has been called "river blindness."
- Diagnosis is made by skin snips or visualizing worms by slit lamp examination of the eyes.
- The treatment of choice is ivermectin, 150 μg/kg orally, as a single dose repeated at 3-month intervals until symptoms resolve.
  - Fever, itching, and an urticarial rash may develop as result of dying microfilariae.

Loiasis (Loa Loa)

- Transmitted by a fly and is found in western and central Africa.
- The microfilariae migrate through the skin, causing localized edema called Calabar swellings.

- Can migrate through the subconjunctiva, causing intense conjunctivitis.
- Active microfilaria migration is associated with marked peripheral eosinophilia.
- Diagnosis is made by daytime blood smear.
- Diethylcarbamazine or ivermectin is recommended as treatment. Diethylcarbamazine can precipitate encephalitis in heavily infected patients.

REFERENCES

General Reading

O'Brien, D, S Tobin, GV Brown, J Torresi: Fever in returned travelers: Review of hospital admissions for a 3-year period. *Clin Infect Dis* 2001; 33:603–9.

Malaria

Aidoo M, Terlouw DJ, Kolczak MS, McElroy PD, ter Kuile FO, et al: Protective effects of the sickle cell gene against malaria morbidity and mortality. Lancet 2002; 359:1311–12.

Angus BJ: Malaria on the World Wide Web. *Clin Infect Dis* 2001; 33:651–61.

Bruneel F, Gachot B, Wolff M, Regnier B, Danis M, Vachon F: Resurgence of black-water fever in long-term European expatriates in Africa: Report of 21 cases and review. *Clin Infect Dis* 2001; 32:1133–40.

Kockaerts Y, Vanhees S, Knockaert D, Verhaegen J, Lontie M, Peetermans W: Imported malaria in the 1990s: A review of 101 patients. *Eur J Emerg Med* 2001; 8:287–90.

Wellems TE, Plowe CV: Chloroquine-resistant malaria. *J Infect Dis* 2001; 184:770–76.

Babesia

Hatcher JC, Greenberg PD, Antique J, Jimenez-Lucho VE: Severe babesiosis in Long Island: Review of 34 cases and their complications. *Clin Infect Dis* 2001; 32:1117–25.

Homer MJ, Aguilar-Delfin I, Telford SR III, Krause PJ, Persing DH: Babesiosis. *Clin Microbiol Rev* 2000; 13:451–69.

White DJ, Talarico J, Chang HG, Birkhead GS, Heimberger T, Morse DL: Human babesiosis in New York State: Review of 139 hospitalized cases and analysis of prognostic factors. *Arch Intern Med* 1998; 158:2149–54.

Leishmania

Berenguer J, Gomez-Campdera F, Padilla B, Rodriguez-Ferrero M, Anaya F, Moreno S, Valderrabano F: Visceral leishmaniasis (kala-azar) in transplant recipients: Case report and review. *Transplantation* 1998; 65:1401–4.

Herwaldt BL: Leishmaniasis. *Lancet* 1999; 354:1191–99.

Murray HW: Treatment of visceral leishmaniasis (kala-azar): A decade of progress and future approaches. *Int J Infect Dis* 2000; 4:158–77.

Rosenthal E, Marty P, del Giudice P, Pradier C, Ceppi C, Gastaut JA, Le Fichoux Y, Cassuto JP: HIV and Leishmania coinfection: A review of 91 cases with focus on atypical locations of Leishmania. *Clin Infect Dis* 2000; 31:1093–95.

Trypansomiasis

de Oliveira RB, Troncon LE, Dantas RO, Menghelli UG: Gastrointestinal manifestations of Chagas' disease. *Am J Gastroenterol* 1998; 93:884–89.

Rassi A, Jr., Rassi A, Little WC: Chagas' heart disease. *Clin Cardiol* 2000; 23:883–89.

Sinha A, Grace C, Alston WK, Westenfeld F, Maguire JH: African trypanosomiasis in two travelers from the United States. *Clin Infect Dis* 1999; 29:840–44.

Intestinal Helminths

Bethony J, Chen J, Lin S, Xiao S, Zhan B, et al: Emerging patterns of hookworm infection: Influence of aging on the intensity of Necator infection in Hainan Province, People's Republic of China. *Clin Infect Dis* 2002; 35:1336–44.

Grencis RK, Cooper ES. Enterobius, Trichuris, Capillaria, and hookworm including ancylostoma caninum. *Gastroenterol Clin North Am* 1996; 25:579–97.

Juckett G. Common intestinal helminths. *Am Fam Physician* 1995; 52:2039–48, 2051–52.

Liu LX, Weller PF: Strongyloidiasis and other intestinal nematode infections. *Infect Dis Clin North Am* 1993; 7:655–82.

Tanowitz HB, Weiss LM, Wittner M: Diagnosis and treatment of common intestinal helminths. II. Common intestinal nematodes. *Gastroenterologist* 1994; 2:39–49.

Strongyloides

Mahmoud AA. Strongyloidiasis. *Clin Infect Dis* 1996; 23:949–52; quiz 953.

Sarangarajan R, Ranganathan A, Belmonte AH, Tchertkoff V: Strongyloides stercoralis infection in AIDS. *AIDS Patient Care STDS* 1997; 11:407–14.

Siddiqui AA, Berk SL: Diagnosis of *Strongyloides stercoralis* infection. *Clin Infect Dis* 2001; 33:1040–47.

Sudarshi S, Stumpfle R, Armstrong M, Ellman T, Parton S, et al: Clinical presentation and diagnostic sensitivity of laboratory tests for *Strongyloides stercoralis* in travelers compared with immigrants in a non-endemic country. *Trop Med Int Health* 2003; 8:728–32.

Trichinella

Bruschi F, Murrell KD: New aspects of human trichinellosis: The impact of new Trichinella species. *Postgrad Med J* 2002; 78:15–22.

Capo V, Despommier DD: Clinical aspects of infection with Trichinella spp. *Clin Microbiol Rev* 1996; 9:47–54.

Clausen MR, Meyer CN, Krantz T, Moser C, Gomme G, Kayser L, Albrectsen J, Kapel CM, Bygbjerg IC: Trichinella infection and clinical disease. *QJ Med* 1996; 89:631–36.

Echinococcus

Balik AA, Basoglu M, Celebi F, Oren D, Polat KY, Atamanalp SS, Akcay MN: Surgical treatment of hydatid disease of the liver: Review of 304 cases. *Arch Surg* 1999; 134:166–69.

Bosanac ZB, Lisanin L: Percutaneous drainage of hydatid cyst in the liver as a primary treatment: Review of 52 consecutive cases with long-term follow-up. *Clin Radiol* 2000; 55:839–48.

Burgos R, Varela A, Castedo E, Roda J, Montero CG, Serrano S, Tellez G, Ugarte J: Pulmonary hydatidosis: surgical treatment and follow-up of 240 cases. *Eur J Cardiothorac Surg* 1999; 16:628–34; discussion 634–35.

Eckert J, Conraths FJ, Tackmann K: Echinococcosis: An emerging or reemerging zoonosis? *Int J Parasitol* 2000; 30:1283–94.

Taenia solium

Garcia HH, Del Brutto OH: Taenia solium cysticercosis. *Infect Dis Clin North Am* 2000; 14:97–119.

Garcia HH, Pretell EJ, Gilman RH, Martinez SM, Moulton LH, et al: A trial of antiparasitic treatment to reduce the rate of seizures due to cerebral cysticercosis. *N Engl J Med* 2004; 350:249–58.

Garg RK: Neurocysticercosis. *Postgrad Med J* 1998; 74:321–26.

White AC, Jr: Neurocysticercosis: Updates on epidemiology, pathogenesis, diagnosis, and management. *Annu Rev Med* 2000; 51:187–206.

Schistosomiasis
Bichler KH, Feil G, Zumbragel A, Eipper E, Dyballa S: Schistosomiasis: A critical review. *Curr Opin Urol* 2001; 11:97–101.

Ross AG, Sleigh AC, Li Y, Davis GM, Williams GM, Jiang Z, Feng Z, McManus DP: Schistosomiasis in the People's Republic of China: Prospects and challenges for the 21st century. *Clin Microbiol Rev* 2001; 14:270–95.

Siddiqui AA, Berk SL: Diagnosis of *Strongyloides stercoralis* infection. *Clin Infect Dis* 2001; 33:1040–47.

Talaat M, El-Ayyat A, Sayed HA, Miller FD: Emergence of *Schistosoma mansoni* infection in upper Egypt: The Giza governorate. *Am J Trop Med Hyg* 1999; 60:822–26.

Whitty CJ, Mabey DC, Armstrong M, Wright SG, Chiodini PL: Presentation and outcome of 1107 cases of schistosomiasis from Africa diagnosed in a nonendemic country. *Trans R Soc Trop Med Hyg* 2000; 94:531–34.

Filariasis
Bockarie MJ, Tisch DJ, Kastens W, Alexander ND, Dimber Z, et al: Mass treatment to eliminate filariasis in Papua New Guinea. *N Engl J Med* 2002; 347:1841–48.

Cunningham NM: Lymphatic filariasis in immigrants from developing countries. *Am Fam Physician* 1997; 55:1199–204.

Dunn IJ: Filarial diseases. *Semin Roentgenol* 1998; 33:47–56.

Shah MK: Human pulmonary dirofilariasis: Review of the literature. *South Med J* 1999; 92:276–79.

Onchocerciasis
Burnham G: Onchocerciasis. *Lancet* 1998; 351:1341–46.

Hall LR, Pearlman E: Pathogenesis of onchocercal keratitis (river blindness). *Clin Microbiol Rev* 1999; 12:445–53.

Malatt AE, and Taylor HR: Onchocerciasis. *Infect Dis Clin North Am* 1992; 6:963–77.

13

ZOONOTIC INFECTIONS

- The natural spread of infection from lower mammals to humans, termed zoonotic infections, has greatly increased over the past three decades.
- Zoonotic infections represent one of the most important classes of emerging infectious diseases.

SPIROCHETES

Lyme Disease (Borrelia burgdorferi)

HIGHLIGHTS

- Transmitted by a small nymph tick.
- Primary disease results in erythema migrans.
- Secondary disease is associated with Bell's palsy, meningitis, and carditis.
- Tertiary disease causes monoarticular arthritis and encephalopathy.
- Diagnosis is usually clinical for primary disease and by ELISA titer for later forms.
- Treatment regimens include doxycycline, penicillin, and ceftriaxone.

Potential severity: Can present acutely or result in a chronic disease that is rarely life-threatening.

EPIDEMIOLOGY, MICROBIOLOGY, AND PATHOGENESIS

- The most common insect-borne disease in the United States. Found in:
  - Northeast United States, Wisconsin, California, and Oregon
  - Temperate regions of Europe, Scandinavia, former Soviet Union, China, Korea, and Japan
- Caused by *Borrelia burgdorferi*, microaerophilic spirochete; grows on BSK-2 media
  - Expresses lipoproteins on its surface (Osps) that help the organism survive in hosts
  - Produces fibronectin-binding protein, flagellar antigen, and 2 heat shock proteins that cross-react with human proteins

287

- Transmitted by *Ixodes* nymph tick, from deer to white-footed mouse to humans
  - Size of a freckle, commonly missed
  - Must attach 36–48 hours to transmit the spirochete
- Begins in the skin, then disseminates
- Induces cell-mediated and humoral immunity
- Can survive for years in the joint fluid, CNS, and skin of untreated humans

CLINICAL MANIFESTATIONS

Just as observed in syphilis (see Chap. 9), Lyme disease can be divided into three stages:

- Primary disease (see Fig. 13-1)
  - Erythema migrans, the hallmark of primary disease, noted in 90% of patients
    - Macular expanding erythematous lesion, central clearing, but also may remain red in the center
    - Begins 1 month after the tick bite
    - Mean diameter 15 cm
    - Painless, can cause itching
- Secondary disease
  - Dissemination associated with small annular lesions and a flu-like illness
    - Generalized lymphadenopathy
    - Migratory joint, tendon, muscle, and bone pain
  - CNS involvement causes waxing and waning headache (10% of cases progress to serious neurologic manifestations if untreated)
    - Meningitis associated with headache and neck stiffness
    - CSF lymphocytosis (100 cells/mm^3)
    - Elevated CSF protein
    - Cranial nerve deficits (Bell's palsy) combined with peripheral neuritis, called Bannworth's syndrome
  - Cardiovascular involvement occurs in 5–8% of untreated cases.
    - Spirochetes infiltrate the myocardium, causing conduction defects.
    - EKG should be ordered in all patients with symptomatic Lyme disease.
    - First-degree heart block is most common; however, second-degree and complete heart block may also develop for a brief period.

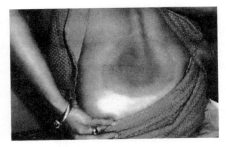

FIGURE 13-1
Erythema migrans of Lyme disease.

- Late disease (tertiary Lyme disease)
  - Symptomatic disease develops months to years after primary disease.
  - Musculoskeletal complaints are most common (60–80% of untreated patients).
    - Migrating arthritis and arthralgias
    - Joint fluid 500–110,000 cells/mm^3, primarily PMN
    - Usually improves with antibiotics
  - CNS—encephalopathy causing mood, cognitive, and sleep disorders
    - Elevated CSF protein and antibody against *B. burgdorferi*
    - Response to antibiotics variable
      - Acrodermatitis chronica atrophicans—a chronic skin infection containing spirochetes
      - Fibromyalgia- or chronic fatigue-like syndrome, controversial, antibiotics not helpful

DIAGNOSIS

- Cultures are rarely positive, and are not recommended.
- Diagnosis is made by combining epidemiology, clinical manifestations, and serology.
- Many patients with Lyme disease deny a tick bite.
- ELISA assay detects IgG and IgM antibodies.
  - Not recommended if classic erythema migrans; this finding is pathognomonic.
  - Titer rise is aborted by early antibiotic treatment.
  - IgM begins to rise at 2 weeks, declines by 2–3 months.
  - IgG rises at 6–8 weeks, persists for life; a negative IgG titer excludes late disease.
  - 3–6% false-positive rate.
- Western blot recommended to confirm all (+) ELISA tests.
  - 23 kDa OspC protein and the 41 kDa flagellar antigen most commonly cross-react.
  - Strict criterion for (+) Western have been established by the CDC.

TREATMENT (SEE TABLE 13-1)

- Primary disease: amoxicillin or doxycycline × 10 days. Longer durations of treatment with doxycycline, or treating with an initial dose of ceftriaxone, followed by 10 days of doxycycline is of no added benefit.
- Disseminated disease with mild carditis (1st-degree heart block) or 7th-nerve palsy: doxycycline × 21 days or IM ceftriaxone × 14 days.
- Meningitis or carditis with high-degree block: IV ceftriaxone or penicillin × 14–30 days.
- Chronic arthritis: doxycycline or amoxicillin × 30–60 days or meningitis regimen.
- Failure to improve on antibiotics suggests another diagnosis.

TABLE 13-1
ANTIBIOTIC TREATMENT OF ZOONOTIC INFECTIONS

Drug	Dose	Relative efficacy	Comments
Lyme disease—Early	Duration 21–28 days		
Amoxacillin (or)	500 mg po TID	First line	
Doxycycline	100 mg po BID		
Cefuroxime	500 mg po BID	Alternative	
—Early disseminated			
Doxycycline (or)	100 mg BID × 21 days		Jarisch-Herxheimer reaction common
Ceftriaxone	2 gm IM QD × 10 days		
—Heart block or meningitis	Duration 14–30 days		
Ceftriaxone (or)	2 gm IV QD		
Penicillin G	4 million units Q4H IV		
—Chronic arthritis	Duration 30–60 days		
Doxycycline (or)	100 mg po BID		
Amoxacillin (or)	500 mg po TID		
Rx of heart block and meningitis			
Leptospirosis—Severe	See text for duration		
Penicillin G (or)	1.5 million units IV Q6H		Jarisch-Herxheimer reaction common
Ampicillin	0.5–1 gm IV Q6H		
—Mild			
Doxycycline (or)	100 mg po BID		
Amoxacillin	500 mg po TID		

Rocky Mountain spotted fever	See text for duration	
Tetracycline (or)	500 mg po Q6H	First line
Doxycycline	100 mg po or IV Q12H	
Chloramphenicol	500 mg po or IV Q6	Alternative
Typhus	See text for duration	
Tetracycline (or)	500 mg po Q6H	First line
Doxycycline	100 mg po or IV Q12H	
Chloramphenicol	500 mg po or IV Q6	Alternative
Add rifampin in areas with resistant strains	600–900 mg po QD	
Erlichia	See text for duration	
Doxycycline	100 mg po or IV Q12H	Also preferred for children
Q fever	See text for duration	
Doxycycline (+)	100 mg po or IV BID	Add hydroxchloroquine for endocarditis
hydroxychloroquine	200 mg po TID	
Bartonella—Lymphatic disease	See text for duration	
Azythromycin (or)	500 mg po × 1, then 250 mg	All equally effective
Clarithromycin (or)	500 mg po BID	
Doxycycline (or)	100 mg po BID	
Ciprofloxacin	500 mg po BID	
—Severe disease	See text for duration	
Azythromycin (+)	500 mg po QD	Efficacy not proven
Rifampin	600 mg po or IV QD	
Brucellosis	See text for duration	
Doxcycline (+)	100 mg po BID	First line
Rifampin	600–900 mg po BID	
Doxycycline (+)	100 mg po BID	Single-drug therapy not recommended
Gentamicin	5 mg/kg IV QD	Alternative

PREVENTION

- When deciding on prophylactic antibiotics, a number of questions should be answered to determine the relative risk of contracting Lyme disease:
  - The size of the tick—Lyme disease is primarily spread by the *Ixodes scapularis* nymph. This tick is very small, about the size of a small freckle. Larger ticks are unlikely to transmit Lyme disease.
  - Attachment—If the tick fails to attach to the skin, it cannot transmit disease.
  - Engorgement—If the tick is engorged with blood, this finding suggests prolonged attachment and an increased risk of disease transmission.
- Prophylactic administration of a single dose of doxycycline (200 mg po) within 72 hours prevents the development of Lyme disease.
  - In areas where the incidence of Lyme disease is approximately 1/100, prophylaxis should be strongly considered.
  - A more targeted approach of administering prophylactic antibiotics to the individual who reports attachment of a small tick for > 24 hours, or finds an engorged tick, may prove more efficacious in areas of low incidence.

Leptospirosis

HIGHLIGHTS

- Contracted after exposure to contaminated fresh water.
- Presents with fever, conjunctivitis, and muscle tenderness.
- Later immunologic phase can cause aseptic meningitis.
- Weil's disease is a rare complication, associated with jaundice, renal failure, and pneumonia.
- Diagnosis is usually presumptive, being confirmed by rising antibody titers.
- Early treatment with penicillin or doxycycline.

Potential severity: Can cause a life-threatening systemic illness. Early diagnosis and treatment reduce the severity of the disease.

EPIDEMIOLOGY

- Found in temperate and tropical climates
  - Rare in United States, except for Hawaii
  - Follows flooding, particularly in Central and South America, Caribbean Islands
- Dogs, livestock, rodents, amphibians excrete in urine, contaminating soil and water
- Trappers, hunters, dairy farmers, livestock workers, veterinarians, military, and sewer workers are at risk.
- Outdoor, fresh water activities predispose to disease.

PATHOGENESIS

- Caused by *Leptospira interrogans*, a tightly coiled spirochete, slow-growing obligate aerobe.
  - 200 serovars of *L. interrogans* and different serovars have a predilection for different animals.
- Penetrates breaks in skin or softened skin after prolonged water exposure, in conjunctiva or mucous membranes, less commonly aerosolized entering via the lungs.
- Disseminates after traveling to the lymphatics and bloodstream.

- Outer surface coated with LPS. Glycoprotein toxin damages endothelial cells.
- Induces IgM and IgG antibodies directed against LPS, killed by macrophages.

CLINICAL MANIFESTATIONS

- Incubation period 5–14 days; severity depends on inoculum and serovar; rat serovars more severe.
- Two phases in less than half of patients:
    ○ Bacteremic phase: Sudden onset, fever, rigors, headache, photophobia, and severe myalgias; dilated conjunctival vessels, marked tenderness of the calf, thighs and midback; macular rash
    ○ Immunologic phase (4–30 days): Conjunctivitis, photophobia, retrobulbar pain, neck stiffness, diffuse lymphadenopathy, hepatosplenomegaly, and aseptic meningitis with CSF lymphocytosis
- Weil's disease rare, severe, mortality 5–40%:
    ○ High direct bilirubin, mild elevation in alkaline phosphatase, mild elevation in transaminase values combined with a high CPK
    ○ Renal failure accompanied by thrombocytopenia
    ○ Hemorrhagic pneumonia

DIAGNOSIS AND TREATMENT

- Usually a clinical diagnosis.
- Can be cultured from blood, CSF, and urine.
    ○ Low yield
    ○ Requires special media: Fletcher's, Ellinghausen's, or polysorbate 80 media
- Serologies helpful for confirming the clinical diagnosis.
    ○ Microscopic agglutination test (only in CDC reference labs), (+) 2 weeks, rises 3–4 weeks, ≥ 4-fold rise diagnostic, titer of ≥ 1:800 + symptoms = active disease, 1:200 suggestive
    ○ ELISA for IgM antibodies commercially available, good sensitivity and specificity
- IV penicillin or ampicillin for severe disease; oral doxycycline or amoxacillin for milder disease for 7 days (see Table 13-1).
- Prophylaxis in endemic areas; doxycyline.

RICKETTSIA AND RELATED INFECTIONS

HIGHLIGHTS

- The majority of cases are tickborne; however, typhus is contracted from lice and fleas and rickettsialpox by the mouse mite.
- Causes a febrile illness associated with headache and myalgias.
- A petechial skin rash is seen in Rocky Mountain spotted fever, but rare with Ehrlichia.
- Thrombocytopenia common with Ehrlichia. Neutropenia seen in the granulocytotropic form.
- Diagnosis is usually based on clinical features and epidemiology, and confirmed by serology.
- Treatment is with doxycycline.

GENERAL

- These organisms are small Gram-negative coccobacilli (0.3-μm diameter coccal forms, 0.3 × 1–2 μm bacillary forms).
- Obligatory intracellular pathogens.
- Clinically the rickettsial family of diseases have been classified into the spotted fever group and the typhus group.

Rocky Mountain Spotted Fever and Other Spotted Fevers

- Potential severity: Untreated Rocky Mountain spotted fever can be fulminant and fatal.

EPIDEMIOLOGY AND PATHOGENESIS

- Found throughout the United States, Mexico, Central and South America
  - Most common in the southeastern and south central United States
  - Areas of Cape Cod, Long Island, and some urban parks
- Injected into the skin by dog and wood ticks in the late spring and summer
- Proliferates in the skin, disseminates via the bloodstream
  - Survives in the host cell cytoplasm, spreads cell to cell, producing plaques of necrotic cells
  - Causes hemorrhage in skin, intestine, pancreas, liver, skeletal muscle, and kidneys

CLINICAL MANIFESTATIONS

- Incubation period 2–14 days.
- Acute onset of nonspecific symptoms: fever, headache, malaise, myalgias, and nausea. Abdominal pain may mimic cholecystitis or appendicitis.
- 5 days after symptoms begin, macular, petechial rash begins on ankles and wrists, spreads to trunk.
  - Spotless infection in 10%; occurs in elderly and African Americans.
  - Urticaria or pruritic rash makes RMSF unlikely.
- Aseptic meningitis, conjunctivitis, funduscopic hemorrhages, ARDS in severe disease.
- Respiratory complaints may become prominent and chest X-ray may reveal alveolar infiltrates or pulmonary edema, indicating ARDS.
- Gangrene of the digits can also develop in severe cases as a sequence of occlusion of small arterioles.
- Laboratory findings tend to be nonspecific.
  - The peripheral white cell count can be normal, elevated, or depressed.
  - Thrombocytopenia is common in more severe cases.
  - Elevations in BUN and serum creatinine may be noted.
  - Transaminase values and bilirubin levels may be elevated as well.
  - If appropriate therapy is not given within the first 5 days, RMSF can progress and cause death within 8–15 days.

DIAGNOSIS AND TREATMENT

- Presumptive diagnosis must be made based on epidemiology and clinical manifestations.
- Culture not recommended.
- Skin biopsy with immunofluorescence staining highly specific.
  - 70% sensitivity and 100% specificity
  - Not recommended if antibiotics given
- Retrospective diagnosis by serology: IFA, latex agglutination, or complement fixation.
- Mistaken for viral syndrome, drug allergy, and meningococcemia.
- Physicians in endemic areas should have a low threshold for treatment.
  - Doxycycline or tetracycline (see Table 13-1)
  - Chloramphenicol for children and pregnant women
  - Usually defervesces within 48–72 hours; continue antibiotics for 2–3 days after afebrile
  - Mortality 22% untreated, 6% with treatment

Other Spotted Fevers

- Boutonneuse fever is caused by *R. conorii*, clinically similar to RMSF.
  - Forms black escar at site of tick bite, called a *tache noire*
  - Found in Europe, Africa, and the Middle East
- Rickettsialpox, caused by *R. akari*, transmitted by a blood-sucking mouse mite.
  - Causes a papulovesicular rash, often mistaken for chickenpox
    - The number of skin lesions varies and they can involve the face, mucous membranes, palms, and soles
  - In the United States found in Boston, Pittsburgh, and Cleveland, as well as in Arizona and Utah
  - Also found in Mexico, South Africa, the Ukraine, Croatia, and Korea
  - Self-limited disease, quickly responds to tetracycline or doxycyline

Typhus

- Potential severity: Patients can become extremely toxic, develop shock and organ failure, and die.
- This group of diseases received the name typhus because the illness caused by these species of Rickettsia clinically mimics typhoid fever (see Chap. 8).

EPIDEMIOLOGY, PATHOGENESIS, AND CLINICAL MANIFESTATIONS

- Louse-borne typhus, caused by *Rickettsia prowazekii*, most serious form
  - Person-to-person spread by lice, common during World War II
  - Now found in Africa, less commonly in South and Central America
  - Rare in eastern and central United States; transmitted by lice or fleas from flying squirrels
  - High fever, severe retro-orbital and bifrontal headache, and myalgias
    - The headache comes on suddenly and is unremitting.
  - Causes small vessel vasculitis, petechial skin rash on trunk, multiorgan failure, peripheral gangrene, encephalitis; 30–70% mortality
- Brill-Zinsser disease is reactivation of *R. prowazeki*, milder, but similar to primary disease

- Flea-borne typhus caused by *R. typhi*, milder form of typhus, worldwide distribution
- Scrub typhus caused by *R. tsutsugamushi* and transmitted by mite larvae (chiggers)
  - Found in Japan, eastern Asia, Australia, and Pacific Islands
  - More gradual onset, black escar at chigger bite site in half of patients, rash common

DIAGNOSIS AND TREATMENT

- Presumptive diagnosis must be made by clinical and epidemiological findings.
- Antibody titers available, immunofluorescence staining of primary lesion helpful.
- Weil-Felix proteus agglutination no longer recommended.
- Treatment with tetracycline, doxycycline, or chloramphenicol for 3 days after became afebrile; may relapse, requiring retreatment (see Table 13-1).

Ehrlichia

- Potential severity: Can cause severe multisystemic disease that is usually not fatal. There are two forms of ehrlichiosis: human monocytotropic ehrlichiosis (HME), and human granulocytotropic ehrlichiosis (HGE).

EPIDEMIOLOGY AND PATHOGENESIS

- Human monocytotopic ehrlichiosis is caused by *E. chaffeensis*.
  - Transmitted by the Lone Star tick found on the white-tailed deer
  - Common Southeast United States; hikers and outdoor workers and golfers at risk
  - Prefers to invade macrophages and monocytes, less commonly entering lymphocytes
  - Reside in phagolysosomes and divide by binary fusion
  - Cluster together, forming intracellular inclusions called morulae
- Human granulocytopic ehrlichiosis is caused by *E. phagocytophila*.
  - Transmitted by Ixodes tick, same tick that transmits Lyme disease and Babesiosis
  - Found in California, Minnesota, Wisconsin, Massachusetts, Connecticut, New York, and Florida
  - Invades polymorphonuclear leukocytes and survives within these cells
- Both pathogens also infect the bone marrow, disrupting normal maturation and blocking production of leukocytes, red blood cells, and platelets.

CLINICAL MANIFESTATIONS, DIAGNOSIS, AND TREATMENT

- Incubation period 7 days, 5% mortality (elderly and immunocompromised)
  - Gradual onset of fever, chills, headache, myalgias, anorexia, and malaise
  - Severe monocytic form: respiratory insufficiency, renal insufficiency, and meningoencephalitis (with CSF lymphocytosis)
  - Severe granulocytic form: respiratory insufficiency, rhabdomyolysis, neutropenia resulting in Gram-negative sepsis
  - Macular, petechial rash in 30–40% of monocytic form, but only 2–11% granulocytic form

- Diagnosis presumptive in most cases
  - Thrombocytopenia and leukopenia common (neutropenia in granulocytic form)
  - Moderate transaminase elevations
  - Peripheral smears—morulae rare in monocytic form, common in granulocytic form (see Fig. 13-2)
  - Retrospective serologies
- Treat with doxycycline for 14 days. Chloramphenicol has no activity in vitro; therefore, doxcline also recommended for children (see Table 13-1).

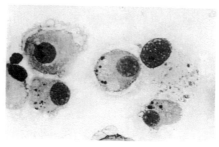

FIGURE 13-2
Granulocyte morulae found in human granulocytotropic ehrlichiosis.

Coxiella burnetti

- Potential severity: Q fever is usually a self-limited disease; however, the rare patient who develops Q fever endocarditis often dies.

EPIDEMIOLOGY AND PATHOGENESIS

- Rare in the United States, more commonly seen in Spain, France, England, Australia, and Canada
- Most commonly transmitted by farm animals: sheep, goats, and cows
  - Excrete in their urine, feces, birth products
  - Placenta highly infectious and aerosolized organisms survive for prolonged periods
- *Coxiella burnetti* is a small, pleomorphic Gram-negative rod; changes its outer lipopolysaccarides
  - Phase II outer antigens are expressed when in the environment
  - Phase I outer antigens are expressed when infecting the host
- Enters the host through the respiratory tract and survives within phagolysosomes of macrophages
  - Induces mononuclear cell infiltration, granuloma formation in the liver
  - Produces areas of focal necrosis and hemorrhage

CLINICAL MANIFESTATIONS, DIAGNOSIS, AND TREATMENT

- Incubation period 3 weeks, usually causing an abrupt flu-like illness with cough
- Less commonly causes a maculopapular rash (10% of cases), other rarer complications:
  - Severe respiratory comprise with ARDS
  - Hepatitis with elevated transaminases, but minimal elevations in bilirubin
  - Mycocarditis and pericarditis
  - Meningitis
  - Chronic endocarditis: negative echo early in the disease, high mortality
- Diagnosis by IgG and IgM antibodies against Phase I and II antigen (blood cultures negative)
  - IgG (titer ≥ 1:200) and IgM (≥ 1:50) anti-Phase II antigens = acute disease
  - IgG (≥ 1:800) and IgA (≥ 1:100) anti-Phase I antigens = chronic disease
- Treatment not as effective as for rickettsial infections (see Table 13-1)
  - Doxycycline × 2 weeks for acute disease; fluoroquinolones may also be helpful.
  - Doxycycline and hydroxychloroquine × 18 months–4 years or life for chronic endocarditis

Cat Scratch Disease, Bacillary Angiomatosis, and Other Diseases Caused by Bartonella

HIGHLIGHTS

- Transmitted by the scratch of a kitten (cat scratch disease) or by lice (bacillary angiomatosis).
- Cat scratch disease (*B. henselae*) causes local lymph node swelling that can become fluctuant.
- Bacillary angiomatosis (*B. quintana*) forms reddish hemangioma-like papules. Seen in indigent AIDS patients.
- Diagnosis is usually clinical. Antibody titers are available. Rarely biopsy is utilized.
- Treatment with azithromycin, clarithromycin, doxycycline, or ciprofloxacin.

Potential severity: Cat scratch disease and bacillary angiomatosis are usually localized diseases that rarely cause serious illness.

EPIDEMIOLOGY OF BARTONELLA INFECTIONS

- Cat scratch disease is caused by *B. henselae*.
  - Transmitted primarily by young cats and less commonly by cat fleas
  - A disease of young people who most commonly contract cat scratches
  - Common throughout North America, higher incidence in warm, humid areas
- Bacillary angiomatosis is caused by *B. henselae* and by *B. quintana*.
  - *B. quintana* transmitted by human body lice
  - Spread in areas with poor sanitation, persons with poor personal hygiene
- *B. bacilliformis* transmitted by the sand fly in the Andes Mountains of South America.
  - Causes Oroya fever and verruga peruana

PATHOGENESIS

- Pleomorphic Gram-negative rods, weakly take up Gram stain, silver stain preferred.
- Enter via the skin, spread to the local lymphatics, rarely disseminate except in AIDS patients.
- Survive within host cell intracellular vacuoles as well as extracellularly.
- Produce an angiogenesis factor that stimulates the growth of new blood vessels.
- Induce both a granulomatous and an acute PMN inflammatory reaction that prevents dissemination.

CLINICAL MANIFESTATIONS

Cat Scratch Disease
- Presents with a warm, tender swollen lymph node 2 weeks after the scratch.
  - Axillary node most common; involved node depends on the site of inoculation.
  - Node can enlarge to 8–10 cm in diameter; however, in most cases the involved node expands to a diameter of 1–5 cm.
  - The primary scratch can often be identified.
  - Low-grade fever is common.
- Rarer manifestations
  - Optic neuritis
  - Encephalopathy that can result in seizures and coma
  - Lytic bone lesions
  - Granulomatous lesions of the liver and spleen
  - Pneumonia
  - Erythema nodosum and thrombocytopenic purpura

Bacillary Angiomatosis
- *B. quintana is* major cause of bacillary angiomatosis (*B. henselae*, less commonly)
  - Seen in indigent AIDS patients with body lice, CD4 usually < 100/mm³.
  - Small reddish papules that coalesce into nodules, bleed profusely.
  - Mistaken for Kaposi's sarcoma, pyogenic granuloma, cherry angiomas, or hemangiomas.
  - Histopathology: multiple small vessels, enlarged endothelial cells, and PMN infiltration.
  - Can also infect the liver and less commonly the spleen, resulting in the formation of discrete blood-filled cystic structures. Called bacillary peliosis.
- Bacteremic illness rare; also called trench fever
  - Seen primarily in the homeless
  - Recurrent 5-day fever (quintan fever)
  - Splenomegaly is common
  - Some patients develop a maculopapular rash
  - Shin pain and malaise

DIAGNOSIS AND TREATMENT OF BARTONELLA INFECTIONS

- Grow on conventional media, slow-growing; clinical laboratory must be alerted.
- Blood cultures frequently falsely negative because organisms adhere to sides of the flask.
- Biopsies frequently unnecessary; Warthin-Starry stain showing black rods is helpful.
- Antibody titers using IFA or EIA, as well as PCR, are now tests of choice.

- Treatment (see Table 13-1): azithromycin, clarithromycin, doxycyline, or ciprofloxacin × 10–14 days.
  - In severe cases, IV azithromycin and rifampin (efficacy not proven)
  - Bacteremia with *B. quintana*, treat 4–6 weeks; endocarditis 6 months
  - Bacillary angiomatosis treat 2–4 months; tissue abscesses 4 months

BRUCELLOSIS

HIGHLIGHTS

- Contracted by contact with domestic or wild animals or by ingestion of unpasteurized milk or cheese.
- Causes a nonspecific febrile illness associated with headache, malaise, and back pain.
- Blood cultures are often positive, but must be held for 21 days. Serology helpful.
- Treatment should include two antibiotics: doxycycline and rifampin or doxycycline and gentamicin.

Potential severity: This febrile illness is often difficult to diagnose, but is rarely fatal.

EPIDEMIOLOGY

- Transmitted to humans by infected domestic and wild animals
  - Cattle, buffalo, camels, yaks, goats, and sheep
  - Swine, wild boars, fox, caribou, antelope, and elk
- Most common in the Mediterranean region, Arab Gulf basin, Indian subcontinent, Mexico, Central and South America. In United States uncommon, mainly in the south and southwest
- Enters via skin break or ingestion of unpasteurized dairy products (milk, cheeses)

PATHOGENESIS

- Aerobic Gram-negative coccobacilli, 3 pathogenic strains: *B. abortis*, *B. suis*, and *B. melitensis*
- Survives in phagolysosomes of PMN and macrophages by producing superoxide dismutase and blocking phagosome-lysosome fusion

CLINICAL MANIFESTATIONS

- 2–4-week incubation period: fever, chills, malaise, anorexia, headache, and back pain
- Important cause of FUO
- Lymphadenopathy and splenomegally only positive physical findings
- Focal infection more common if treatment is delayed for 30 or more days:
  - Osteomyelitis and arthritis, particularly sacroilieitis
  - Hepatic involvement is common
  - Lymphocytic meningitis
  - Endocarditis usually requires valve replacement
  - Positive urine culture common, orchitis in 20% of men
  - Bone marrow suppression, granulomas found
  - Pulmonary disease rare

DIAGNOSIS

- Blood cultures are positive in 70% of cases; hold for 21 days
- Bone marrow cultures often positive
- Serologic diagnosis frequently helpful
  - Serum agglutination or ELISA, IgM and IgG antibody titers
  - Titer > 1:160 or 4-fold rise between acute and convalescent samples

TREATMENT (SEE TABLE 13-1)

- Doxycyline plus rifampin, or doxycycline plus gentamicin or streptomycin × 6 weeks
  - Alternative for children: trimethoprim-sulfa plus rifampin
- Meningitis or endocarditis: doxycycline plus rifampin plus trimethoprim-sulfa × months-years
- Never use a single drug; high risk of relapse

REFERENCES

Lyme Disease

Kalish RA, Kaplan RF, Taylor E, Jones-Woodward L, Workman K, Steere AC: Evaluation of study patients with Lyme disease, 10–20-year follow-up. *J Infect Dis* 2001; 183:453–60.

Klempner MS, Hu LT, Evans J, et al: Two controlled trials of antibiotic treatment in patients with persistent symptoms and a history of Lyme disease. *N Engl J Med* 2001; 345:85–92.

Massarotti EM: Lyme arthritis. *Med Clin North Am* 2002; 86:297–309.

Nadelman RB, Nowakowski J, Fish D, et al: Prophylaxis with single-dose doxycycline for the prevention of Lyme disease after an *Ixodes scapularis* tick bite. *N Engl J Med* 2001; 345:79–84.

Sigal LH: Lyme disease: A clinical update. *Hosp Pract* (Off Ed) 2001; 36:31–32, 35–37, 41–42, 47.

Smith RP, Schoen RT, Rahn DW, et al: Clinical characteristics and treatment outcome of early Lyme disease in patients with microbiologically confirmed erythema migrans. *Ann Intern Med* 2002; 136:421–28.

Wormser GP, Ramanathan R, Nowakowski J, McKenna D, Holmgren D, et al: Duration of antibiotic therapy for early Lyme disease: A randomized, double-blind, placebo-controlled trial. *Ann Intern Med* 2003; 138:697–704.

Leptospirosis

Ko AI, Galvao Reis M, Ribeiro Dourado CM, Johnson WD, Jr, Riley LW: Urban epidemic of severe leptospirosis in Brazil. Salvador Leptospirosis Study Group. *Lancet* 1999; 354:820–25.

Sejvar J, Bancroft E, Winthrop K, Bettinger J, Bajani M, et al: Leptospirosis in "Eco-Challenge" athletes, Malaysian Borneo, 2000. *Emerg Infect Dis* 2003; 9:702–7.

Rickettsial Diseases

Comer JA, Diaz T, Vlahov D, Monterroso E, Childs JE: Evidence of rodent-associated Bartonella and Rickettsia infections among intravenous drug users from Central and East Harlem, New York City. *Am J Trop Med Hyg* 2001; 65:855–60.

Holman RC, Paddock CD, Curns AT, Krebs JW, McQuiston JH, Childs JE: Analysis of risk factors for fatal Rocky Mountain spotted fever: Evidence for superiority of tetracyclines for therapy. *J Infect Dis* 2001; 184:1437–44.

Masters EJ, Olson GS, Weiner SJ, Paddock CD: Rocky Mountain spotted fever: A clinician's dilemma. *Arch Intern Med* 2003; 163:769–74.

Paddock CD, Holman RC, Krebs JW, Childs JE: Assessing the magnitude of fatal Rocky Mountain spotted fever in the United States: Comparison of two national data sources. *Am J Trop Med Hyg* 2002; 67:349–54.

Reynolds MG, Krebs JS, Comer JA, Sumner JW, Rushton TC, et al: Flying squirrel–associated typhus, United States. *Emerg Infect Dis* 2003; 9:1341–43.

Watt G, Kantipong P, Jongsakul K, Watcharapichat P, Phulsuksombati D, Strickman D: Doxycycline and rifampicin for mild scrub-typhus infections in northern Thailand: A randomised trial. *Lancet* 2000; 356:1057–61.

Ehrlichiosis

Glushko GM: Human ehrlichiosis. *Postgrad Med* 1997; 101:225–30.

Ijdo IJ, Meek JI, Cartter ML, et al: The emergence of another tickborne infection in the 12-town area around Lyme, Connecticut: Human granulocytic ehrlichiosis. *J Infect Dis* 2000; 181:1388–93.

Wallace BJ, Brady G, Ackman DM, et al: Human granulocytic ehrlichiosis in New York. *Arch Intern Med* 1998; 158:769–73.

Q Fever

Caron F, Meurice JC, Ingrand P, et al: Acute Q fever pneumonia: A review of 80 hospitalized patients. *Chest* 1998; 114:808–13.

Bernit E, Pouget J, Janbon F, et al: Neurological involvement in acute Q fever: A report of 29 cases and review of the literature. *Arch Intern Med* 2002; 162:693–700.

Raoult D, Houpikian P, Tissot Dupont H, Riss JM, Arditi-Djiane J, Brouqui P: Treatment of Q fever endocarditis: Comparison of 2 regimens containing doxycycline and ofloxacin or hydroxychloroquine. *Arch Intern Med* 1999; 159:167–73.

Bartonella Infections

Brouqui P, Lascola B, Roux V, Raoult D: Chronic *Bartonella quintana* bacteremia in homeless patients. *N Engl J Med* 1999; 340:184–89.

Fournier PE, Lelievre H, Eykyn SJ, et al: Epidemiologic and clinical characteristics of *Bartonella quintana* and *Bartonella henselae* endocarditis: A study of 48 patients. *Medicine (Baltimore)* 2001; 80:245–51.

Loutit JS, Bartonella infections: Diverse and elusive. *Hosp Pract* (Off Ed) 1998; 33:37–38, 41–44, 49.

Zangwill KM, Hamilton DH, Perkins BA, et al: Cat scratch disease in Connecticut: Epidemiology, risk factors, and evaluation of a new diagnostic test. *N Engl J Med* 1993; 329:8–13.

Brucellosis

Chomel BB, DeBess EE, Mangiamele DM, et al: Changing trends in the epidemiology of human brucellosis in California from 1973 to 1992: A shift toward foodborne transmission. *J Infect Dis* 1994; 170:1216–23.

Colmenero JD, Reguera JM, Martos F, et al: Complications associated with *Brucella melitensis* infection: A study of 530 cases. *Medicine (Baltimore)* 1996; 75:195–211.

CHAPTER

14

BIOTERRORISM

- Potential severity: Biologic weapons are intended to kill and terrorize their victims. Treatment must be immediate and public health measures need to be instituted quickly and efficiently to prevent additional casualties.
- A biologic weapon is defined as the use of microbial agents for hostile purposes or in armed conflict. The "ideal" biologic agents should be:
  1. Able to reliably cause permanently debilitating or fatal disease in a high percentage of victims
  2. Capable of being targeted precisely to the enemy, and not cause a worldwide epidemic that could harm friendly soldiers or civilians
  3. Capable of being produced in large quantities at reasonable cost
  4. Capable of being stored for prolonged periods without losing potency
  5. Capable of being readily aerosolized to allow rapid delivery over a broad geographic area
- Only a restricted number of biologic pathogens fulfill most of these criteria. Four agents are of particular concern at the present time: anthrax, plague, tularemia, and smallpox are the top four potential biologic weapons.
- Other organisms that could be used as biologic weapons include botulinum toxins, brucellosis, Q fever, alpha viruses (Venezuelan equine encephalitis, Eastern and Western encephalitis), and viral hemorrhagic fevers (Ebola virus and Marberg agent).
- Medical personnel must be aware of the clinical manifestations, modes of transmission, appropriate diagnostic tests, and available treatment and prophylactic options for managing a biologic attack.

ANTHRAX

HIGHLIGHTS

- This Gram-positive rod forms spores that can be readily aerosolized.
- Inhalation disease causes two phases of illness:
  1. A flu-like febrile illness accompanied by a normal physical exam.
  2. Sudden onset of respiratory distress accompanied by meningitis in half of cases. CXR shows a widened mediastinum and may be accompanied by pleural effusions and/or an infiltrate.
- Cutaneous disease usually consists of a single nonpainful lesion in an exposed area. Develops into a black eschar with edematous margins.
- Diagnosis: In early phase the diagnosis is presumptive, based on epidemiology. In second phase, by culture and Gram stain.

- Treatment of inhalation disease: rapid initiation of IVciprofloxacin combined with second antibiotic. For cutaneous disease, oral ciprofloxacin; avoid surgical manipulation.
- Prophylaxis: ciprofloxacin or doxycycline $\times$ 60 days.

MICROBIOLOGY, PATHOGENESIS, AND EPIDEMIOLOGY

- *B. anthracis* is an aerobic Gram-positive rod, nonhemolytic on blood-agar plates.
- Under poor nutrient conditions forms spores.
  - Resist heat, high salinity, alkaline pH, and many disinfectants
  - When aerosolized enter the lung, are ingested by macrophages and transported to the mediastinum
- Spores germinate in the mediastinum and bacteria produce 3 exotoxins.
  - Protective antigen that binds to host cell receptors, allows lethal and edema factor entry
  - Lethal factor and edema factor cause cell lysis and tissue necrosis
- Naturally transmitted by animal products: wool, goat hair, and animal hides.
- Anthrax spores have been a favorite agent for use as a biologic weapon.
  - The devastating effects of aerosolized anthrax spores are illustrated by two events:
    - Accidental release of anthrax spores from a bioweapons plant in Sverdlovsk (now Yekaterinburg), Russia, in 1979 caused 96 inhalation cases and 64 deaths.
    - The introduction of anthrax spores into 5 letters sent through the U.S. Postal Service caused 22 cases of anthrax, 11 with inhalation disease and 11 cutaneous cases, and resulted in 5 fatalities.
      - Postal workers were at particular risk, because spores can be released from sealed envelopes during mail processing.
      - Cross-contamination of mail also occurred, killing 2 unsuspecting victims.
  - These recent events emphasize the importance of training public health and law enforcement personnel on proper handling of potentially contaminated samples, decontamination, and prophylaxis.

CLINICAL MANIFESTATIONS

- Health care personnel must be familiar with the clinical manifestations of anthrax.
  - Early recognition and treatment can be lifesaving.
  - Diagnosis of anthrax should raise the possibility of bioterrorist attack and warrant immediate notification of the proper authorities, to allow countermeasures to be emergently activated.
- An exposure and occupational history are very helpful in focusing on the possibility of anthrax in patients with a febrile illness or cutaneous lesions of unclear etiology.

CUTANEOUS ANTHRAX (SEE FIG. 14-1)

- Usually a single lesion develops on an exposed area of the body; arm most common.
- Develops 1–7 days after inoculation; begins as a papule.
- Progresses over 3–4 days to a vesicle filled with organisms; margin edematous.
- Lesion then ruptures and forms a black escar.
  - Origin of the name anthrax, which is the Greek name for coal

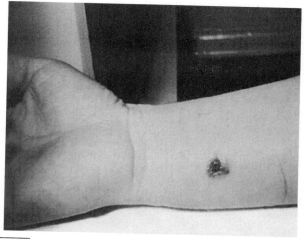

FIGURE 14-1

Typical cutaneous anthrax lesion. Note the black eschar and the edematous margins.

- Not painful, often itches.
- Lymphangitis, lymphadenopathy, fever, and malaise may accompany skin infection.
- Spontaneously heals over several weeks, leaving a scar.

INHALATION ANTHRAX (WOOLSORTERS' DISEASE) (SEE FIG. 14-2)

- Important that the clinician be aware of the biphasic presentation of inhalation anthrax.
- Recognition of the possibility of anthrax and treatment during the first phase can abort the fulminant and fatal second phase.
- First phase lasts 2–4 days.
  - Viral-like syndrome
  - Chest heaviness may be described.
  - Other less commonly described symptoms in U.S. cases:
    - Sweats, may be drenching
    - Sore throat
    - Nausea and vomiting
    - Abdominal pain
    - Headache and confusion
  - Physical exam usually unremarkable other than a few rhonchi on chest exam.
  - Symptoms and signs that favor anthrax over a viral respiratory syndrome include:
    - Neurologic symptoms in the absence of headache
    - Dyspnea
    - Nausea and vomiting
    - Abnormal pulmonary auscultation

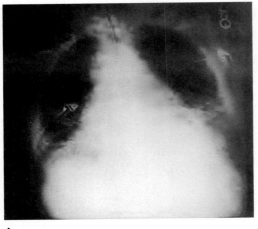
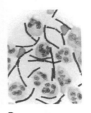

A **B**

FIGURE 14-2

Pulmonary anthrax. (A) Chest X-ray showing a widened mediastinum. (B) CSF Gram stain demonstrating boxcar-like Gram-positive rods. (From *N Engl J Med* 2001; 345:1607–10.)

- ○ Symptoms that favor respiratory viral syndrome over anthrax:
    - ▪ Rhinorrhea
    - ▪ Sore throat
- • Second phase follows phase 1 after a brief asymptomatic period.
    - ○ Sudden onset of severe respiratory distress
        - ▪ Fever
        - ▪ Tachycardia
        - ▪ Tachypnea
    - ○ Rales on chest exam
    - ○ CXR (see Fig. 14-2).
        - ▪ Widened mediastinum
        - ▪ Infiltrates may be seen
        - ▪ Pleural effusion frequently observed
    - ○ Thoracentesis: hemorrhagic fluid, positive Gram stain and culture
    - ○ Confusion in half of cases
        - ▪ CSF: PMN, positive Gram stain (see Fig. 14-2), and culture
    - ○ Blood cultures positive, and Gram stain of the peripheral blood may reveal Gram-positive bacilli.
    - ○ Death usually within 24 hours. Death can occur "in midsentence."

GASTROINTESTINAL ANTHRAX

- • A rare disease occurs primarily in developing countries.
- • Follows ingestion of contaminated meat.
- • Incubation period is usually 3–5 days.
- • Followed by sever gastrointestinal symptoms, including severe abdominal pain, hematemesis, and bloody diarrhea.
- • Death within 2–5 days.

DIAGNOSIS

- Epidemiologic history is important and the diagnosis is often presumptive.
  - In natural cases, a history of contact with herbivores or products from these animals, particularly if the products come from outside the United States.
  - In the setting of a possible bioterrorist attack, an employment history and history of being present in a contaminated area are important clues.
- Nasal swabs are helpful for determining the physical parameters of exposure, but not for deciding individual prophylaxis.
- Gram stain and cultures of skin lesions are often positive.
- Positive blood and CSF cultures usually accompany a fatal outcome.
- ELISA assays for antibodies against lethal and edema toxins are available. A 4-fold rise in titers over 4 weeks or a single titer of 1:32 is considered positive.
- A Laboratory Response Network has been established in the United States to specifically identify bioweapons pathogens. All suspected samples should be referred to one of these laboratories for confirmatory diagnosis.

TREATMENT AND PROPHYLAXIS
(SEE TABLE 14-1)

- Inhalation anthrax
  - Threshold must be very low in the setting of a bioterrorist attack.
  - Antibiotics must be given immediately in a symptomatic patient.
  - Intravenous ciprofloxacin (400 mg Q12H) or doxycycline (100 mg Q12H) combined with 1 or 2 additional antibiotics with activity against the pathogen.
  - Penicillin, ampicillin, rifampin, chloramphenicol, clindamycin, vancomycin, and clarithromycin all demonstrate in vitro activity.
  - Because anthrax strains may have constitutive as well as inducible β-lactamases, monotherapy with penicillin or ampicillin is not recommended.
  - When meningitis is suspected, doxycycline should not be used because of its poor central nervous system penetration.
  - Once the patient has stabilized, oral antibiotics can be given, ciprofloxacin (500 mg BID) or doxycyline (100 mg BID) being the treatments of choice.
  - Because of the risk of delayed germination of spores within the host, therapy should be continued for 60 days.
- Cutaneous anthrax
  - Oral ciprofloxacin or doxycyline for 60 days is recommended.
  - Avoid excision of skin lesions; danger of precipitating bacteremia.
- Prophylaxis for all individuals suspected of exposure:
  - Fluoroquinolone (ciprofloxacin, levofloxacin, or ofloxacin), alternative doxycyline × 60 days
  - Vaccine, inactivated exotoxin: military personnel and workers at risk of exposure, 6 doses for immunity followed by annual booster
  - Decontaminate exposed areas and personal items with 0.5% hypochlorite (1 part household bleach to 10 parts water)

TABLE 14-1
ANTIBIOTIC TREATMENT OF BIOTERRORIST BACTERIAL AGENTS

Drug	Dose	Relative efficacy	Comments
Anthrax—Prophylaxis	Duration 60 days		
Ciprofloxacin	500 mg po BID	First line	
Doxycycline	100 mg po BID	Alternative	
—Treatment	Duration 60 days		
Ciprofloxacin (or)	400 mg IV Q12H	First line	
Doxycycline	200 mg, followed by 100 mg IV Q12H		
In serious disease can be combined with:		Alternatives (see text)	
Penicillin G (or)	4 million units IV Q4H		
Rifampin (or)	600 mg po or IV QD		
Vancomycin (or)	1 gm IV Q12H		
Imipenam (or)	500 mg IV Q6H		
Clindamycin (or)	600–900 mg IV Q8H		
Clarithromycin	500 mg po BID		
Plague			
—Prophylaxis			
Doxycycline	100 mg BID × 7 days		

308

—Treatment Treat 10–14 days

Streptomycin (or)	15 mg/kg IM Q12H	First line	Equally effective
Gentamicin (or)	5 mg/kg IV QD		
Doxycycline	200 mg, then 100 mg IV Q12H		
Ciprofloxacin	400 mg IV BID	Alternative	Likely to be effective, but little clinical experience
Chloramphenicol	500 mg IV Q6H		Treatment for meningitis

Tularemia

—Prophylaxis Take for 2 weeks

Ciprofloxacin	500 mg po BID
Doxycycline	100 mg po BID

—Treatment Treat 10–14 days

Gentamicin	5 mg/kg IV QD	First line
Streptomycin	10–15 mg/kg IM Q12H	Alternatives
Doxycycline	200 mg, followed by 100 mg IV Q12H	

PLAGUE (YERSINIA PESTIS)

HIGHLIGHTS

- This Gram-negative rod can be aerosolized, resulting in pneumonia.
- Natural infection is spread by rhodent fleas and causes bubonic plague.
- Inhalation disease results in bloody sputum production, chest pain, and dyspnea. CXR shows bronchopneumonia.
- Diagnosis by sputum and/or buffy coat Gram stain.
- Treatment must be immediate with streptomycin, gentamicin, or doxycycline.
- Respiratory isolation × 48 hours after initiation of treatment.

EPIDEMIOLOGY, MICROBIOLOGY, AND PATHOGENESIS

- Usually spread by rhodent fleas; rare cases in the southwestern United States.
  - In the United States most common reservoirs are squirrels and prairie dogs.
- Soviet Union and the United States developed methods to aerosolize.
- A Gram-negative bacillus that grows aerobically on standard nutrient plates, including blood and MacConkey agar.
  - Grows slowly, often requiring 48 hours.
  - Colonies are small and grayish.
- Produces endotoxin and other virulence factors, including a coagulase and a fibrinolysin.
- Ingested by PMN and monocytes; able to replicate in monocytes.
  - Results in acute inflammation and tissue necrosis
  - Spreads to regional lymph nodes to form fluctuant bubos
  - Readily enters the bloodstream

CLINICAL MANIFESTATIONS

- Flea transmitted form, incubation of 2–8 days associated with:
  - Fever, chills, weakness, and headache
  - Followed by bubo formation; nodes very painful
    - Bubos are usually egg shaped 1–10 cm in length.
  - Within 2–4 days septic shock leads to peripheral gangrene and death.
- Pneumonic plague expected in a bioterrorist attack
  - Incubation period 2–4 days, chills, fever, myalgias
  - Within 24 hours:
    - Bloody sputum production (caused by bacterial coagulase, fibrinolysin, and tissue necrosis)
    - Chest pain
    - Followed by dyspnea and cyanosis
    - Also develop abdominal pain, nausea, vomiting, and diarrhea
  - Without antibiotic treatment, death occurs from circulatory collapse within 18 hours.

DIAGNOSIS

- A biologic attack with *Y. pestis* should be considered if large numbers of patients present to the ER with hemoptysis and severe rapidly progressive pneumonia.
- CXR demonstrates bilateral bronchopneumonia.
- Readily diagnosed by sputum or lymph node aspirate.
  - Gram stain usually reveals Gram-negative bacilli.
  - Gram stain of a buffy coat from peripheral blood reveals Gram-negative bacilli and strongly suggests the diagnosis.
  - Cultures usually require 48 hours.
  - A sensitive PCR method is under development.

TREATMENT AND PREVENTION (SEE TABLE 14-1)

- If pneumonic plague is not considered and conventional antibiotic treatment for community-acquired pneumonia is mistakenly begun, the disease will progress.
- Treatment must be rapid; a delay of greater than 24 hours results in 100% fatality.
- Streptomycin or gentamicin or doxycycline × 14 days.
  - Streptomycin considered the drug of choice.
  - Ciprofloxacin may be effective.
  - Chloramphenicol recommended for meningitis (crosses the blood-brain barrier).
- Surgical debridement of bubos should not be performed; high risk of spreading the infection to others (needle aspiration can be performed for diagnosis).
- Early treatment of pneumonic plague reduces mortality to 60%.
- Overall mortality for bubonic plague is 14%; however, early treatment is usually curative.
- Prevention:
  - Respiratory precautions required for pneumonic plague.
    - Can spread from person to person by aerosol
    - Respiratory isolation until 48 hours of antibiotic treatment has been completed
  - Doxycyline × 7 days for respiratory exposure
  - Vaccine under development

TULAREMIA
(FRANCISELLA TULARENSIS)

HIGHLIGHTS

- This Gram-negative coccobacillus usually causes ulcers, and glandular fever following skinning of an infected wild animal.
- Can be aerosolized resulting in bronchopneumonia similar to aerosolized plague. Cough is dry and nonbloody and patients may experience typhoid fever-like symptoms.
- Diagnosis usually presumptive, and later confirmed by serology.
- Treatment immediately with gentamicin, doxycycline, or streptomycin.
- Respiratory isolation is not required.

EPIDEMIOLOGY, MICROBIOLOGY, AND PATHOGENESIS

- Usually cutaneously spread from infected rabbits, muskrats, beavers, squirrels, and birds; hunters contract following skinning, dressing, and eating infected animals.
- Also spread by leaf blowers. In endemic areas consider tularemia in landscapers with an unexplained febrile illness.
- An aeorosolized form can be manufactured for bioterrorism.
- A small Gram-negative coccobacillus requires cysteine-supplemented media.
  - High fatty-acid content cell wall, LPS endotoxin, less potent than *E. coli.*
  - Intracellular pathogen induces acute inflammation and granuloma formation.
  - Low inocula causes disease (10–50 organisms), very dangerous.

CLINICAL MANIFESTATIONS

- Similar clinically to plague, incubation period 3–5 days
  - Abrupt onset of fever, headache, malaise, myalgias, abdominal pain, and diarrhea
  - A severe generalized headache is often a prominent complaint.
  - Ulceroglandular form: painful ulcer with raised borders, regional lymphadenopathy
  - 20% present with typhoid fever–like illness without lymphadenopathy
- Bronchopneumonia expected with bioterrorist attack, similar to plague except:
  - Dry, hacking cough, hemoptysis rare
  - May present with typhoid fever–like symptoms

DIAGNOSIS

- The presentation of a large number of patients with severe bronchopneumonia and a nonproductive cough should suggest a bioterrorist attack with *F. tularensis*
- CXR
  - Bronchopneumonia in 50% of cases after inhalation
  - Pleural effusions may be noted in 15%
- Pleural fluid tap reveals lymphocytes suggesting tuberculosis.
- Gram stain of sputum and skin ulcers usually negative.
- May be identified in lymph nodes by silver stain.
- Tissue and blood cultures may be positive, but:
  - Require special media containing a sulfhydryl compound.
  - A risk to laboratory personnel and must be handled in BSL-3 containment facility
- Diagnosis is usually presumptive; antibody titers rise after 2 weeks.
  - >1:160 antibody titer considered significant

TREATMENT AND PREVENTION
(SEE TABLE 14-1)

- Gentamicin the drug of choice; doxycycline and streptomycin alternatives
  - A streptomycin-resistant strain was developed in the 1950s as a weapon
- Person-to-person spread has not been reported, and respiratory precautions are not required
- Prophylaxis within 24 hours of exposure with ciprofloxacin or doxycycline × 14 days
- Vaccine under development
- Mortality is 30%; a less deadly agent than anthrax or plaque

SMALLPOX

HIGHLIGHTS

- This small double-stranded DNA poxvirus was eradicated in 1977.
- Spread from person to person by airborne droplets.
- Clinically differs from chickenpox in 3 ways:
  1. Has a more severe febrile prodrome than chickenpox.
  2. Skin lesions are synchronous is progression, while chickenpox lesions are found in all stages of development.
  3. Lesions are centripetal in spread, beginning on the extremities and spreading to the trunk. Chickenpox lesions spread centrifugally.
- Managed by strict respiratory isolation and supportive care.
- Rapid vaccination within 7 days of exposure is preventive.

GENERAL

- Endemic smallpox was eradicated in 1977 and smallpox vaccinations were discontinued for civilians in 1980 and for military recruits in 1989.
- A high percentage of the world's population is now without immunity to this deadly virus.
- Stocks of virus were kept in the United States and Russia raising concerns that this virus could be used in a bioterrorist attack.

EPIDEMIOLOGY

- Humans are the only reservoir for disease.
- Incubation period 7–17 days.
- Infectious with the onset of the rash, until all scabs separate from the skin (3–4 weeks).
  - Transmitted from person to person by coughing or skin particles
    - Most infectious if patient coughing or has the hemorrhagic form of disease
  - Spread within households and to hospital personnel
  - Virions can survive in the environment; inactivated by chlorine, ammonia, iodine, and autoclaving.

VIROLOGY AND PATHOGENESIS

- Variola is a double-stranded DNA virus.
- Replicates in the cytoplasm of host cells; infectious particles bud from the cell surface.
- Enters the lung via airborne droplets; spreads to regional nodes, then to bloodstream.
  - Disseminates to all tissues
  - Epithelial cells very susceptible; skin develops perivascular infiltration
  - Ballooning degeneration and inclusion body formation (Guarnieri bodies), followed by cell necrosis

CLINICAL MANIFESTATIONS

- The clinician must be able to differentiate from chickenpox (varicella-zoster virus).
- A prominent febrile prodrome for 2–4 days associated with high level viremia. Fever is accompanied by:
  - ◦ Rigors
  - ◦ Malaise, vomiting
  - ◦ Headache and backache
  - ◦ Delirium in 15% of cases
  - ◦ Virus can be readily cultured from the blood at this time
  - ◦ Chickenpox usually has a mild prodrome; patients often feel well prior to the onset of rash

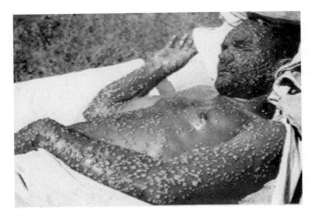

A

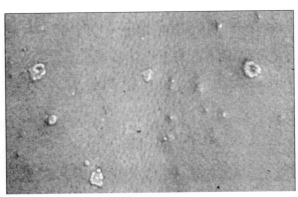

B

FIGURE 14-3

(A) Adult with severe smallpox skin lesions (from www.coldcure.com). (B) Close-up of individual raised skin lesions all at a similar stage of progression. (From Henderson DA: Smallpox: Clinical and epidemiologic features. *Emerg Infect Dis* 1999; 5:537–39.)

- Skin lesions have a centripetal spread (extremities to trunk) versus centrifugal spread in chickenpox (see Fig. 14-3 and Chap. 15).
  - Initially most prominent on the face and forearms
  - Subsequently spreads to the lower extremities
  - After a week spreads to the trunk
- Synchronous development versus asynchronous in chickenpox
  - Progress from macular to papular to vesicular to crusting; leaves scars
  - Lesions feel shotty, deep, and are uniform in size,
  - Chickenpox lesions are irregular in shape and size
    - Softer and superficial
    - Do not scar

DIAGNOSIS, TREATMENT, AND PREVENTION

- Readily diagnosed clinically
  - Can be confirmed by viral culture
  - PCR diagnostic techniques are under development
- Supportive care is the only therapy available. The key is to prevent disease.
  - Cidofovir may prove helpful, but there is no clinical experience with this agent.
  - Overall mortality for smallpox is 30% in unvaccinated and 3% in vaccinated patients. Mortality is highest in the very young and very old.
- Infected patients should be strictly isolated: negative pressure rooms, masks, gloves, gowns.
- Need to recognize and isolate partially immunized individuals with minimal symptoms, who can shed the virus and spread disease.

PREVENTIVE STRATEGIES

- Vaccine protective if given within 7 days of exposure.
  - The vaccine is a preparation of live vaccinia virus (cowpox virus) given by intradermal inoculation.
  - Successful vaccination should result in a vesicle formation at the site of inoculation followed by scar formation (scarification).
  - Disseminated vaccinia is a rare complication. Contraindicated in persons at increased risk for dissemination
    - HIV infection
    - Patients receiving immunosuppressants
    - History or presence of eczema
    - Persons who have close contact with individuals at risk
  - In preparation for an anthrax attack, risk benefit analysis favors vaccination of health care personnel, but not the general population.
  - Vaccinia immune globulin is protective, but impractical for mass prophylaxis.
    - Requires large volume IV injections (0.6 cc/kg IV or 42 ml in a 70-kg person)

REFERENCES

General

USAMRIID Medical Management of Biological Casualties Handbook, U.S. Army Medical Research Institute of Infectious Diseases. Frederick, MD: Fort Detrick, February 2001.

Anthrax

Borio L, Frank D, Mani V, et al: Death due to bioterrorism-related inhalational anthrax: Report of 2 patients. *JAMA* 2001; 286:2554–59.

Bush LM, Abrams BH, Beall A, and CJ: Index case of fatal inhalational anthrax due to bioterrorism in the United States. *N Engl J Med* 2001; 345:1607–10.

Centers for Disease Control and Prevention: Investigation of bioterrorism-related anthrax and interim guidelines for clinical evaluation of persons with possible anthrax. *JAMA* 2001; 286:2392–96.

Guarner J, Jernigan JA, Shieh WJ, Tatti K, Flannagan LM, et al: Pathology and pathogenesis of bioterrorism-related inhalational anthrax. *Am J Pathol* 2003; 163:701–9.

Hupert N, Bearman GM, Mushlin AI, Callahan MA: Accuracy of screening for inhalational anthrax after a bioterrorist attack. *Ann Intern Med* 2003; 139:337–45.

Inglesby TV, O'Toole T, Henderson DA, et al: Anthrax as a biological weapon, 2002: Updated recommendations for management. *JAMA* 2002; 287:2236–52.

Mayer TA, Bersoff-Matcha S, Murphy C, et al: Clinical presentation of inhalational anthrax following bioterrorism exposure: Report of 2 surviving patients. *JAMA* 2001; 286:2549–53.

Plague

Boisier P, Rahalison L, Rasolomaharo M, et al: Epidemiologic features of four successive annual outbreaks of bubonic plague in Mahajanga, Madagascar. *Emerg Infect Dis* 2002; 8:311–16.

CDC Imported plague—New York City, 2002. *MMWR* 2003; 52:725–28.

Gage KL, Dennis DT, Orloski KA, et al: Cases of cat-associated human plague in the Western US, 1977–1998. *Clin Infect Dis* 2000; 30:893–900.

Krishna G, Chitkara RK: Pneumonic plague. *Semin Respir Infect* 2003; 18:159–67.

Tularemia

CDC Tularemia—Oklahoma, 2000. *MMWR* 2001; 50:704–6.

Feldman KA, Enscore RE, Lathrop SL, et al: An outbreak of primary pneumonic tularemia on Martha's Vineyard. *N Engl J Med* 2001; 345:1601–6.

Feldman KA, Stiles-Enos D, Julian K, Matyas BT, Telford SR III, et al: Tularemia on Martha's Vineyard: Seroprevalence and occupational risk. *Emerg Infect Dis* 2003; 9:350–54.

Limaye AP, Hooper CJ: Treatment of tularemia with fluoroquinolones: Two cases and review. *Clin Infect Dis* 1999; 29:922–24.

Perez-Castrillon JL, Bachiller-Luque P, Martin-Luquero M, Mena-Martin FJ, Herreros V: Tularemia epidemic in northwestern Spain: Clinical description and therapeutic response. *Clin Infect Dis* 2001; 33:573–76.

Smallpox

Bozzette SA, Boer R, Bhatnagar V, Brower JL, Keeler EB, et al: A model for a smallpox-vaccination policy. *N Engl J Med* 2003; 348:416–25.

Frey SE, Couch RB, Tacket CO, et al: Clinical responses to undiluted and diluted smallpox vaccine. *N Engl J Med* 2002; 346:1265–74.

Frey SE, Newman FK, Cruz J, et al: Dose-related effects of smallpox vaccine. *N Engl J Med* 2002; 346:1275–80.

Joklik WK, Moss B, Fields BN, Bishop DH, Sandakhchiev LS: Why the smallpox virus stocks should not be destroyed. *Science* 1993; 262:1225–26.

SERIOUS ADULT VIRAL ILLNESSES OTHER THAN HIV

Potential severity: Most adult viral illnesses, with the exception of varicella, influenza, hantavirus, and SARS, can cause severe illness, but are not life-threatening.

VARICELLA ZOSTER VIRUS (VZV)

HIGHLIGHTS

- Spread by respiratory droplets with high efficiency from person to person.
- Chickenpox skin lesions are at various stages of development. They begin on the trunk and spread to the extremities.
- Herpes zosters usually develops in those > 50 years old and affects specific dermatomes.
- Treat adults with chickenpox and all cases of herpes zoster with acyclovir, valacyclovir, or famciclovir.

EPIDEMIOLOGY

- Chickenpox infects 3–4 million/year in the United States.
  - ○ Primarily a disease of children
  - ○ 10% of cases develop in adults
- Circulates exclusively in humans and there are no other known reservoirs of infection.
- Becomes epidemic in the susceptible population in winter and early spring, affecting both genders and all races equally.
- Highly infectious, attack rates of 70–90% in susceptible family members
  - ○ Spreads person to person by air droplets
- Herpes zoster herpes zoster affects primarily the elderly, 500,000/year in the United States.
  - ○ Caused by reactivation of latent VZV in those who have previously had chickenpox.
  - ○ Develops in up to 1% of people over 60 years of age.
  - ○ 75% of cases occur in those over age 45.

Based on Chapter 15 by Dr. Sankar Swaminathan in *Infectious Diseases in 30 Days*, F. Southwick (Ed.).

- ○ Not associated with exposure to others with chickenpox or zoster, but patients with zoster are capable of transmitting the virus to susceptible individuals.

PATHOGENESIS AND CLINICAL MANIFESTATIONS

- Double-stranded DNA virus
    - ○ Enters via the respiratory tract.
    - ○ Subsequently causes viremia and disseminates.
    - ○ Seeds the skin, as well as internal organs and the nervous system.
    - ○ Lifelong latent infection in the dorsal root ganglia is then established.
- Primarily infects the skin in chickenpox:
    - ○ Lesions begin on the trunk and face, spread outward to the arms and legs (centrifugal spread, see Chap. 14 for comparison to smallpox).
    - ○ Lesions in all stages (maculopapules, vesicles, and scabs) are present at the same time (asynchronous).
- Zoster or shingles
    - ○ Localized eruption along the course of one or more dermatomes.
        - ■ Most commonly the thoracic or lumbar dermatomes
        - ■ Begins as erythematous papules that evolve into vesicles
    - ○ The rash is often preceded by localized pain.
        - ■ In thoracic dermatomes can mimic an acute abdomen
    - ○ Involvement of certain nerves can be more serious.
        - ■ Opthalmicus (fifth cranial nerve, opthalmic branch)
            - • Infects the cornea, can be sight-threatening
        - ■ Ramsay-Hunt syndrome (fifth, ninth, and tenth cranial nerves)
            - • Facial palsy
            - • Loss of taste
            - • Lesions in external auditory canal

DIAGNOSIS

- Diagnosis is generally made based on the skin rash morphology.
- Rarely herpes zoster can be mistaken for herpes simplex infection.
- Vesicles can be cultured for virus.
- PCR is highly specific and sensitive.

COMPLICATIONS

- Pneumonia in adults can be fatal.
    - ○ More severe in pregnant women
    - ○ Severity often correlates with extent of the skin lesions
    - ○ Worse in smokers
- Encephalitis is rare, 20% mortality.
    - ○ Headache
    - ○ Often develop seizures
    - ○ Obtundation
- Herpes zoster is associated with multiple complications.
    - ○ Postherpetic neuralgia in up to 50% of patients. More common if > 50 years old
    - ○ Guillain-Barré syndrome, transverse myelitis, and encephalitis
    - ○ Ophthalmic branch keratitis, iridocyclitis, blindness, also granulomatous cerebral angiitis
    - ○ Dissemination in immunosuppressed patients is often fatal.
- 250 deaths/year from chickenpox in the United States, 15 × higher in adults

TREATMENT AND PREVENTION

- Acyclovir recommended for adolescents and adults with chickenpox. Serious infection should receive high-dose intravenous therapy.
  - Most effective when given within 24 hours of the appearance of the rash
  - Acyclovir 800 mg po 5 × /day for 5 days
  - For serious disease, acyclovir 10 mg/kg IVQ8H × 7–10 days
- Antiviral treatment for all cases of herpes zoster (acyclovir: 800 mg po 5 × /day, famciclovir: 500 mg po TID or valacyclovir 1 gm po TID × 7 days)
  - Reduces acute neuritis and accelerates healing
  - Prevents dissemination in the immunocompromised host
  - May reduce postherpetic neuralgia
  - Efficacy of concurrent treatment with corticosteroids to reduce postherpetic neuralgia is controversial
- Live attenuated vaccine highly efficacious (nearly 100% effective)
  - Recommended for all susceptible individuals > 12 months of age
  - Impact on herpes zoster not clarified
- Varicella zoster immune globulin effective at preventing active disease
  - Give within 96 hours of exposure
  - Recommended for all exposed pregnant women and immunocompromised patients

EPSTEIN-BARR VIRUS

HIGHLIGHTS

- Shed in the oral secretions of asymptomatic adults, allowing spread to unexposed individuals.
- Fever, sore throat, and lymphadenopathy are the hallmarks of mononucleosis.
- Diagnosis by heterophile antibody and IgM anti-VCA antibody titer.
- Therapy is usually supportive. Antibiotics should be avoided; 90% develop a rash with ampicillin.

EPIDEMIOLOGY, PATHOPHYSIOLOGY, AND CLINICAL MANIFESTATIONS

- Transmitted by the presence of virus in oropharyngeal secretions of asymptomatic shedders; 95% of adults carry the virus.
  - In the United States 50% of children are seropositive by age 5.
  - A second period of seroconversion occurs in early adulthood.
- Infects B cells; manifestations due to vigorous T- and NK-cell inflammatory responses.
- Fever, sore throat, and lymphadenopathy are the classic triad of mononucleosis.
  - Pharyngitis may be exudative and severe.
  - The enlarged lymph nodes are usually not tender.
  - Other findings include splenomegaly, hepatitis, palatal petechiae, jaundice, and rash.
  - Ampicillin almost always causes a rash.
- The differential diagnosis for mononucleosis should include acute HIV infection.
- The Monospot test may be negative, especially early in the disease.

COMPLICATIONS

- Acute complications:
  - Splenic rupture
  - Neurologic involvement
  - Airway obstruction
  - Less commonly hepatitis, hemolytic anemia, thrombocytopenia, and neutropenia
- Chronic complications:
  - Hairy leukoplakia
  - B-cell lymphoma and NK-cell lymphoma
  - Young adults who have EBV mononucleosis are at increased risk for EBV-positive Hodgkins lymphoma
  - Gastric adenocarcinoma and leiomyosarcomas
- X-linked lymphoproliferative syndrome (XLP) or Duncan's syndrome is prone to overwhelming lethal primary infection with Epstein-Barr virus.

DIAGNOSIS

- Heterophile antibody agglutination test (+) 90% of primary disease
- Monospot less sensitive in children, often needs to be repeated
- IgM antibody to VCA (viral capsid antigen) most sensitive and specific
  - Often elevated at the time of presentation
  - Declines quickly, absent by 4–8 weeks, positive IgM VCA = recent EBV infection
  - IgG VCA persists for life
- EBNA (nuclear antigen) begins to rise after 4 weeks, rising titer = recent EBV infection
- Antibodies to early EBV antigens are usually not helpful
- Quantitative PCR viral load is primarily experimental

THERAPY

- Acute mononucleosis is generally given supportive care
  - Avoid antibiotics when possible.
  - Prednisone (1 mg/kg/day of prednisone with tapering over 1–2 weeks) for airway obstruction, thrombocytopenia, or hemolytic anemia.
  - High dose acyclovir or ganciclovir may be helpful in very severe cases.
- Chronic active EBV infection
  - Very high antibodies to early antigens, no EBNA antibody production
  - Severe end organ involvement
  - May benefit from antiviral therapy
- Chronic fatigue syndrome—antiviral therapy of no benefit
- Oral hairy leukoplakia in HIV-infected patients due to lytic EBV infection
  - Acyclovir (800 mg po 5×/day) can control the infection.
  - Relapse often occurs when treatment is discontinued.

HANTAVIRUS

HIGHLIGHTS

- Humans are infected by aerosolized rodent saliva and urine.
- Begins with a mild fever followed by ARDS
- Diagnosis by PCR and immunofluorescence staining
- No treatment available other than supportive care

EPIDEMIOLOGY

- Spread by rodents that excrete the virus in their saliva and urine; aerosol inhaled by humans
- Risk factors include cleaning or entering any buildings that harbor rodents
- Found in the New Mexico, Arizona, Colorado, Utah four corners area, New England, and the Midwest

CLINICAL MANIFESTATIONS AND DIAGNOSIS

- Initially a mild febrile illness with abdominal pain that over a few days progresses to fulminant respiratory failure
  - Virus causes a pulmonary capillary leak syndrome with ARDS.
  - Severe hypoxia, hemoconcentration, immature white blood cells, thrombocytopenia, increased PTT, and LDH
- Diagnosis: Serology almost always positive at the time of admission
  - PCR and immunohistochemical stains can identify the virus in tissues.
  - If diagnosis suspected, CDC should be notified.

THERAPY

- Supportive care
- Cautious fluid administration
- If survive ARDS, fully recover

PREVENTION

- Avoid inhalation of aerosolized material contaminated by rodents
- General measures to decrease rodent infestation

SEVERE ACUTE RESPIRATORY SYNDROME (SARS)

HIGHLIGHTS

- First epidemic originated in China.
- Efficiently spread by aerosolized droplets, particularly by "superspreaders." Hospital personnel are at high risk for secondary infection.
- Begins with a febrile prodrome followed in 3–7 days by dry cough and dyspnea.

- Diagnosis: CXR patchy interstitial infiltrate combined with positive antibody to SARS coronavirus.
- Supportive care and strict respiratory isolation.

EPIDEMIOLOGY

- In March 2003 the World Health Organization orchestrated a worldwide effort to control a sudden outbreak of a progressive respiratory illness termed severe acute respiratory syndrome (SARS).
- First arose in Gunadon Province of China, and quickly spread to Hong Kong, Vietnam, Singapore, and Canada.
- In February 2003, an infected business man traveling from China stayed in a hotel in Hong Kong.
  ○ Infected 10 other individuals staying on the same floor
  ○ These individuals spread the illness to 5 different countries including: Hong Kong, Singapore, Vietnam, Thailand, and Canada
- Primarily spread to close contacts
  ○ Family members and hospital personnel not maintaining respiratory precautions
  ○ Transmitted in closed spaces, including airplanes

ETIOLOGY AND PATHOGENESIS

- A single-stranded RNA virus called coronavirus (similar to influenza and measles)
- SARS strain has a unique genomic sequence, being most closely related to bovine and avian coronaviruses and distantly related to human corona viruses
- An enveloped virus that does not withstand drying
- Attaches to cells in the respiratory tract and enters the cytoplasm of cells, where it multiplies
- Released from dead cells and also extruded from living cells
- Tissue damage thought to be primarily due to the host's immune response
- Primarily spread by respiratory droplets produced by coughing
  ○ "Superspreaders," individuals who produce small droplets and more efficiently spread the virus to others
- Excreted in the gastrointestinal tract
- Survives on surfaces and hands for approximately 3 hours

CLINICAL MANIFESTATIONS

- Adults aged 25–70 years previously healthy
- Few suspected cases < 15 years
- Incubation period typically 2–7 days (as long as 10 days)
- Prodrome of fever (> 100.4°F [> 38.0°C]) often high, can have chills and rigors with:
  ○ Headache, malaise, and myalgia
  ○ Mild respiratory symptoms
  ○ Absent—rash and neurologic or gastrointestinal findings
  ○ Diarrhea in some cases
- 3–7 days later lower respiratory phase:
  ○ Onset of a dry, nonproductive cough
  ○ Dyspnea
  ○ Hypoxemia
  ○ 10–20% require intubation and mechanical ventilation

LABORATORY FINDINGS

- Absolute lymphocyte count often decreased
- WBC normal or decreased
- Leukopenia and thrombocytopenia or low-normal platelet counts (50,000–150,000/µL) at the peak of the respiratory illness in 50%
- CPK (up to 3,000 IU/L) and hepatic transaminases (2–6 × normal) increased early in the respiratory phase
- LDH elevated 70–80%
- Renal function remains normal

CXR

- Normal during the febrile prodrome
- Abnormal during the respiratory phase
  - Early focal interstitial infiltrates
  - Progress to more generalized, patchy, interstitial infiltrates
  - Late stages can develop areas of consolidation
  - Pulmonary pathology: pulmonary edema, desquamation of type 2 pneumocytes

DIAGNOSIS USES THE WHO DEFINITIONS

- Suspected case:
  - Fever > 38°C (≥ 100.5°F) **plus**
  - Cough or difficulty breathing **plus**
  - Residence in an area with recent local transmission of SARS within 10 days of the onset of symptoms
- Probable case:
  - A suspected case with CXR findings of pneumonia or ARDS **or**
  - A suspected case with a positive test for SARS **or**
  - A suspected case with an unexplained respiratory illness leading to death with autopsy demonstrating the pathology of ARDS without a defined cause

TREATMENT AND OUTCOME

- Meticulous supportive care
- No specific treatment has proved to be efficacious. Therapies attempted:
  - Antibiotics (may prevent bacterial superinfection). Considered later in the disease based on Gram stain findings (see Chaps. 1 and 4)
  - Oseltamivir or intravenous ribavirin
  - Ribavirin and corticosteroids (some patients have worsened as corticosteroids have been tapered)
- Fatality Rate 8% worldwide; poorer prognosis with
  - Older age (≥ 60 years, 43% mortality in Hong Kong cases)
  - High LDH or high PMN count

PREVENTION

- Strict respiratory isolation of all suspected cases
  - Isolate hospitalized patients in negative pressure rooms.
  - N-95 respirator masks should be worn, gowns, globes, protective eye wear.
  - Health care workers are at particular high risk if present during intubation of an infected patient (can be mistaken for CHF).

- Possible infected patients who do not require hospitalization
  - Should not leave home until asymptomatic for 10 days
  - Should use separate utensils, towels, etc.
  - Contacts may leave home as long as they are asymptomatic
- Travel advisories by WHO for areas where multiple active cases are reported

---

INFLUENZA

HIGHLIGHTS

- Influenza A and B can cause epidemics and influenza A pandemics.
- Spread efficiently from person to person by aerosolized respiratory secretions.
- Present with high fever, headache, myalgias, rhinorrhea, and nonexudative pharyngitis.
- Can be complicated by severe pneumonia.
- Commercial immunodetection methods available, only 60% sensitivity.
- Treat within 48 hours with amantadine or rimantidine for Influenza A and the neuramidase inhibitor oseltamivir for influenza A and B.
- Influenza vaccine recommended for groups at increased risk for complications and persons with increased risk of transmitting infection to others.

EPIDEMIOLOGY

- Influenza A and B cause epidemics; influenza A also causes pandemics
- Epidemics every 1–3 years, occur in the winter
- Antigenic drift = changes in hemagglutinin and neuraminidase proteins by genetic mutation
- Antigenic shift = reassortment, or exchange of genomic segments with avian influenza species
  - Occurs in influenza A
  - Causes pandemics
  - Reassortment may occur in pigs and possibly birds
- Virus is spread by aerosols from respiratory secretions.
- In United States, 15 million infections annually in the young, 4 million in older adults

PATHOPHYSIOLOGY AND CLINICAL MANIFESTATIONS AND COMPLICATIONS

- Infects the respiratory epithelium and kills host cells as it replicates.
  - Virus multiplies rapidly, leading to the production of large numbers of infectious virus in the respiratory secretions.
  - Causes diffuse inflammation and damage
  - In severe cases, causes extensive necrosis
- Abrupt onset of high fever and shaking chills associated with:
  - Headache
  - Myalgias
  - Rhinorrhea and nonexudative pharyngitis with cervical adenopathy

- Recovery can be prolonged, taking up to 3 weeks or even longer.
  - Persistent cough and fatigue
  - Pulmonary function can remain abnormal for weeks.
- Complications:
  - Viral pneumonia can progress to fatal ARDS and pulmonary hemorrhage.
    - The leading cause of death
  - Superinfection with *S. aureus*, *H. influenzae*, or *S. pneumoniae*
    - Appear to be recovering from influenza, but then suddenly develop fever and typical signs of bacterial pneumonia (see Chap. 4)
  - Reye's syndrome associated with aspirin use
    - Fatty infiltration of the liver
    - Lethargy or even delirium and coma, associated with cerebral edema

DIAGNOSIS

- With influenza as opposed to other respiratory illnesses there is a predominance of the systemic symptoms.
  - Epidemic nature of the disease in the community is helpful.
  - When influenza is circulating in a community, an adult displaying the symptoms described above is highly likely to have influenza.
- Commercial immunodetection methods able to make rapid diagnosis
  - Depends on the adequacy of samples
  - Sensitivity can be as low as 60%.
  - Viral culture confirmatory

TREATMENT

- For influenza A give amantadine (200 mg po QD) or rimantandine (200 mg po QD), which bind the viral membrane and block replication (see Chap. 1).
  - Give to all influenza A–infected patients.
  - Early treatment is more effective. Continue for 5 days.
- For both influenza A and B, give the viral neuramindase inhibitors zamanavir (10 mg intranasally) or oseltamivir (75 mg po QD) for 5 days.
  - Give early, best results within 48 hours of onset of symptoms.
  - Zamanavir commonly precipitates bronchospasm, limiting its usefulness.
- Mortality highest in those over 65 years old (1–2% in this age group).

PREVENTION

- Influenza vaccine is a trivalent inactivated vaccine directed against both types A and B influenza.
  - Target strains are selected for each year's vaccine based on what was circulating worldwide the year before.
  - Effectiveness depends on the success of the match between the vaccine and the currently circulating strains.
  - Vaccination decreases disease severity as well as the infection rate.

- Groups recommended for vaccination:
  - A. Groups at increased risk for influenza complications
    1. Persons 65 or older
    2. Residents of nursing homes or other chronic care facilities
    3. All persons with chronic pulmonary or cardiovascular disease (including asthma)
    4. All those under 18 on chronic aspirin therapy
    5. Women who will be in the second or third trimester of pregnancy during the influenza season
  - B. Those with increased risk of transmitting influenza to high-risk individuals
    1. Health care personnel
    2. Employees of nursing homes or other chronic care facilities who have patient contact
    3. Home care providers and household contacts of those at high risk

HERPES SIMPLEX VIRUS

HIGHLIGHTS

- Spread by direct contact with infected skin or mucous membranes.
- Primary HSV-1 infection can result in gingivostomatitis, while secondary infection usually results in vesicular lesions of the lips.
- Primary HSV-2 often causes extensive genital lesions with painful adenopathy and can also result in aseptic meningitis.
- Diagnosis usually by skin appearance. Immunostaining and viral culture are diagnostic. PCR used for detection in the CSF.
- Treatment of primary disease with acyclovir, valacyclovir, or famciclovir.

EPIDEMIOLOGY

- HSV-1 causes herpes labialis; over 90% of individuals worldwide have been infected.
- HSV-2 causes genital herpes; the incidence varies from 10 to 80%, depending on sexual activity.
  - The higher the number of sexual partners and other STDs, the higher the likelihood of HSV-2 infection.
- Transmitted from person to person due to contact with infected skin or muosa.

PATHOGENESIS

- Virus replicates in the epithelium and infects a nerve ending and then replicates in nerve ganglia; periodically reactivates causing recurrent infection
  - HSV-1 resides in the trigeminal ganglion
  - HSV-2 in the sacral ganglion

CLINICAL MANIFESTATIONS

- HSV-1
  - Initial infection with HSV-1 is often subclinical and many people never experience clinical reactivation.
    - Others experience gingival-stomatitis, especially small children.
    - Lesions are usually ulcerative and exudative and may involve extensive areas of the lips, oral cavity, pharynx, and perioral skin.
    - Healing over several days to 2 weeks and is usually complete without scarring.
  - Secondary episodes of HSV-1 result in fever blisters, typical vesicular and ulcerative lesions of the lips, occasionally other areas of face or in the mouth.
    - Triggered by sunlight exposure, stress, and viral infections
    - Usually much less severe than primary disease
- HSV-2 causes genital herpes in both women and men.
  - Primary infection can result in an aseptic meningitis and fever.
    - Inflammation can lead to temporary bladder or bowel dysfunction.
  - Lesions may be vesicular, pustular, or ulcerative, involving the penis in men and vagina and cervix in women.
  - Pain, itching, dysuria, and vaginal or urethral discharge. Symptoms of primary infection tend to be more severe in women.
- Less common forms of skin infection:
  - Herpetic whitlow, usually found in health care workers, mistaken for a bacterial infection
  - Herpes gladiatorum, develops in wrestlers at sites of skin abrasions
- Complications can be serious:
  - Herpes encephalitis (HSV-1) (see Chap. 6)
  - Herpes keratitis—a leading cause of blindness (see Chap. 5)
  - Cutaneous dissemination in eczema patients
  - Tracheobronchitis in intubated debilitated patients, occasionally progresses to pneumonia

DIAGNOSIS AND TREATMENT

- Diagnosis is usually made clinically.
  - Immunofluorescence of skin lesions available
  - Tzanck prep demonstrates multinucleated giant cells, not specific
  - Viral culture quickly grows from vesicular lesions.
  - Encephalitis
    - CSF PCR for encephalitis
    - MRI of the brain and EEG localizing abnormalities in temporal areas
- Treatment
  - Recommended for primary skin infections
    - Acyclovir (400 mg po TID) × 5–7 days or
    - Famciclovir (250 mg po BID) × 5–7 days or
    - Valacyclovir (500 mg–1 g po QD) × 5–7 days
  - Efficacy of treatment of recurrent episodes more controversial
    - Can attempt treatment during the prodrome (skin tingling)
    - Suppressive therapy may be used for recurrent genital herpes.
  - Encephalitis or disseminated disease, intravenous acyclovir (10 mg/kg Q8H × 14 days)

CYTOMEGALOVIRUS

HIGHLIGHTS

- A high percentage of children are infected and young children are the primary source of adult infection, being spread by urine, feces, or mucous secretions.
- Can cause a mononucleosis syndrome, and causes more serious disease in immunocompromised hosts.
- Diagnosis by IgM anti-CMV titer or CMV serum antigen test.
- A self-limited disease in normal hosts. Requires ganciclovir treatment in the immunocompromised host.

EPIDEMIOLOGY

- A common worldwide infection. In the United States 40–80% of children positive
- Young children are the primary source of infection for adults.
- Transmitted by blood, urine, saliva, cervical secretions, semen, feces, and breast milk

CLINICAL MANIFESTATIONS

- Many infections are subclinical
- Responsible for 10% of mononucleosis cases
  - The leading cause of heterophile-negative mononucleosis
- In immunocompromised host, causes (see Chap. 16):
  - Retinitis
  - Hepatitis
  - Pneumonitis
  - GI disease (gastric and esophageal ulcers and colitis)
  - Polyradiculopathy

DIAGNOSIS

- IgM anti-CMV titer usually indicates acute disease; a 4-fold rise in IgG anti-CMV titer is also diagnostic of acute disease. Serum CMV antigen indicates active viral replication.
- Viral culture not useful in normal individuals because the virus can be intermittently shed in the urine many years after primary infection.
- Diagnosis in immunocompromised patients is more complex (see Chap. 16).

TREATMENT

- A self-limited disease in the normal host.
- Ganciclovir (5 mg/kg IVQ12H) or foscarnet (60 mg/kg IVQ8H) treatment required to control organ infections in immunocompromised patients.

REFERENCES

CDC: Revised U.S. surveillance case definition for severe acute respiratory syndrome (SARS) and update on SARS cases—United States and worldwide, December 2003. *MMWR* 2003; 52:1202–6.

Cohen JI, Corey GR: Cytomegalovirus infection in the normal host. *Medicine* 1985; 64:100–14.

Couch RB: Drug therapy: Prevention and treatment of influenza. *N Engl J Med* 2000; 343:1778.

Duchin JS, et al: Hantavirus pulmonary syndrome: A clinical description of 17 patients with a newly recognized disease. *N Engl J Med* 330:949–55.

Hjalgrim H, Askling J, Rostgaard K, Hamilton-Dutoit S, Frisch M, et al: Characteristics of Hodgkin's lymphoma after infectious mononucleosis. *N Engl J Med* 2003; 349:1324–32.

Ksiazek TG, Erdman D, Goldsmith CS, Zaki SR, Peret T, et al: A novel coronavirus associated with severe acute respiratory syndrome. *N Engl J Med* 2003; 348:1953–66.

Lee N, Hui D, Wu A, Chan P, Cameron P, et al: A major outbreak of severe acute respiratory syndrome in Hong Kong. *N Engl J Med* 2003; 348:1986–94.

Nichol KL, Nordin J, Mullooly J, Lask R, Fillbrandt K, et al: Influenza vaccination and reduction in hospitalizations for cardiac disease and stroke among the elderly. *N Engl J Med* 2003; 348:1322–32.

Poutanen SM, Low DE, Henry B, Finkelstein S, Rose D, et al: Identification of severe acute respiratory syndrome in Canada. *N Engl J Med* 2003; 348:1995–2005.

Swaminathan S, Wang F: Antimicrobial therapy of Epstein-Barr virus infections, in: *Antimicrobial Therapy and Vaccines*, V Yu, TC Merigan, S Barriere, et al: (eds.). Baltimore: Williams & Wilkins, 2002.

Vazquez M, LaRussa PS, Gershon AA, Steinberg SP, Freudigman K, Shapiro ED: The effectiveness of the varicella vaccine in clinical practice. *N Engl J Med* 2001; 344:955–60.

16

INFECTIONS IN THE IMMUNOCOMPROMISED HOST

HIGHLIGHTS

- Management of the immunocompromised host depends on the type of immunodeficiency.
- For neutropenic patients, emergent diagnosis and treatment is required.
  - Monotherapy (cefepime or imipenam) is equivalent to dual antibiotic therapy.
  - Vancomycin should be avoided when possible.
  - Antifungal therapy indicated if fever persists despite 7 days of antibiotic treatment.
- For patients with depressed cell-mediated immunity, extensive workup of fever including biopsies to determine the etiology. Acute therapy usually not required.
  - CMV antibody recipients or those receiving CMV-positive organs require prophylaxis early in transplant with ganciclovir or valganciclovir.
  - HSV-antibody-positive patients also require prophylaxis with acyclovir or ganciclovir.

Potential severity: Rapid evaluation and empiric antibiotics are required in the febrile neutropenic patient, high-grade, life-threatening bacteremia being common.

FORMS OF IMMUNODEPRESSION

- Immunocompromised hosts primarily include:
  - Those with leukemias, lymphomas, and solid tumors who are receiving cytotoxic chemotherapy
  - Those with bone marrow transplants, including stem cell transplants
  - Those with solid organ transplants
  - Patients receiving immunosuppressive agents and immune modulators for inflammatory disorders
- Three main types of immunocompromise:
  1. Neutropenia ($< 500\,\text{mm}^3$) often accompanied by mucosal damage
     - Risk of infection increases as the cell number decreases.
       - Incidence inversely related to absolute neutrophil number $< 500\,\text{mm}^3$
         - Higher incidence observed $< 200\,\text{mm}^3$
       - Incidence also increases the longer the duration of neutropenia.
         - 7–10 days of neutropenia, lower risk of infection
         - > 10 days, high risk of infection
     - Usually caused by cancer chemotherapy that depresses the bone marrow

2. Depressed cell-mediated immunity
   ○ Associated with high-dose corticosteroids
   ○ Follows immunosuppression for organ transplantation
3. Combined neutropenia and depressed cell-mediated immunity.
   ○ Bone marrow transplant patients in the early stages are neutropenic
   ○ After the bone marrow repopulates they have depressed cell-mediated immunity

PATHOGENS ASSOCIATED WITH NEUTROPENIA AND MUCOSITIS

- Infecting organisms primarily arise from the skin, oral cavity, and GI tract
- Bacteria include:
  ○ Gram-positive aerobic organisms most frequent:
    - *Staphylococcus epidermidis* and *S. aureus*
    - *Streptococcus viridans*, enterococcus
  ○ Gram-negatives second in frequency:
    - *E. coli*
    - Klebsiella spp.
    - *Pseudomonas aeruginosa*
    - Others include: Enterobacter, Proteus, Acinetobacter, Stenotrophomonas, Citrobacter
  ○ Anaerobes less common, can occur with severe mucositis
- Fungal infections develop after antibiotic therapy has had time to reduce the bacterial flora (usually a minimum of 7 days, unless a history of prior fungal infections):
  ○ Candida spp.
  ○ Aspergillus spp.

INFECTIONS ASSOCIATED WITH DEPRESSED CELL-MEDIATED IMMUNITY

- First month after transplant can be infected by the same hospital-acquired pathogens as other hosts.
- Over 6 months post transplant. At this time immunosuppressants are decreased and most patients are infected with the same community-acquired pathogens as normal hosts.
- From 1 to 6 months post transplant is associated with the widest variety of opportunistic infections.
  ○ Mycobacteria spp.
    - Patients can reactivate untreated *M. tuberculosis* and may present as having miliary tuberculosis (see Chap. 4).
    - Atypical mycobacteria are also a concern.
  ○ *Listeria monocytogenes*
    - Contracted from contaminated food
    - All foods should be freshly cooked or reheated at high temperature
    - Usually presents as bacteremia or meningitis
  ○ Nocardia spp.
    - Pneumonia often involving upper lobes
    - Brain abscess also a common presentation, can mimic brain metastasis (see Chaps. 4 and 6)
  ○ *Legionella pneumophila* (see Chap. 4)

- Fungal infection is often life-threatening and may be difficult to diagnose.
  - Cryptococcus most common (see Chap. 5)
  - Aspergillus spp., Fusarium spp., and the Mucor/Rhizopus group
  - Candida spp. within the first month
  - Histoplasmosis, coccidiomycosis depending on geographic location
  - Dematiacious fungi or black mold
- Reactivation of old viral infections a major concern
  - CMV the most common infection post transplant, due to reactivation, blood transfusion, or infected organ transplant
    - Depends on the recipient and donor CMV status
      - CMV antibody-negative recipient, CMV Ab-positive donor: high risk
      - CMV Ab-positive recipient and CMV Ab-positive donor or CMV Ab-negative donor: intermediate risk
      - CMV Ab-negative recipient and CMV Ab-negative donor: lowest risk
    - Diagnosis of active CMV infection utilizes two tests that are also used to monitor response to therapy:
      - CMV antigen test always correlates with active replication.
      - CMV PCR can detect latent as well as active infection; higher copy number is indicative of active invasive infection.
  - EBV less common
    - Actively replicates in 20–30% of transplant recipients
    - Can cause a lymphoproliferative syndrome
- Other pathogens include:
  - *Pneumocystis carinii* (see Chap. 17)
  - Toxoplasmosis (see Chap. 17)
  - Disseminated strongyloidiasis (see Chap. 12)

INFECTIONS ASSOCIATED WITH MIXED DEFICITS FOUND IN BONE MARROW TRANSPLANTATION

- Phase I (days 0–30 post transplant): Neutropenic phase, and patients are managed similarly to other neutropenic patients.
- Phase II (days 30–100 post transplant): Similar to other organ transplant patients with compromised cell-mediated immunity. CMV particularly common, as is graft versus host disease (GVDH).
- Phase III (> 100 days post transplant): Often continued defects in cell-mediated immunity, as well as depressed humor immunity resulting in continued suscepti-bility to:
  - CMV and herpes-zoster virus
  - Epstein-Barr virus–related lymphoproliferative disorders
  - Infections with encapsulated bacteria S. pneumoniae and H. influenzae due to:
    - Functional hyposplenism after total body irradiation
    - Chronic GVHD
    - Decreased IgG2 and specific pneumococcal antibody production

DIAGNOSIS AND TREATMENT OF THE NEUTROPENIC PATIENT

- If neutropenia is the consequence of recent cytotoxic chemotherapy, the onset of significant fever (temp. $\geq 38.3°C$ or $101°F$) warrants emergent diagnostic studies and antibiotic therapy.
- The progression of infection in neutropenic patients can be rapid.

- Infection cannot be readily differentiated from noninfectious causes of fever.
  - The usual manifestations of infection are often absent.
    - Skin infections lack erythema, warmth, and purulence.
    - CXR is often normal in bacterial pneumonia.
    - CSF may have minimal PMN in bacterial meningitis.
- Initial workup of fever should include:
  - Physical examination looking for sites of infection—lungs, skin, and mucous membranes
  - Biopsy and culture any skin lesions
  - Blood, urine, and any other suspicious sites cultured
  - Chest radiograph
    - High-resolution CT may detect infiltrates in 1/2 of normal CXRs in neutropenic patients with fever.
    - If an infiltrate is detected, because of the wide variety of potential pathogens, bronchoscopy with lavage should be performed.
- Begin empiric antibiotic therapy
  - Regimen depends on the severity of illness
    - Low severity defined as:
      - Fever $< 39°C$ and nontoxic appearance
      - Absolute neutrophil and monocytes count $\geq 100\,mm^3$
      - Normal CXR
      - Nearly normal LFTs and renal function
      - Neutropenia < 7 days and expected recovery by < 10 days
      - No evidence for intravascular device infection
      - Malignancy in remission
      - No neurologic deficits
      - No abdominal pain
      - No comorbid conditions (hypotension, vomiting, diarrhea, evidence for deep organ infection)
      - Low severity score of ≥ 21 (see Table 16-1)

TABLE 16-1
SCORING INDEX FOR IDENTIFICATION OF LOW-RISK FEBRILE
NEUTROPENIC PATIENT AT THE TIME OF PRESENTATION OF FEVER

Characteristic	Score
Extent of illness*	
No symptoms	5
Mild symptoms	5
Moderate symptoms	3
No hypotension	5
No chronic obstructive pulmonary disease	4
Solid tumor or no fungal infection	4
No dehydration	3
Outpatient at the time fever onset	3
Age < 60 years[†]	2

Note: the highest score is 26. Score of ≥ 21 indicates low risk for complications and morbidity. * Choose one item only. [†] Does not apply to children < 16 years.
SOURCE: From Hughes et al: 2002 IDSA Guidelines for Use of Antimicrobial Agents in Neutropenic Patients with Cancer. *Clin Infect Dis* 2002; 34:730–51.

- ○ Oral antibiotics if low severity
  - ▪ Ciprofloxacin (500 mg BID) plus amoxicillin-clavulanate (875 mg BID)
- ○ Intravenous antibiotics if higher severity; can also be used for low-severity cases
  - ▪ Monotherapy has been found to be comparable to dual therapy
    - • Cefepime, 2 gm Q12H or
    - • Imipenam, 500 mg Q6H
  - ▪ Dual therapy without vancomycin (all regimens equivalent) (aminoglycosides should be avoided if the patient is receiving other nephrotoxic or otoxic drugs, or drugs that cause neuromuscular blockade, and in patients with significant renal dysfunction)
    - • Cefepime, 2 gm Q12H, + gentamicin (5–6 mg/kg first dose) or tobramycin (5–6 mg/kg first dose) or amikacin (15 mg/kg first dose), then dose by levels (or)
    - • Ticarcillin-clavulinate, 3 gm Q4H, (or) piperacillin-tazobactam, 3 gm Q6H, + aminoglycoside (see above) (or)
    - • Imipenam, 500 mg Q6H, + aminoglycoside (see above)
    - • Piperacillin-tazobactam + ciprofloxacin, 400 mg IV, may be equivalent
  - ▪ Vancomycin (1 gm Q12H) should be avoided for routine empiric therapy because of the increased risk of selecting for vancomycin-resistant enterococci; however, should be added if:
    - • An intravascular device infection is suspected
    - • Known colonization with methicillin-resistant *S. aureus* or penicillin-resistant enterococcus
    - • Positive blood cultures with Gram-positive cocci prior to final identification and sensitivity testing
    - • Hypotension or other evidence of cardiovascular compromise
- ○ Adjustments in empiric antibiotic therapy
  - ▪ If afebrile in 3–5 days and a positive culture is obtained:
    - • Adjust antibiotics to the least toxic regimen, but maintain broad-spectrum coverage to prevent breakthrough bacteremia
    - • Continue for ≥ 7 days
    - • Continue until clinically responded and cultures negative
    - • Usually continue until neutrophils ≥ 500/mm^3
  - ▪ If afebrile in 3–5 days and cultures are negative:
    - • For low-risk patients can switch to oral ciprofloxacin and amoxicillin-clavulinate
    - • For high-risk patients continue intravenous antibiotics
    - • Continue for ≥ 7 days and usually until neutrophils ≥ 500/mm^3
  - ▪ If the patient remains febrile after 3–5 days:
    - • Reassess: review cultures, repeat physical exam, examine intravenous catheters, consider additional imaging studies, check antibiotic serum levels (particularly aminoglycosides), and repeat cultures
    - • Persistent fever for ≥ 5 days:
      - ○ If nontoxic, no new findings, and neutrophil count expected to recover quickly, continue same antibiotics.
      - ○ If clinical worsening or persistent toxicity, alter antibiotics:
        - ▪ Switch from monotherapy to dual therapy

- Consider adding vancomycin if appropriate criteria (see above)
- Add antifungal therapy if the neutropenia expected to persist for > 5–7 days
  - Liposomal amphotericin, B 5 mg/kg/day, IV (or)
  - Voriconazole, 400 mg po Q12H or 6 mg/kg IV Q12H first day followed by 4 mg/kg Q12H
- Duration of antibiotic therapy
  - Afebrile after 3–5 days of therapy and neutrophil count ≥ 500/mm^3 × 2 days, can discontinue after afebrile × 48 hours
    - Neutrophil count < 500/mm^3
      - Initially low risk and now nontoxic, discontinue when afebrile for 5–7 days
      - Initially high risk, neutrophil count < 100/mm^3, mucositis, and unstable signs, continue antibiotics
  - Persistent fever
    - Neutrophil count ≥ 500/mm^3, stop antibiotics after the neutrophil count has been at this level for 4–5 days and reassess
    - Neutrophil count < 500, continue × 2 weeks and then reassess; if no disease and clinically stable, can stop
- Antiviral therapy is not indicated in neutropenic patients unless a specific viral infection is documented.

DIAGNOSIS AND MANAGEMENT OF THE FEBRILE NONNEUTROPENIC COMPROMISED HOST

- Empiric antibiotics are generally not recommended.
- The number of possible organisms is very large and diagnosis requires:
  - Careful history, including:
    - Details of onset of the fever
    - Recent illnesses in the family
    - The underlying reason for immunosuppression, the dose and length of time on immunosuppressive therapy
    - Epidemiology, including travel or previous residence
      - Ohio River valley: consider reactivated histoplasmosis
      - Southwest: consider reactivation of coccidioidomycosis
  - Biopsy specimens and other samples for microscopic analysis and culture
  - Studies to exclude viral infections using CMV serum antigen, and herpes simplex cultures (see Chap. 15)
- Emergent management required for:
  - CNS symptoms such as headache and confusion. Consider:
    - Cryptococcosis
    - Listeriosis
  - Empiric antibiotics for infected central lines and urinary tract infections
  - Infiltrate on CXR:
    - If the patient is producing sputum, a sample should be cultured and sent for Gram, acid fast, and silver stains.
    - If there is no sputum, order urgent pulmonary consultation; often requires bronchoscopy.
- Complexity of care of these patients requires the early input of a subspecialist.

PREVENTION

- Bacterial infections
  - Intravenous IgG may be given to patients with IgG levels <400 mg/DL to prevent sinus and pulmonary infections due to *S. pneumoniae*.
- CMV
  - All transplant patients and donors should have CMV IgG serum titers.
    - Recipient negative and donor negative
      - Do not require prophylaxis
      - Require CMV negative or leukocyte-cleansed blood and platelet transfusions to prevent transfusion-associated CMV
    - Recipient positive and/or donor CMV positive requires either:
      - Oral prophylaxis for the first 100 days
        - Ganciclovir (1000 mg po TID) (or)
        - Valganciclovir (900 mg po QD)
      - Preemptive therapy preferred for CMV positive recipient with CMV negative donor (lower incidence of active disease)
        - Periodic screening for CMV serum antigen or quantitative PCR. If positive treat with:
          - Ganciclovir, 5 mg/kg IV Q12H × 14–21 days
          - Valganciclovir, 900 mg po BID induction, then 900 mg QD; may prove to be efficacious
- HSV
  - All transplant recipients should have anti-HSV IgG titers measured before transplantation.
  - Bone marrow transplant patient with a positive titer should receive prophylaxis during the induction phase and during the first 30 days after transplant (Phase I) with:
    - Valacylovir (1000 mg po BID or TID) (or)
    - Valganciclovir (900 mg po BID) if also require CMV prophylaxis
  - Other transplant patients undergoing high-level immunosuppression should be considered for prophylaxis.
- VZV
  - The recipient and all family members should be vaccinated at least 4 weeks prior to transplant with the live attenuated vaccine.
- Fungal infections
  - Allogeneic bone marrow transplant patients have a high incidence of *Candida albicans* infection during Phase I.
  - Fluconazole, 200 mg po QD, is recommended as prophylaxis.
- *Pneumocystis carinii*
  - Transplant patients are at risk throughout the period of immunosuppression.
  - Trimethoprim-sulfa (1 DS po 3 times per week or 1 single-strength po QD) is recommended.

REFERENCES

Bodey GP, Buckley M, Sathe YS, Freireich EJ: Quantitative relationships between circulating leukocytes and infection in patients with acute leukemia. *Ann Intern Med* 1966; 64:328–40.

Fishman JA, Rubin RH: Infection in organ-transplant recipients. *N Engl J Med* 1998; 338:1741–51.

Hughes WT, Armstrong D, Bodey GP, Bow EJ, Brown AE, Calandra T, Feld R, Pizzo PA, Rolston KV, Shenep JL, Young LS. 2002 guidelines for the use of antimicrobial agents in neutropenic patients with cancer. *Clin Infect Dis* 2002; 34:730–51.

Koh A, Pizzo PA: Empirical oral antibiotic therapy for low risk febrile cancer patients with neutropenia. *Cancer Invest* 2002; 20:420–33.

Sickles EA, Greene WH, Wiernik PH: Clinical presentation of infection in granulocytopenic patients. *Arch Intern Med* 1975; 135:715–19.

Walsh TJ, Pappas P, Winston DJ, et al. Voriconazole compared with liposomal amphotericin B for empirical antifungal therapy in patients with neutropenia and persistent fever. *N Engl J Med* 2002; 346:225–34.

Winston DJ, Yeager AM, Chandrasekar PH, Snydman DR, Petersen FB, et al: Randomized comparison of oral valacyclovir and intravenous ganciclovir for prevention of cytomegalovirus diseases after allogeneic bone marrow transplantation. *Clin Infect Dis* 2003; 36:749–58.

CHAPTER

17

HIV INFECTION

HIGHLIGHTS

- 30 million cases in Africa, 1 million in the United States.
- Risk of contracting: 100% from contaminated blood, 1/300 from a needle stick, 30% infected mother to neonate, and 0.01–1% for vaginal or anal intercourse.
- The virus enters by dendritic cells and attacks CD4 T cells.
- Average incubation period to AIDS is 10 years.
- Primary infection results in the abrupt onset of fever, nonexudative pharyngitis, and lymphadenitis. Also develop a maculopapular rash, headache, and aseptic meningitis.

Potential severity: Management of HIV is challenging and complex. The associated opportunistic infections are often difficult to diagnosis and are often life-threatening.

EPIDEMIOLOGY

- Highest incidence is in Africa, where the virus originated.
  - 3–4 million new infections per year
  - 30 million living with AIDS
  - Heterosexual transmission, incidence in men = women
- In North America and Europe, lower incidence and prevalence
  - The United States approaching prevalence of 1 million.
  - Incidence has slightly increased since 1998 owing to a change in attitude caused by HAART.
- Risk of contracting HIV infection
  - Very high with a contaminated blood transfusion (probably 100%)
    - Risk of receiving contaminated blood now < 1/500,000
  - 1/300 for needle stick
  - Mother to newborn without treatment = 30%
    - Antiretroviral therapy reduces the risk to < 1%
  - Vaginal or anal intercourse 0.01–1%
    - Genital ulcers increase risk 10 ×
    - Condoms prevent transmission
- Preventive measures very cost-effective as compared to treatment

Based on Chapter 17, "HIV Infection" by Dr. Bernard Hirschel in *Infectious Diseases in 30 Days*, F. Southwick (ed.).

PATHOGENESIS OF HIV INFECTION

- Dendritic cells in the mucosa transport the virus to CD4 T cells in the lymph nodes.
- Early infection caused by monocytotrophic virus, later infection by lymphocytrophic virus
  - The primary receptors for HIV entry are CD4 molecules on the cell membrane surface.
  - A coreceptor is also necessary for infection.
    - Coreceptor CCR5 is used by monocytotrophic or non-syncytium-inducing (NSI) virus and predominates in early infection.
    - Coreceptor CXCR4 is used by lymphocytotrophic virus, is syncytium-inducing (SI), and predominates in later infection.
  - CD4 lymphocytes proliferate and are preferentially infected and destroyed.
    - Loss of CD4 lymphocytes may explain the specific immune deficiency associated with HIV infection.
- Millions of viral particles enter the bloodstream during primary infection.
- Anti-HIV antibodies develop; cytotoxic T cells proliferate, controlling infection.
  - The viral load usually drops to a plateau level of 50–5,000 viral particles/mm^3.
  - The higher the plateau level, the faster the development of AIDS.
- CD4 count drops from 1,000/mm^3, then returns to normal and subsequently drops 70/mm^3 per year.
- Average incubation period until AIDS develops is 10 years.
  - When the CD4 count <200/mm^3, opportunistic infections begin and development of one of these infections indicates progression to AIDS (see Table 17-1 and later sections).
  - Progression is affected by:
    - Age: older patients usually progress more rapidly.
    - Genetic factors (example: mutations in the CCR5 receptor slow progression).
- Active infection is associated with the production of 10^9 to 10^{11} viral particles/day, and destruction of 10^{11} CD4 cells/day.

CLINICAL MANIFESTATIONS OF PRIMARY HIV INFECTION

- Abrupt onset of fever 2–4 weeks after exposure, can be as long as 10 weeks.
- Accompanied by:
  - Nonexudative pharyngitis and lymphadenitis
  - Painful ulcers may develop in the oral or genital mucosa
  - Red macular-papular skin rash on the head, neck, and upper torso
  - Headache and aseptic meningitis
    - Headache may be retro-orbital and be made worse by eye movements
    - CSF has lymphocytes, normal glucose, and mild protein elevation
  - Anorexia, nausea, diarrhea
  - Peripheral WBC normal or slightly depressed with decreased CD4 lymphocytes and increased CD8, CD4/CD8 ratio usually < 1
- The acute illness usually lasts 2 weeks. Lethargy and fatigue can persist for several months.

TABLE 17-1
INDICATOR CONDITIONS IN THE CASE DEFINITION OF AIDS (ADULTS)*

Candidiasis, of esophagus, trachea, bronchi, or lungs—3,846 (16%)
Cervical cancer, invasive—144 (0.6%)
Coccidioidomycosis, extrapulmonary—74 (0.3%)
Cryptococcosis, extrapulmonary—1,168 (5%)
Cryptosporidiosis with diarrhea > 1 month—314 (1.3%)
Cytomegalovirus of any organ other than liver, spleen, or lymph nodes; eye—1,638 (7%)
Herpes simplex with mucocutaneous ulcer > 1 month or bronchitis, pneu monitis, esophagitis—1,250 (5%)
Histoplasmosis, extrapulmonary—208 (0.9%)
HIV-associated dementia: disabling cognitive and/or other dysfunction interfering with occupation or activities of daily living—1,196 (5%)
HIV-associated wasting: involuntary weight loss > 10% of baseline plus chronic diarrhea (≥ 2 loose stools/day ≥ 30 days) or chronic weakness and documented enigmatic fever ≥ 30 days—4,212 (18%)
Isospora belli infection with diarrhea > 1 month—22 (0.1%)
Kaposi's sarcoma—1,500 (7%)
Lymphoma, Burkitt's—162 (0.7%), immunoblastic—518 (2.3%), primary CNS—170 (0.7%)
M. avium, disseminated—1,124 (5%)
M. tuberculosis, pulmonary—1,621 (7%), extrapulmonary—491 (2%)
Nocardiosis < 1%
P. carinii pneumonia—9,145 (38%)
Pneumonia, recurrent-bacterial (≥ 2 episodes in 12 months)—1,347 (5%)
Progressive multifocal leukoencephalopathy—213 (1%)
Salmonella septicemia (nontyphoid), recurrent—68 (0.3%)
Strongyloidosis, extraintestinal (none)
Toxoplasmosis of internal organ—1,073 (4%)
Wasting syndrome due to HIV (18%)

* The numbers and percentages behind the diagnoses indicate the frequencies of occurrence in the database of the Swiss HIV cohort registry of more than 11,000 patients.

LABORATORY EVALUATION OF HIV INFECTION

HIGHLIGHTS

- Diagnosis is made by HIV antibody testing, highly sensitive and specific with 50% positive rate within 20 days of exposure and > 95% by 90 days.
- Viral load and CD4 counts are monitored to decide on and monitor treatment as well as to determine prognosis.
- Staging of HIV is based on CD4 count and clinical events.
- Antiviral-resistant genotype testing is helpful in determining when to discontinue a drug.

DIAGNOSIS OF HIV INFECTION

- Diagnosis of HIV is made by measuring anti-HIV antibodies in the serum.
- HIV antibody tests highly specific and sensitive (exceeds 99%).
  - ○ To exclude clerical errors should confirmed by a second antibody test
  - ○ Remains positive for life in most cases
- 5% seroconvert within 7 days, 50% within 20 days, and > 95% within 90 days.
- "Window" period = viremia with a negative serology; lasts a few days to several weeks.
- "Indeterminant" test usually false positive; should be confirmed by Western blot analysis.
- PCR-based tests not recommended for diagnosis.

TESTS USED FOR MONITORING OF TREATMENT AND PROGNOSIS

- Two values are usually measured, viral load and CD4 lymphocyte count.
- Level of viremia correlates with speed of progression.
  - ○ Viral load is determined by PCR, which measures the copies of RNA copies/mm^3, ranges from 500 to 1 million prior to antiretroviral treatment.
  - ○ Treatment should reduce viral load to undetectable (< 5 to < 50, depending on the test used) within 2–6 months.
  - ○ Individual tests vary by 2-fold.
  - ○ A small temporary rise or "blip" in viral load from undetectable to 100 copies is not significant and does not warrant a change in the therapeutic regimen.
- CD4 count is the most reliable determinant of prognosis.
  - ○ Patients with CD4 < 200/mm^3 are at risk of opportunistic infections and tumors.
    - ■ Below this value, incidence rises exponentially.
    - ■ Very unusual for patients to die of AIDS with CD4 counts above 50/mm^3.
  - ○ CD4 count varies up to 10–30% between counts; therefore, small variations are not significant and should not be overinterpreted.

TESTS FOR ANTIRETROVIRAL RESISTANCE

- Used to guide the discontinuation of ineffective drugs.
- Genotype testing detects specific mutations.
  - ○ Sequences the HIV reverse transcriptase and protease genes to detect resistance mutations
    - ■ The occurrence of a single mutation usually does not predict a specific resistance phenotype.
    - ■ Combinations of many mutations must be considered. The prediction of resistance from a combination of mutations is called the "virtual phenotype."
    - ■ Predicts but does not prove resistance.
  - ○ Less expensive and most commonly used
- Phenotypic testing inserts viral genes into a standardized viral strain.
  - ○ Directly measures sensitivities of these viral constructs
  - ○ Time-consuming and expensive

CLASSIFICATION

- Classification is based on CD4 count and clinical symptoms (see Table 17-2).
- The United States and Europe have different definitions of AIDS.
  - USA = CD4 < 200 or an AIDS-defining illness (Table 17-1)
  - Europe = AIDS-defining illness (Table 17-1)
- The stage of HIV infection is defined by:
  - The CD4 lymphocyte count (biological stage 1, 2, or 3).
  - Clinical events (A, B, or C).
  - Occurrence of a type C disease defines AIDS.
  - In the United States, AIDS is also defined by a CD4 count of less than 200/mm^3 (categories C1, C2, C3, A3, or B3).

TABLE 17-2
STAGES OF HIV INFECTION

	CLINICAL CATEGORIES*		
CD4 cell categories	A Asymptomatic, or PGL or Acute HIV infection	B Symptomatic (not A or C)	C AIDS indicator conditions (1987)
>500/mm^3 (≥29%)	A1	B1	C1
200–499/mm^3 (14–28%)	A2	B2	C2
<200/mm^3 (<14%)	A3	B3	C3

Clinical signs associated with clinical stage A:
  primary HIV infection; generalized persistent lymphadenopathy; lack of symptoms (asymptomatic patients).
Clinical signs and symptoms associated with clinical stage B:
  oral candidiasis; relapsing vaginal candidiasis; herpes zoster; localized neoplasia of the cervix; any other clinical manifestations not defined by categories A and C.
Clinical category C:
  corresponds to the occurrence of a so-called AIDS-defining opportunistic disease listed in Table 17-1.

*Dark shaded areas represent the stages that are defined as AIDS in the US.

OPPORTUNISTIC DISEASES

GENERAL CONSIDERATIONS

- Many AIDS-defining illnesses result from reactivation latent infections:
  - Bacteria (*M. tuberculosis*)
  - Herpes viruses (e.g., cerebral lymphoma due to Epstein-Barr virus, retinitis due to cytomegalovirus)
  - Papovavirus JC (the agent of progressive multifocal leukoencephalopathy)
  - Fungi (*Pneumocystis carinii* pneumonia)
  - Parasites (*Toxoplasma encephalitis*)
- Other infections may be newly acquired:
  - *S. pneumoniae*
  - Salmonella
  - Cryptococcosis
- Several infections can be present at the same time, greatly complicating diagnosis and treatment.
- HAART has dramatically reduced the number of opportunistic infections.
  - In the United States and Europe advanced stages of AIDS with chronic diarrhea, cachexia, central nervous system, and pulmonary manifestations are now rare.

PRIMARY AND SECONDARY PROPHYLAXIS

- Primary prophylaxis prevents the first occurrence of a disease.
- Secondary prophylaxis prevents relapses after the first episode.
- Latent infections often activate as cell-mediated immunity wanes.
- Serologic and skin testing are used to detect latent infections on initial evaluation and guide primary prophylaxis. Examples:
  - Presence of IgG against *Toxoplasma gondii* in a patient whose CD4 count is below 100 identifies a high risk of cerebral toxoplasmosis.
  - Positive PPD in an HIV-infected individual warrants immediate INH prophylaxis (see Chap. 4).
- Prophylaxis for most opportunistic infections is recommended for CD4 < 200.
- After treatment of active infections, secondary prophylaxis is often necessary to prevent relapse.
- Prophylaxis can be discontinued on HAART, when the CD4 is durably > 200.
- Table 17-3 summarizes the common preventive regimens.

TABLE 17-3
PROPHYLAXIS OF OPPORTUNISTIC INFECTIONS

Disease	Indications	Drugs and dosage	Comments
***P. carinii* pneumonia** PCP	Primary prophylaxis if CD4 counts less than 200/μl, or after an episode of PCP	Trimethoprim-sulfamethoxazole, 960 mg, 1 double-strength tablet 3 times a week or 480 mg/day Pentamidine aerosols, 300 mg, once monthly Dapsone, 50 mg/day plus pyrimethamine 50 mg/day	Most effective. Protects also against cerebral toxoplasmosis Does not protect against cerebral toxoplasmosis Add folinic acid 2 times 15 mg/week
Cerebral toxoplasmosis	Primary prophylaxis if CD4 count below 100 Secondary prophylaxis	Trimethoprim-sulfamethoxazole, 960 mg 3 times weekly or 480 mg qd Sulfadiazine, 2 g/day, or clindamycin, 3 times 600 mg/day **plus** pyrimethamine, 25 mg/day	Protects also against pneumocystosis
Mycobacteria other than tuberculosis	Primary prophylaxis if CD4 count less than 50/μl	Azithromycin, 1,200 mg/week or rifabutin 300 mg/day	Rifabutin has many drug interactions in particular with protease inhibitors
Tuberculosis	Primary prophylaxis if more than 5 mm skin induration with a 5 U tuberculin test	Isoniazid, 5 mg/kg/day (maximum 300 mg/day) during 6 month with 40 mg/day of vitamin B6po	The skin reaction is difficult to interpret with moderate to advanced immune deficiency
Cryptococcosis	Primary prophylaxis if CD4 count is below 50 Secondary prophylaxis after an episode of cryptococcosis	Fluconazole, 400 mg per week or 200 mg 3 times weekly Fluconazole, 200 mg/day	
Cytomegalovirus retinitis	Primary prophylaxis if CD4 count below 50 and secondary prophylaxis after an episode of retinitis	Valganciclovir, 450 mg/day po	Only in regions with a high incidence

PULMONARY INFECTIONS

See Chap. 4, Tables 17-4 through 17-6.

HIGHLIGHTS

- *Pneumocystis carinii* is the most common infection when CD4 < 200/mm³, usually presenting with dyspnea and fever, interstitial butterfly pattern on CXR, and a high serum LDH. Trimethoprim-sulfa is the treatment of choice.
- Bacterial pneumonias are frequent, particularly *S. pneumoniae*. Treated with third- or fourth-generation cephalosporins.
- Tuberculosis can occur at any CD4 count, but CXR often atypical when CD4 count is low. HIV patients with pneumonia should be placed in respiratory isolation until TB is excluded. Miliary tuberculosis is always a concern in the severely immunosuppressed HIV patient.
- Rarer forms of pneumonia include: *M. kansansii*, Kaposi's sarcoma, interstitial lymphoid pneumonia, histoplasmosis, coccidioidomycosis, nocardiosis, aspergillosis, and rhodococcus.

GENERAL CONSIDERATIONS

- Possible etiologies depend on (see Table 17-4):
  - Patient history
    - Presence of intravenous drug abuse
    - Previous episodes of bacterial pneumonia
    - Exposure to tuberculosis
    - Epidemiology
      - Residence in a developing country (increased risk of tuberculosis)
      - Environmental and animal exposures (example, horse exposure increases risk of Rhodococcus)
  - CD4 lymphocyte count
    - Pneumocystis most common when CD4 < 200/mm³
    - Bacterial pneumonias, including tuberculosis, can occur at any CD4 level.
  - Use of preventive therapy
- Relative frequency of different pulmonary infections
  - Prior to the use of trimethoprim-sulfamethoxazole, *P. carinii* pneumonia was the initial opportunistic infection in 1/3 of the cases of AIDS.
  - Bacterial pneumonia, particularly due to *S. pneumoniae*, is 10–100 times more frequent than in HIV-negative patients.
- General approach to the HIV patient with pneumonia
  - If the CD4 count is > 200/mm³ and a lobar infiltrate, the presumptive diagnosis is bacterial pneumonia.
  - If CD4 count < 200/mm³, *P. carinii* pneumonia is most likely, except if the patient has faithfully taken trimethoprim-sulfamethoxazole prophylaxis.
  - The chest X-ray pattern is helpful in narrowing the diagnostic possibilities (see Table 17-5).
  - A definite diagnosis usually requires bronchoalveolar lavage.

TABLE 17-4
LUNG DISEASES LINKED TO HIV

Diagnosis	Signs and symptoms	Laboratory results	Radiology	Initial treatment
Bacterial pneumonia due to *S. pneumoniae*	Rapid onset of fever, dyspnea, cough, and sputum production	Leukocytosis with neutrophilia, blood cultures often positive	Lobar or diffuse infiltrate	Amox. clav. or cephalosporin
P. carinii pneumonia	Fever, dyspnea, cough for several weeks. Auscultation is usually normal	Hypoxemia, elevated LDH, diagnosis through bronchoalveolar lavage	Diffuse reticulonodular interstitial infiltrate	Trimethoprim-sulfamethoxazole
Tuberculosis	Weight loss, fever, cough, night sweats, lymphadenopathy	Positive sputum smear by Ziehl stain; positive sputum and blood cultures; typical histopathology of lymph nodes	Mediastinal adenopathy. Variable pulmonary infiltrate; cavitary upper lobe lesions are rare	Isoniazide + rifampin + pyrazinamide + ethambutol
Kaposi's sarcoma	Usually associated with skin or mucosal lesions	Typical lesions seen on bronchoscopy	Nodular infiltrates with perihilar location	Treatment for HIV, rarely radiotherapy or chemotherapy
Interstitial lymphoid pneumonia	Transitory fever and dyspnea	No specific findings	Reticulonodular infiltrates	Possibly steroids. Diagnosis by exclusion!

347

TABLE 17-5
CHEST X-RAY AND POSSIBLE ETIOLOGIES

Chest X-ray	Etiology
Normal	Bronchitis PCP
Lobar or other focal infiltrates	Bacterial pneumonia TB, PCP, cryptococcosis
Diffuse interstitial infiltrates	PCP TB Bacterial pneumonia Atypical pneumonia Interstitial lymphocytic pneumonia
Pleural effusion	Bacterial pneumonia TB Kaposi's sarcoma
Mediastinal adenopathy	TB Atypical mycobacteria Lymphoma Kaposi's sarcoma
Cavities	Lung abscess *M. kansasii* *R. equi* TB *S. aureus*
Cysts or bullae	PCP

TABLE 17-6
TREATMENT OF *P. CARINII* PNEUMONIA:
TRIMETHOPRIM-SULFAMETHOXAZOLE AND ALTERNATIVES

Substances	Dosage	Side effects
Trimethoprim- sulfamethoxazole	Two 800/160 mg pills Q8H or 20 mg/kg/iv/d Q6H	Skin rash, nausea and vomiting, anemia, leukopenia
Dapsone plus	100 mg po/qd	Rash, nausea and vomiting. Hemolytic anemia in patients with G6PD deficiency
Trimethoprim	1.2 g po/qd	
Clindamycine plus	3 × 600 mg po/qd	
Primaquine	30 mg po/qd	
Atovaquone	2 × 750 mg po/qd	Skin lesions, nausea, vomiting and diarrhea. Less efficacious, but better tolerated than sulfonamides

PNEUMOCYSTIS CARINII PNEUMONIA (PCP)

- Occurs in immunosuppressed patients
  - CD4 count $< 200/mm^3$
  - Patients on high-dose steroids or other immunosuppressives after organ transplantation
  - Severely malnourished individuals
  - Neonates or infants
- Subacute or acute onset of:
  - Shortness of breath
    - Initially, shortness of breath on exertion
    - Later, shortness of breath at rest
    - Caused by fluid accumulation in the alveoli
  - Dry cough
  - Fever should always be present
  - Weight loss and fatigue
- Lung auscultation is usually normal.
- CXR may be normal, but usually demonstrates an interstitial butterfly pattern.
  - Reticulonodular bilateral infiltrate can be asymmetric.
  - Can mimic pulmonary edema associated with left-sided congestive heart failure.
  - Less commonly can form cystic lesions or cause a pneumothorax.
  - Patients receiving pentamidine inhalation prophylaxis usually have asymmetric infiltrates limited to the lung apices.
- Gallium-67 citrate scan shows increased uptake in infected areas of the lung
  - Very sensitive.
  - Expensive and time consuming. Recommended only for patients with normal CXR and a high suspicion for PCP.
- LDH elevated in over 90%
  - Higher values and a persistent elevation despite therapy are associated with a poorer prognosis.
- Oxygen saturation may be depressed, particularly after any physical activity. An arterial blood gas should be performed in patients being considered for hospital admission.

Diagnosis
- Bronchoalveolar lavage or
- Induced sputum after inhalation of 3% NaCl over 30 minutes
  - Yield varies from 50 to 90%, depending on the institution
- Samples subjected to cytologic analysis after methenamine silver and Giemsa stains
  - Newer methods also available (PCR, immunofluorescence)
- If suspicion is high, treatment should not be delayed. Lavage samples remain positive for 1–3 days after initiation of treatment.

Treatment:
- Trimethroprim-sulfa is the drug of choice.
  - Two double-strength DS tablets po Q8H for 21 days (1,600 mg of sulfamethoxazole and 320 mg of trimethoprim)
  - Administer intravenously if patient severely ill
  - Alternatives are less effective and often more toxic (see Table 17-6). May be required if the patient develops a severe allergic reaction

- ○ Addition of folinic acid not recommended; reduces efficacy of trimethoprim-sulfa.
- ○ Needs to be followed by secondary prophylaxis (see Table 17-3 and below)
- When the pO_2 < 70 mm, prednisone is given before anti-PCP therapy; can prevent the need for intubation. Give prednisone 1 mg/kg/day × 5 days, then 40 mg/day × 5 days, followed by 20 mg/day × 11 days.

Prevention (see Table 17-6)
- 20% per year incidence of PCP in HIV patients with CD4 < 200 if they do not receive prophylaxis
- Trimethoprim-sulfa, 1 DS (960 mg) po 3 times per week or 1 single-strength (480 mg) daily, is the drug of choice.
  - ○ Efficacious, inexpensive, and also prevents toxoplasmosis
  - ○ 50% of patients will develop signs of cutaneous intolerance
    - ▪ Desensitizing permits readministration in the majority of cases.
    - ▪ Mechanisms of intolerance are not well understood.
      - • Dose dependent
      - • Probably not an allergy
      - • Up to 60% of patients with cutaneous intolerance do not relapse when re-exposed
- Alternatives are not as effective.
  - ○ Dapsone (100 mg po QD) does not cover toxoplasmosis; must add pyrimethamine
    - ▪ If a positive Toxoplasma IgG titer give:
      - • 50 mg dapsone + 50 mg of pyrimethamine po QD (or)
      - • 200 mg of dapsone + 75 mg pyrimethamine po once per week
      - • Both regimens are nearly equivalent to trimethoprim-sulfa
  - ○ Aerosolized pentamidine (Respirgard nebulizer, 300 mg every 4 weeks)
    - ▪ May be associated with cough and asthma
    - ▪ Preventive use of bronchodilators may be helpful
  - ○ Atovaquone, 750 mg/day po BID. Well tolerated, but expensive

BACTERIAL PNEUMONIA
- Produces the same symptoms and signs as pneumonias in HIV-negative patients (see Chap. 4)
  - ○ Sudden onset of fever, chills, cough, and dyspnea
  - ○ Most frequent cause is *S. pneumoniae*, less commonly:
    - ▪ *H. influenzae* (particularly in smokers)
    - ▪ *S. aureus*
    - ▪ *P. aeruginosa* found more frequently than in non-HIV patients
  - ○ Bacteremia and relapses are frequent.

Empirical Treatment
- Outpatient: Amoxicillin-clavulanate (875 mg po Q12H) (or)
- Usually require hospitalization and should receive
  - ○ Ceftriaxone (1–2 gm IV QD) or Cefotaxime (2 gm IV Q8H)
  - ○ If suspect Pseudomonas, use Cefepime (2 gm IV Q8-12H) or a fluoroquinolone with Gram-positive coverage (Levofloxacin, 500 mg IV QD, or Gatifloxacin, 400 mg IV QD)
- Treatment duration is 10–14 days (see Chap. 4).

TUBERCULOSIS

- Usually a subacute disease with weight loss, cough, fever, night sweats, and lung lesions
  - With normal or moderately depressed CD4 count, CXR shows typical apical cavitary lung lesions.
  - In patients with lower CD4 counts, CXR may be atypical resulting in:
    - Middle or lower lung field infiltrates
    - Mediastinal node enlargement
- With severe immunosuppression HIV patients can present as miliary disease (see Chap. 4).
  - Interstitial lung disease
  - Meningitis
  - Negative sputum AFB smears, but positive blood cultures

Diagnosis

- AFB stains and cultures of the sputum
  - May release large numbers of organisms in the absence of cavitary lung lesions
  - All HIV patients with an abnormal CXR should be placed in respiratory isolation and assumed to have tuberculosis until AFB smears are negative.
  - AFB sputum smears and cultures are often negative in miliary disease.
  - Liquid media results in more rapid growth (10–14 days) and presumptive identification can be made by nucleic acid probes.
- Blood cultures are more frequently positive in HIV patients and should be drawn.
- Susceptibility testing critical
  - Multiresistant TB is associated with 50% mortality in AIDS.

Therapy

- 4-drug therapy recommended (see Chaps. 1 and 4):
  - Isoniazid (300 mg po QD)
    - Liver functions should be monitored particularly if on HAART therapy.
    - Vitamin B_6 should also be given.
  - Rifampin (600 mg po QD)
    - Contraindicated in patients receiving protease inhibitors or nonnucleoside inhibitors because of rifampin's interference with hepatic clearance.
    - Alternative is streptomycin (500 mg IM Q12H); different QD regimens are also used, and should be adjusted for weight.
  - Pyrazinimide (15–30 mg/kg po QD)
  - Ethambutol (15 mg/kg po QD)
    - 25 mg/kg recommended only when a multiresistant strain is suspected.
    - Color vision should be monitored Q4–6 weeks when using 25 mg/kg.
- Duration of therapy
  - 4 drugs for first 2 months followed by INH and rifampin for 7 months.
  - Therapy should be continued for 6 months after sputum smear is negative for AFB.
  - If the response to therapy is slow, therapy needs to be prolonged.
  - Paradoxic worsening may occur at the beginning of therapy.
    - Results in higher fever, lymphadenopathy, and worsening CXR
    - In absence of systemic toxicity, treatment should not be modified.
- Multidrug-resistant tuberculosis is associated with > 50% mortality in HIV and requires management by a physician who specialize in the management of tuberculosis.

- Delay HAART therapy because of the potential for:
  - Multiple drug-drug interactions
  - Overlapping toxicities
  - Difficulties in differentiating paradoxic responses to antituberculous therapy from reconstitution syndrome associated with HAART therapy

MYCOBACTERIUM KANSASII

- In HIV-positive patients causes a disease resembling classic TB.
  - Fever, cough, weight loss
  - Pulmonary infiltrates predominating at the apex; usually without cavitation
- Isoniazid, rifampin, and ethambutol are efficacious (see above).

MYCOBACTERIA OTHER THAN TUBERCULOSIS (MOTT)

- Includes *Mycobacterium avium intracellulare* and other similar mycobacteria.
- Usually do not cause pulmonary disease.
- Cause a systemic illness with fever, weight loss, night sweats, and liver involvement.
- MOTT are frequently found in sputum, where their pathogenic significance remains uncertain.

PULMONARY KAPOSI'S SARCOMA

- Pulmonary involvement seen in patients with obvious cutaneous Kaposi's sarcoma (KS).
  - Mucosal surfaces are invaded in 30–50% of cutaneous cases.
  - Usually asymptomatic
- CXR shows:
  - Reticulonodular infiltrates with a perihilar distribution
  - Hilar lymphadenopathy
  - Less commonly, pleural effusions
- Treatment by radiotherapy or chemotherapy is indicated for relief of cough or dyspnea.
- Lung lesions, as well as other manifestations of Kaposi's sarcoma, improve on antiretroviral combination therapy.

OTHER RARE PULMONARY DISEASES

INTERSTITIAL LYMPHOID PNEUMONIA

- Diagnosis by exclusion
- More frequent in children
- Presents with fever and dyspnea
- CXR shows reticulonodular infiltrates, which may vary and disappear spontaneously
- Pathogenesis is unknown, but may be due to HIV itself
- Treatment with corticosteroids

HISTOPLASMOSIS (SEE CHAP. 4)

- In AIDS the disease is often disseminated, presenting with:
  ○ Lymphadenopathy and hepatosplenomegaly
  ○ Gastrointestinal involvement with ulcers
  ○ Skin lesions
  ○ Anemia
- Diagnosis is made by blood cultures and bone marrow culture as well as histopathology.
- Treatment:
  ○ Amphotericin B (0.7–1 mg/kg IV QD) initially for life-threatening illness
  ○ Followed by lower-dose amphotericin B (0.4–0.5 mg/kg IV QD) or switch to itraconazole (400 mg po QD) when the patient has defervesced.

COCCIDIOIDOMYCOSIS (SEE CHAP. 4)

- Restricted to the southwestern United States and Central America
- Symptoms include:
  ○ Fever and cough
  ○ CXR reticular nodular pattern
- Diagnosis is made by sputum culture or culture of bronchoalveolar lavage fluid
- Treatment: amphotericin B (0.5–1 mg/kg/day) or fluconazole (400–800 mg/day)

DISSEMINATED TOXOPLASMOSIS

- Pulmonary involvement is rare.
  ○ Seen only in the presence of extreme immunosuppression (CD4 count below 20)
  ○ 5% incidence in France among HIV patients
- Clinical presentation can be similar to PCP, with CXR showing interstitial infiltrates.
- Lactate dehydrogenase (LDH) is extremely elevated.
- Diagnosis by bronchoalveolar lavage, Toxoplasma organisms being seen on microscopic analysis.
- Treatment same as for cerebral toxoplasmosis (see below).
- Rapidly fatal if not diagnosed and treated.

NOCARDIA ASTEROIDES (SEE CHAP. 4)

- Can cause chronic pneumonia with nodular pulmonary lesions on CXR.
- Can disseminate to other organs including the skin, kidneys, and brain.
- Diagnosed by direct stain of the sputum or skin biopsy
  ○ Delicate, Gram-labile, branched filaments are detected. Modified acid-fast positive
  ○ Seen by methenamine silver and Brown-Brenn stains on histopathology

Treatment
- Prolonged administration of trimethoprim-sulfamethoxazole (2.5–10 mg/kg of the trimethoprim component).
  ○ High doses for at least 6 weeks
  ○ Lower doses for 6–12 months
- Anecdotal responses to imipenem and the newer fluoroquinolones have been described.

INVASIVE ASPERGILLOSIS

- Often a terminal complication with disastrous prognosis in hospitalized patients.
  - Most commonly associated with high-dose corticosteroids or neutropenia
- Cardiac and central nervous system lesions may be associated with pneumonia.
- Voriconazole, 6 mg/kg IV Q12H, loading dose followed by 4 mg/kg IV Q12H is now the drug of choice. Amphotericin B at maximal doses can also be used.

RHODOCOCCUS EQUII

- A Gram-positive rod that causes acute cavitary pneumonias in AIDS patients
- Found in soil; high concentrations found in horse manure
  - Half of patients have contact with horses.

Diagnosis
- CXR cavitary lesions similar to tuberculosis, Nocardia, and fungal pulmonary infections
- May require bronchoscopy
- Blood cultures frequently positive
- Modified acid-fast-positive organisms may be identified in the sputum.

Treatment
- Vancomycin (1 gm IV Q12H) combined with
- Rifampin (600 mg po QD)
- Erythromycin (1 gm IV Q6H) may also be added
- Other drugs that can be used include:
  - Imipenam (0.5–1 gm IV Q6H)
  - Ciprofloxacin (500–750 mg po or 400 mg IV Q12H)
  - Amikacin (15 mg/kg IV QD divided into Q12H or Q8H doses)
- Mortality 15% in HIV patients; however, half of patients are never cured.

GASTROINTESTINAL SYSTEM

See Chap. 8 and Table 17-7.

HIGHLIGHTS

- Oral candidiasis and esophagitis are common with significant immunosuppression. Treated with low-dose fluconazole.
- Aphthous ulcers, oral hairy leukoplakia, and Kaposi's sarcoma also found in the oral cavity.
- Diarrhea often a major problem in HIV disease and can be caused by antiretroviral drugs, conventional bacteria, *M. tuberculosis* and atypical mycobacteria, CMV, and protozoa.
- Rectal and anal lesions are often sexually transmitted and can be caused by syphilis, gonorrhea, papilloma virus, and herpes simplex.
- Tumors can result from Kaposi's sarcoma and lymphoma.
- Coinfection with hepatitis C and hepatitis B is common. Hepatitis can also be caused by antiretroviral drugs.

TABLE 17-7
GASTROINTESTINAL DISEASES

Where	Disease	Etiology	Signs and symptoms	Diagnosis
Oral cavity	Thrush	Candida stomatitis (C. albicans)	Whitish plaques	Inspection
	Leukoplakia	Epstein-Barr virus	Whitish spots with irregular surface on margin of tongue	Inspection and biopsy
	Aphthous ulcers	Herpes simplex CMV, idiopathic or unknown	Painful erosions of around 5 mm	Culture or biopsy
Esophagus	Candida esophagitis	C. albicans	Dysphagia, retrosternal pain with coexisting Candida stomatitis	Clinical signs and symptoms, endoscopy
	Ulcers and erosions	Cytomegalovirus or herpes simplex	Dysphagia and retrosternal pain	Endoscopy (longitudinal ulcers) and histology
Stomach	Gastritis	Candida, CMV, herpes, H. pylori?	Various signs and symptoms Frequently pH is elevated	Endoscopy and biopsy
Small intestine	Malabsorption	Cryptosporidium Isospora belli E. bieneusii	Chronic watery diarrhea Loss of weight Malabsorption	Examination of feces
		Salmonella, Shigella, Campylobacter	Acute or subacute diarrhea and fever	Culture of feces and blood
	Malignant lymphoma		Loss of weight Intestinal obstruction Perforation	CT scan and biopsy
Biliary system	Cholangitis	CMV? Cryptosporidium? HIV? Microsporidium?	Epigastric pain, nausea, anorexia, weight loss	Endoscopy or X-ray examination showing segmental stenosis without gallstones
Liver	Hepatitis	M. avium intracellulare	Fever Weight loss Abdominal pain	Biopsy or blood culture
Colon	Colitis	CMV or herpes simplex	Diarrhea Abdominal pain Tenesmus	Biopsy

ORAL CAVITY AND ESOPHAGUS

Candidiasis
- Develops in all HIV patients with serious immunocompromise
- Typically see white plaques
  - Detach when scraped; often called oral thrush
  - Red spots on the tongue and palate may also be seen
  - Also can present as angular cheilitis
- Often accompanied by esophagitis
  - Patients complain of dysphagia and retrosternal pain
  - Esophagitis is an AIDS-defining illness, i.e., Class C, while stomatitis only Class B
  - Diagnose by endoscopy with esophageal scraping and biopsy

Diagnosis
- Usually a clinical diagnosis
- Scrapping showing pseudohyphae is helpful
- Throat cultures are not helpful because Candida normally colonizes the mouth

Treatment
- Fluconazole the initial drug of choice
  - First episode cured with a single dose of 150–400 mg po
  - HAART with reversal of immunosuppression prevents relapses.
  - Under conditions where immunosuppression cannot be reversed:
    - Treat relapses (or)
    - Prophylaxis with 50 mg/day or 150 mg/week
    - Either approach eventually leads to resistance and more frequent relapse.
- Fluconazole-resistant strains can be treated with:
  - Low-dose amphotericin B (20–30 mg/day iv)
  - Other uzoles (voriconazole, itraconazole solution, or ketoconazole is effective in some cases)
  - Caspofungin also a possible treatment

Mouth Ulcers and Aphthous Stomatitis
- Superficial lesions of the oral esophageal mucosa cause pain and dysphagia
- Differential diagnoses includes:
  - Herpes simplex
  - Cytomegalovirus
  - Side effects of drugs (zalcitabine)
  - Idiopathic ulcers
  - Persistent lesions should be biopsied for viral culture and immunofluorescence

Oral Hairy Leukoplakia
- A whitish lesion with irregular borders in the lateral part of the tongue, often bilateral
- Caused by Epstein-Barr virus
- Histology shows epithelial hyperplasia
- Treatment is not necessary, but in resistant cases:
  - Topical application of podophyllotoxin can be effective.
  - Acyclovir can also be administered but usually only causes temporarily regression of the lesions (see Chap. 15).

Tumors
- Kaposi's sarcoma frequently involves the oral cavity
- Produces painless macules or nodules with characteristic purple coloration on the palate, gingivae, or tongue

Salivary Glands
- Benign lymphoepithelial lesions and cystic hyperplasia involve mostly the parotid gland
- Can be associated with xerostomia
- Clinically similar to Sjögren's syndrome
- The parotid lesions are frequent in children, and are attributed to HIV itself

Differential Diagnosis of Esophagitis
- Candida most frequent; however, when esophageal symptoms occur in a patient who does not have clear evidence of candida stomatitis, other causes must be sought:
  - Cytomegalovirus causes longitudinal ulcers.
    - Biopsy, showing the characteristic viral inclusions in endothelial, epithelial, or smooth muscle cells
  - Herpes simplex type 1 causes small discrete lesions. Less commonly caused by herpes type II or by herpes zoster.
    - Diagnosis is made by biopsy plus immunofluorescence and/or culture.
  - Idiopathic ulcers
    - Diagnosis by exclusion
    - Treatment by thalidomide may bring relief

SMALL AND LARGE INTESTINE

Diarrhea
- Associated with weight loss, particularly in Africa, where it is called "slim disease"
- HIV infection alone can cause diarrhea
- Drugs
  - Antiretroviral drugs
    - Protease inhibitors most common (nelfinavir, ritonavir, amprenavir, lopinavir, indinavir)
    - Didanosine
  - Antibiotics can result in *C. difficile*–associated diarrhea (check *C. difficile* toxin)
- Salmonella, Shigella, and Campylobacter
  - Salmonella gastroenteritis is more commonly associated with bacteremia in HIV patients
  - Bacteremia most common with *Salmonella typhimurium* and *Salmonella enteritidis*
- Gastrointestinal *M. tuberculosis*
  - Difficult to differentiate from abdominal lymphoma
  - Laparascopic biopsy may be required for diagnosis
- Atypical mycobacteria (MOTT)
  - Most common with *M. avium*
  - Systemic illness with fever, weight loss, abdominal pain, and diarrhea
  - Diagnosis
    - Blood cultures often positive
    - Biopsies: submucosa may be filled with characteristic acid-fast bacilli

- CMV colitis in patients with CD4 < 50
  - Severe diarrhea, abdominal pain, tenesmus, and fever
  - May also cause cholangitis and pancreatitis
  - Colonoscopy shows multiple erosions, and biopsies reveal the characteristic intranuclear inclusions
- Protozoa (see Chap. 8)
  - Cryptosporidium, microsporidia, and isospora belli
  - Search for oocysts; trichrome stain for microsporidia

RECTUM AND ANUS

- Sexually transmitted disease common in this area including (see Chap. 9):
  - Gonococcal proctitis
  - Syphilis
  - Venereal warts
  - Herpes simplex can cause:
    - Rectitis with tenesmus and bleeding
    - Persistent and debilitating ulcerations
    - May require hospital admission and IV high-dose acyclovir
      - Resistance to acyclovir may require treatment with foscarnet.
- Cytomegalovirus less commonly causes anal ulcerations.
- Anal and rectal carcinomas are more frequent in homosexual patients.
  - Often related to the human papilloma virus
  - Screening papilloma virus in homosexual patients should be considered.

TUMORS OF THE DIGESTIVE SYSTEM

Kaposi's Sarcoma
- Gastric or intestinal involvement is found in about one half of the cases.
- Usually asymptomatic.
- Involvement of the gastrointestinal tract without involvement of skin is rare.
- Rare complications include bleeding, obstruction, invagination, and perforations.

Lymphoma
- AIDS-associated lymphomas involve preferentially the gastrointestinal tract (and the brain).
- Symptoms of lymphoma are difficult to distinguish from those of opportunistic infections.
  - Cause diarrhea, abdominal pain, fever and, weight loss
- Chemotherapy may be effective, but often is very difficult to administer to these severely immunosuppressed patients.

LIVER (SEE CHAP. 8)

Viral Hepatitis
- Hepatitic C coinfection with HIV
  - Hepatitis C and HIV are transmitted parenterally
    - HIV-HCV coinfection is particularly frequent in IV drug addicts and hemophiliacs.
  - Coinfected patients tend to have unfavorable prognostic indices for hepatitis C:
    - Higher incidence of infection with HCV type 1
    - Higher incidence of cirrhosis
    - Higher levels of HCV viremia

- Coinfection also adversely affects HIV.
    - CD4 response to HAART is less vigorous.
- Treatment with interferon and ribovirin now recommended (see Chap. 8)
    - History of depression a relative contraindication for interferon
    - Anemia a contraindication for ribovirin
- Coinfection with hepatitis B and HIV
    - Hepatitis B is sexually transmitted and is very common among men having sex with men.
    - Lamivudine (3-TC) is active against both HIV and hepatitis B and HAART using lamivudine diminishes HBV viremia.
    - The risk of development of HBV resistance to lamivudine is high with prolonged therapy.
    - Tenofovir a new alternative for lamivudine-resistant HBV.
- Liver damage induced by antiretroviral drugs
    - Most antiretroviral drugs may cause liver damage. The nature of that damage differs:
        - The nucleoside reverse transcriptase inhibitors (NRTIs) rarely cause severe steatosis associated with elevated plasma lactate levels.
            - More frequent with stavudine
        - Protease inhibitors
            - Indinavir and BMS-632232 cause asymptomatic hyperbilirubinemia (pseudo-Gilbert's syndrome).
            - Ritonavir and nelfinavir rarely cause cholestasis and hepatitis.
        - Nonnucleoside retrotranscriptase inhibitors (NNRTIs) can cause toxic hepatitis.
            - Neviripine in women has resulted in death or required liver transplantation.
            - Severe cases have not been reported with efavirenz.

CENTRAL NERVOUS SYSTEM

See Table 17-8 and Chap. 6.

HIGHLIGHTS

- HIV can cause aseptic meningitis in association with primary infection and encephalopathy resulting in dementia later in the course of infection.
- CMV can also cause encephalitis in patients with CD4 counts $< 50/mm^3$.
- Focal cortical lesions are a common CNS complication.
    - Toxoplasmosis is most common and results in multiple ring-enhancing lesions.
    - CNS lymphoma is the second most common and usually results in a single irregular contrast-enhancing lesion.
    - Progressive multifocal leukoencephalopathy shows distinct hyperintense lesions on MRI.
    - Rarer causes include cryptococcoma, tuberculoma, septic emboli, syphilitic gumma, and VZV encephalitis.
- Meningitis is most commonly caused by Cryptococcus when the CD4 count $< 200/mm^3$.
- Peripheral neuropathies are common and can be caused by HIV, autoimmunity, antiretroviral drugs, and malnutrition.

TABLE 17-8
CENTRAL NERVOUS SYSTEM

Diagnosis	Symptoms and signs	Laboratory/CSF findings	CT/IRM/PET-SPECT	Treatment of choice	Evolution
Cerebral toxoplasmosis	Focal deficit, headache, fever, seizures	<200 CD4 cells. Presence of IgG anti-toxo antibodies. PCR pos. if untreated	Multiple cortico-medullary lesions with contrast enhancement and edema. PET scan: hypodense lesions	Sulfadiazine + pyrimethamine + folinic acid	>80% response to treatment. 2° pro-phylaxis until immune reconstitution
Primary cerebral lymphoma	Slow onset of ↓ conciousness, headache, or focal deficits	<100 CD4. CSF: PCR "always" positive for EBV. Rarely cytology +	Variable number of lesions, periventricular contrast enhancement, lesions are + in the PET scan	Radiotherapy ± chemotherapy	Very serious prognosis
Progressive multifocal leukoencephalopathy	Progressive ↓ of superior cerebral functions, focal lesions	<100 CD4 cells. CSF: usually positive for papovavirus JC	CT: ↓ density of white substance, no contrast enhancement or edema. MRI: ↑ T2 signal without gadolinium enhancement	No specific treatment, cidofovir? intensify anti-HIV treatment	Has improved since HAART

	Clinical features	CSF/Lab findings	Imaging	Treatment	Prognosis
Cryptococcal meningitis	Fever, headache. Meningeal signs can be present or absent	<100 CD4. Blood and CSF + for cryptococcal antigen. Direct stain of CSF	No useful information	Amphotericin B ± flucytosine or fluconazole	>80% response. Prophylaxis with fluconazole until immune reconstitution
HIV encephalopathy and dementia	Cognitive and motor impairment	<200 CD4 HIV↑ in the CSF. Moderate ↑ in CSF cells and proteins	Cortico-subcortical atrophy. MRI shows ↑ signal in T2	Intensify the antiretroviral treatment	Progressive dementia within a few months
Aseptic meningitis	Headache, neck stiffness, photophobia, nausea during PHI	Moderate or no immunosuppression. CSF: moderate cell ↑	Normal	No specific treatment	Spontaneous resolution
CMV encephalitis	Confusion, lethargy, cranial nerve palsies, nystagmus	<50 CD4 PCR in the CSF is positive	Periventricular contrast enhancement	Foscarnet and ganciclovir	Bad prognosis

PET/SPECT = positron emission tomography/single photon emission computed tomography. CSF = cerebrospinal fluid. PHI = primary HIV infection.

DISORDERS CAUSED BY HIV AND CMV VIRUSES

Aseptic Meningitis in Association with Primary HIV Infection
- Half of patients with the acute retroviral syndrome complain of headaches.
- 5–20% have clinical signs of meningitis.
  - Neck stiffness and/or photophobia
  - CSF: 5–200/mm^3 lymphocytes, mildly elevated protein, normal CSF glucose
  - Cranial nerve involvement may occur.
  - Symptoms usually disappear spontaneously.
- Encephalitis is rare in primary HIV infection.

HIV Encephalopathy
- A diagnosis of exclusion
- Dementia symptoms
  - Problems with memory, mental slowness, and lack of precision are the first signs
  - Later accompanied by apathy and withdrawal; can be mistaken for depression
- Findings on exam:
  - Poor comprehension and coordination
  - Abnormal gait
  - Nystagmus and archaic reflexes
- CSF shows a variable increase in proteins and mononuclear cells.
- MRI: cerebral atrophy and increased T2 signal in the subcortical white matter in parasagittal regions.
- HAART has dramatically decreased the incidence of HIV dementia.
  - The effects of HAART on symptomatic encephalitis are variable, but can result in spectacular improvement.

Cytomegalovirus Encephalitis
- In addition to encephalitis CMV causes polyradicular myelitis and peripheral neuropathy in HIV-infected patients.
- Encephalitis usually seen when CD4 count < 50/mm^3.
- Clinical manifestations
  - Confusion and lethargy
  - Cranial nerve palsies and nystagmus
- MRI or CT shows periventricular contrast enhancement.
- Diagnosis
  - Exclude other causes
  - CSF PCR 80% sensitive, and specificity
- Treatment with ganciclovir or foscarnet.
- Prognosis is unfavorable despite treatment.

FOCAL CNS LESIONS
- Cerebral toxoplasmosis, primary cerebral lymphoma, and progressive multifocal leucoencephalopathy account for 90% of focal lesions.
- Differential diagnosis relies on:
  - CT scan and nuclear magnetic resonance.
  - The polymerase chain reaction to amplify DNA of putative infectious agents in the cerebrospinal fluid.
  - Cerebral biopsy remains an option in exceptional cases.

Toxoplasma Encephalitis

- Latent infection is present in 10% (United States) to 90% (developing countries and France)
- Usually presents with:
  - Confusion
  - Headaches may be localized
  - Fever
  - A focal deficit; for instance, hemiplegia
  - Convulsions
- Occurs with CD4 < 200

Diagnosis

- IgG toxo antibody (+)
  - Consider another diagnosis if negative or if taking trimethoprim-sulfa
- MRI or CT scan (MRI detects smaller lesions and lesions in the brain stem)
  - Multiple abscesses
  - Preferentially located at the corticomedullar junction and basal ganglia
  - Annular contrast or gadolinium enhancement
  - Marked edema common
- CSF PCR confirmatory, but L.P. should be avoided when significant cerebral edema

Treatment

- Empiric treatment indicated if anti-IgG antibody is positive and MRI findings typical.
- Sulfadiazine (1–1.5 g po QID) and pyramethamine (200 mg po the first day, then 50 mg every 6th day)
  - Also give folinic acid (10 mg/day) to prevent bone marrow toxicity
  - Continued for 4–6 weeks
- Dexamethasone (4 mg IV Q6H) may administered to diminish the cerebral edema.
- Follow-up CT or MRI at 2 weeks should demonstrate improvement.
- After treatment, secondary prophylaxis required: sulfadiazine 2 gm/day po and pyrimethamine 25 mg/day po
- Alternatives may be required because of toxicity.
  - Sulfadiazine can cause cutaneous, renal, or hepatic toxicity.
  - Pyrimethamine can result in bone marrow toxicity.
  - Alternatives
    - Clindamycin (600 mg po Q6H, then 600 mg Q12H) combined with pyrimethamine
      - Better tolerated
      - Efficacy is reduced.
    - Atovaquone suspension (750 mg po Q12H or Q8H) combined with pyrimethamine

Primary Brain Lymphoma

- B-cell lymphoma consisting of large immunoblastic lymphocytes that always contain EBV virus DNA
- Progression of headache, focal signs, and confusion over several weeks
- MRI or CT scan shows:
  - 1–2 irregular enhancing lesions
  - Preferentially localized in the periventricular regions
- Positron emission tomography (PET) and single photon emission computed tomography (SPECT) scans helpful in differentiating from toxoplasmosis and PML

- CSF
  - May contain lymphocytes
  - PCR is almost always positive for EBV.
- Sensitive to radiation and chemotherapy, but prognosis poor if CD4 $< 200/mm^3$

Progressive Multifocal Leukoencephalopathy
- Caused by reactivated JC papovavirus
  - 75% of the population is seropositive
  - Infects oligodendrocytes and causes demyelinization
- Starts insidiously with:
  - Loss of memory
  - Dysphasia
  - Visual disturbances
  - Aphasia or motor signs
  - Convulsions less common
- MRI shows hyperintense T2 images in the subcortical regions.
- CT lesions are not contrast enhancing and are not associated with cerebral edema.
- CSF
  - No inflammatory cells
  - PCR (+) for JC papovavirus
- Treatment with HAART can stabilize the illness and in some cases lead to clinical improvement.

Other Rare Focal Cerebral Lesions
- Cryptococcoma
  - Cryptococcal antigen test in CSF and blood can be negative.
- Tuberculoma
- Septic emboli may be associated with cerebral abscesses and mycotic aneurisms in IV drug abusers.
- Other lesions that may cause generalized CNS lesions or, less commonly, focal lesions:
  - Varicella zoster virus encephalitis
  - Secondary or tertiary syphilis

MENINGITIS

Cryptococcal Meningitis (see Chap. 6)
- The most common cause of meningitis in HIV-infected patients; CD4 usually $< 200/mm^3$
- Headache and fever the most common complaints; neck stiffness is usually absent.
  - A cause of FUO in AIDS patients
- CSF required to make the diagnosis
  - Lymphocytosis usual; may have decreased CSF glucose and elevated protein
    - CSF formula may be minimally abnormal.
  - India ink positive in 60% of cases
  - CSF latex antigen test positive
    - Titers are often high (1:32 to $> 1:1024$)
    - Serum antigen almost always positive
  - CSF and blood cultures are usually positive
- CT and MRI usually are not helpful.

Treatment
- Amphotericin B (0.7 IV mg/kg QD) for at least 2 weeks
- Addition of flucytosine (25 mg/kg Q6H) recommended by some
  - Associated with gastrointestinal and bone marrow toxicity
  - Renal excreted requiring reduction as serum creatinine increases
- After 2 weeks, fluconazole, 400 mg po or IV QD for 6–10 weeks
- Secondary prophylaxis required until CD4 > 200/mm^3 with fluconazole 200 mg po QD
- Fluconazole 400 mg po QD for less severe cases (without intracranial hypertension, normal mental status, cryptococcal antigen in the CSF at less than 1:1,000 dilution)
- Itraconazole not recommended; does not efficiently cross the blood-brain barrier

CEREBROVASCULAR DISEASES

- Cerebrovascular accidents are much more frequent in the HIV-infected than in comparable populations of the same age.
- Pathogenesis is uncertain, but a direct involvement of HIV in vasculitis is suspected.
  - Meningovascular syphilis should be excluded.
- Transient ischemic attacks have also been described.

PERIPHERAL NEUROPATHY

Distal Symmetric Polyneuropathy
- Causes painful paresthesia and dysesthesia in hands and feet
- Associated with:
  - Diminished reflexes and motor weakness in the legs
  - Autonomic dysfunction

Treatment
- Very difficult to manage
- Amytriptiline or carbamezepine may be useful
- Aggravated by vitamin deficiencies, diabetes, and alcohol abuse
- Drugs can also exacerbate
  - Dapsone, vincristine, and isoniazide.
  - Antiviral drugs, stavudine, and zalcitabine cause neuropathy, and less commonly didanosine and lamivudine. Should be replaced by other nucleosides.

Inflammatory Demyelinating Polyneuropathy
- Usually occurs during early stages of HIV infection.
  - In some cases associated with CMV infection
- Presentation is similar to Guillain-Barré syndrome.
- Treatment with corticosteroids, plasmaphereses, or IV immunoglobulins.
- Outcome is usually favorable.

Mononeuritis Multiplex
- Sudden nerve palsies involving one or several nerves, including cranial and laryngeal nerves
- Can occur at any stage of HIV infection
- Varicella zoster virus can be a cause in advanced immunodeficiency

Myelopathy
- Presents with gait disturbance, ataxia, spastic paraparesis, and urinary or fecal incontinence.
- MRI scan is usually normal but edema or even enhancing lesions may be seen.
- Autopsy findings show vacuolization of myelin and an accumulation of macrophages.
- Exclude reversible causes:
  - Epidural abscess
  - Toxoplasmosis
  - Infections with HTLV1
  - Herpes simplex, zoster, or cytomegalovirus
  - Vitamin B_{12} deficiency
- No treatment available

OPHTHALMOLOGY

See Chap. 5.

HIGHLIGHTS

- HIV retinopathy is frequent, but does not interfere with vision.
- CMV retinitis the most common cause of sight-threatening infection in HIV; usually associated with a CD4 count $< 50/mm^3$. Requires treatment with ganciclovir, valganciclovir, or foscarnet. Cidofovir for ganciclovir-resistant virus.
- Retinal necrosis is caused by VZV and requires emergency treatment with IV acyclovir to prevent the rapid development of blindness.

HIV RETINOPATHY

- Frequent, benign, and does not necessitate treatment
- Cotton wool exudates are characteristically observed.
  - Correspond to focal lesions of ischemia
- Other lesions include intraretinal hemorrhages, telangiectases, and microaneurysms.
  - Must be distinguished from retinal lesions caused by diabetes or hypertension
- Does not interfere with vision

CYTOMEGALOVIRUS RETINITIS

- Occurs in patients with profound immunosuppression <50 CD4 cells/mm^3
  - IgG CMV antibodies are invariably present.
  - Before HAART became available, 25–30% of patients with AIDS developed retinitis.
- All patients with HIV should be repeatedly questioned about changes in vision. More specifically:
  - Blurring of vision
  - Loss of central vision or other blind spots
  - Floaters or flashing lights
- A subacute disease with visual deficits progressing within a few weeks
- Diagnosis is easily made by examining the retina, which has a mixture of:
  - Exudates that often sheath the vessels
  - Hemorrhages
  - Atrophy

- Without treatment:
  - ○ Retinal detachment and progressive loss of vision occur.
  - ○ Often, both eyes are involved.
  - ○ Involvement of other organs occurs, including the colon, the esophagus, or the brain.

Treatment (see Chaps. 1 and 15)
- Ganciclovir (5 mg/kg IV Q12H) the drug of choice
  - ○ Valgancilovir (450 mg po BID) higher bioavailability than oral ganciclovir, may be efficacious for treatment as well as for maintenance
  - ○ Oral ganciclovir or valganciclovir recommended for primary and secondary prophylaxis
- Foscarnet (60 mg/kg IV Q8H) an alternative for patients with marrow toxicity from ganciclovir
- Treatment with IV ganciclovir and/or foscarnet necessitates use of a permanent catheter.
- Cidofovir (5 mg/kg IV once weekly during 2 weeks, then 5 mg/kg every 2 weeks) recommended only for CMV that is resistant to ganciclovir and foscarnet
- Duration of initial therapy 14–21 days
  - ○ Doses then lowered:
    - ▪ Oral valganciclovir, 450 mg QD, or ganciclovir, 1,000 mg TID
    - ▪ Ganciclovir, 6 mg/kg/day IV 5 days per week
    - ▪ Foscarnet, 100 mg/kg/day IV 5 days per week
    - ▪ Cidofovir, 5 mg/kg every 2 weeks

Outcome
- Relapses occur within 29–120 days, depending on the regimen.
- HAART therapy, achieving a durable rise of CD4 counts above 100, allows discontinuation of treatment without risk of relapse.

Prevention
- Oral ganciclovir diminishes the incidence of CMV retinitis by 50%
- Expense, inconvenience, and side effects make prophylaxis impractical
- Prevented by effective HAART therapy

RETINAL NECROSES
- A medical emergency necessitating treatment within hours
- Caused by varicella zoster virus
- Two clinical presentations can be distinguished:
  - ○ Acute retinal necrosis (ARN)
    - ▪ Orbital pain
    - ▪ Inflammation visible in the anterior ocular segment with hypopyon
    - ▪ Simultaneous peripheral retinal necrosis with vasculitis
    - ▪ Without treatment, progression is rapid with retinal detachment and blindness
  - ○ Progressive outer retinal necrosis (PORN)
    - ▪ Does not cause pain
    - ▪ Marked loss of visual acuity
    - ▪ Often preceeded by a recent episode of herpes zoster
    - ▪ The anterior segment demonstrates no evidence of inflammation
    - ▪ Peripheral lesions of retinal necrosis are observed
    - ▪ Without treatment, major risk of rapid loss of vision

- Treatment the same for both disorders
  - High doses of intravenous acyclovir (10 mg/kg Q8H)
  - Ganciclovir if there is a possibility of CMV retinitis

OTHER INFECTIOUS EYE DISEASES

- *P. carinii* may rarely involve the retina.
- Cryptococcal meningitis may be complicated by papillary edema.
- *Candida albicans* and bacteria that enter the bloodstream may cause retinitis in IV drug abusers.
- Rifabutin can cause uveitis, particularly when rifabutin levels are boosted by coadministration of macrolides or protease inhibitors.

SKIN DISEASES

See Table 17-9.

HIGHLIGHTS

- The development of a new skin rash often warrants immediate action. Can be a manifestation of primary HIV infection, opportunitistic infection, or a drug reaction.
- Even benign skin diseases may have a major psychologic impact when they reveal the patient's HIV status to the outside world.
- Primary HIV skin lesions consist of erythematous macules or papules on the chest, back, and face.
- Chronic herpes simplex-1 and -2 may persist when the CD4 count is low.
- Herpes zoster has a 20× higher incidence in HIV patients and may disseminate.
- Kaposi's sarcoma due to HHV-8 is found predominantly in homosexual men and may be difficult to differentiate from bacillary angiomatosis (caused by Bartonella).
- Seborrheic dermitis may be severe in HIV patients.
- Syphilitic skin lesions must always be exluded by serology.
- Drug reactions can be severe, resulting in erythroderma and desquamation.

SKIN LESIONS ASSOCIATED WITH PRIMARY HIV INFECTION

- Erythematous macules or papules with ill-defined margins.
- Symmetric distribution, on the front and back, the face, and sometimes on palms and soles
- Skin lesions neither itch nor hurt.
- Resemble pityriasis, secondary syphilis, a viral exanthema (due to Epstein-Barr virus, cytomegalovirus, rubella), or a toxic or allergic reaction to drugs.
- Lesions persist for a median of 2 weeks, then fade spontaneously.
- Less commonly, painful mucosal ulcers occur.

OPPORTUNISTIC INFECTIONS WITH SKIN OR MUCOSAL INVOLVEMENT

Chronic Herpes Simplex
- Herpes simplex type 1 or 2 may cause persisting genital, perianal, or perioral ulcerations in severely immunocompromised patients.
- Other etiologic agents should be excluded:

- ○ Fungi
- ○ Mycobacteria
- ○ Cytomegalovirus or varicella zoster virus
- ○ Malignant skin tumors
- Biopsy and immunofluorescence or by culture of virus
- Preferred treatment
  - ○ Valaciclovir, 500 mg po Q12H, or famciclovir, 125 mg po Q12H
  - ○ May become resistant to acyclovir and its derivatives, necessitating alternative treatment with foscarnet

Herpes Zoster
- Caused by reactivation of varicella zoster virus
- Occurs almost 20 times more frequently in HIV-positive than in HIV-negative patients of the same age
- Can present at any stage of immunosuppression
- In the severely immunosuppressed may:
  - ○ Extend beyond one or two dermatomes
  - ○ Causes atypical, ulcerated, and painful lesions that are difficult to treat
- In atypical cases, biopsy with direct immunofluorescence establishes the diagnosis.
- Treatment
  - ○ Milder cases, valaciclovir, 1 g po Q8H, or famciclovir, 500 mg po Q12H
  - ○ With severe immune suppression, intravenous acylovir 10 mg/kg Q8H

Kaposi's Sarcoma
- Associated with HHV-8 virus
- In United States and Europe found in HIV-infected homosexual men
- Can occur at almost any level of immunosuppression. Immune suppression greatly increases the risk.
- Clinical characteristics
  - ○ Often multifocal from the start
  - ○ Macules, papules, or nodules, purple color
  - ○ Usually on extremities, the tip of the nose, and the palate
  - ○ Lesions usually are slowly progressive.
  - ○ Do not cause pain
  - ○ Rarely aggressive with limb edema, GI and pulmonary involvement
- Histopathology: vascular proliferation and fusiform cells

Treatment: May be refractory to therapy
- HAART usually induces remissions.
- Local disease, cryo- or radiotherapy
- Severe disease
  - ○ Liposomal adriamycin (40 mg per m^2 Q2–3 weeks) (or)
  - ○ Bleomycin plus vincristine is also effective (or)
  - ○ Alpha-interferon (up to 50×10^6 units IV 5 days per week) if CD4 > 200 /μl

Bacillary Angiomatosis (see Chap. 13)
- Infection with *Bartonella quintana* and less commonly *B. henselae* causes papules and nodules with red to violet color.
  - ○ Present in variable numbers
  - ○ Not painful
  - ○ May ulcerate
- Usually febrile and extremely immunosuppressed indigent AIDS patients.

TABLE 17-9
SKIN DISEASES IN HIV

	Signs and symptoms	Diagnosis	Treatment	Comments
Acute HIV infection	Reddish macules on the trunk, face, palms, and soles of feet	↑ viremia and P24 antigenemia	HAART	Standard screening test for HIV can still be negative
Oral leukoplasia	Whitish plaques on lateral aspect of the tongue	Clinical diagnosis	No treatment	Associated with advancing immunodeficiency
Kaposi's sarcoma (due to HHV8)	Macules, papules, or nodules of purple to dark blue color. Edema and ulcers are possible	Inspection and histology	HAART. Local treatment. Cryotherapy, radiotherapy, and systemic chemotherapy	
Bacillary angiomatosis (B. henselae)	Red to violet papule or nodule	Histology (culture is difficult)	Antibiotics (macrolides, quinolones, and tetracyclines)	Rare, associated with advanced immunodeficiency
Herpes zoster	Vesicles on a red surface, necrosis, dermatomal distribution	Through inspection possibly confirmed by culture and immunofluorescence	Valaciclovir or famciclovir or acylovir po In serious cases IV acylovir	Chronic and disseminated forms are possible in advanced immunodeficiency

Seborrheic dermatitis (mold Malassezia?)	Red and squamous plaques on the face and trunk	Inspection	Topical ketoconazole	Prevalence > 30%
Acute condylomata	Wart-like papules ressembling a "rooster's comb"	Inspection or histology and typing of HPV	Curettage, podophylline, electrocoagulation, or laser	Treat sexual partner at the same time
Molluscum contagiosum (poxvirus)	Umbilicated papules	Inspection and histology	Curettage or electrocoagulation	
Herpes simplex	Painful vesicles or ulcers, which can become very large	Inspection, culture, and immunofluorescence	Valaciclovir or famciclovir, possibly acylovir iv	The lesions are primarily perianal, vulvar, or peribuccal
Prurigo nodularis	Isolated, very itchy squamous papules	Histology	Symptomatic treatment	Possibly with UV irradiation

- Biopsy with silver impregnation stains can show the Bartonella and differentiate the disease from Kaposi's sarcoma.
- A serologic test is also available.
- Treatment prolonged (2–4 months)
  ○ Clarithromycin, 500 mg po BID (or)
  ○ Azithromycin, 500 mg first day followed by 250 mg po QD (or)
  ○ Ciprofloxacin 500 mg po BID

Seborrheic Dermatitis
- Seborrheic dermatitis is more severe in HIV-infected patients.
- Reddish plaques covered by small scales appear on the face (nose, between the eyebrows), the scalp, and the sternum.
- Ketaconazole cremes and shampoos are efficacious.

SEXUALLY TRANSMITTED DISEASES
(SEE CHAP. 9)

Syphilis
- Serologic tests for syphilis are sensitive in the HIV-infected patient.
- Recommended treatment regimens for secondary or latent tertiary syphilis: 2.4 million units of benzathine penicillin IM at week 0, 1, and 2.
- Neurosyphilis requires a prolonged course of high dose of intravenous penicillin or ceftriaxone.

Drug Reactions
- Drug rashes are very frequent during HIV infection.
- Can constitute an emergency.
- Alarming signs necessitating hospitalization:
  ○ Conjunctivitis or lesions of the buccal mucosa
  ○ Generalized erythroderma
  ○ Detachment of the skin
- Can often treat through mild drug rashes and the rash will disappear
  ○ Particularly true of early reactions to efavirenz and nevirapine

MODERN ANTI-HIV THERAPY

HIGHLIGHTS

- The timing of therapy initiation must balance the long-term toxicity and cost versus the benefit of maintaining the viral load below detectable levels.
- The course of HIV has been likened to a train speeding toward a fallen bridge. The speed of the train is analogous to the viral load and the distance to the damaged bridge (AIDS) determined by the CD4 count.
- Therapy should be started and changed by a physician who specializes in HIV care.
- Three or more drugs should always be used and viral load should reduced to undetectable by 6–9 months to minimize the likelihood of selecting for resistant virus.
- The usual initial regimen recommended based on control trials is 2 NRTIs (AZT and 3TC) combined with 1 NNRTI (efavirenz).
- Side effects and drug-drug interactions are a major problems and must be closely monitored.
- 95% compliance is critical for successful treatment. Cures have not been achieved, and treatment must be lifelong.

INTRODUCTION: THE TEN COMMANDMENTS OF ANTIVIRAL TREATMENT (TABLE 17-10)

- Highly active antiretroviral therapies (HAART) can produce:
  - Durable suppression of viral replication with undetectable plasma levels of HIV-RNA in over half of the patients
  - Recovery of immunity
  - An 80% reduction in morbidity and mortality
- HAART also produces problems.
  - Does not completely eradicate HIV
  - Often, patients cannot comply with long-term combination treatment
  - Causes unexpected and ill-understood side effects
- Starting and maintaining HAART is complex.
  - A physician specializing in HIV care should be consulted whenever HAART is started or changed.
  - Mismanagement of antiretroviral therapy can lead to untoward toxicities and the development of resistant virus that can no longer be treated.
- Therapy is guided by 10 basic principles (see Table 17-10).

TABLE 17-10
10 PRINCIPLES FOR HAART

1. *Indication.* The presence of HIV infection establishes theoretically the indication for treatment, but treatment does not usually start until sub clinical immune deficiency is apparent.
2. *Combination.* Antiretroviral treatment consists of at least 3 drugs.
3. *First chance = best chance.* The choice of drugs during a first treatment course determines what possibilities still remain when a second and different treatment becomes necessary later. Chances for success are best first. Later, alternatives are limited by selection of resistant mutants.
4. *Complexity.* Antiretroviral treatment is complex, in particular because of drug interactions and side effects.
5. *Resistance.* Selection of resistant quasispecies occurs frequently. Within substance classes, cross-resistance is complete among available NNRTIs and partial among PIs and NRTIs.
6. *Information.* Starting and maintaining an effective antiretroviral treatment is time-consuming, because the information needs of physician and patients are considerable.
7. *Motivation and compliance.* The patient's willingness to take the drugs regularly at prescribed times and dosages will largely determine the success of treatment. Patients must understand the relation between insufficient compliance and drug resistance.
8. *Monitoring.* Efficacy of antiretroviral treatment is established by regular measures of viral RNA and of CD4 counts.
9. *Goals of treatment.* The goal of treatment is durable suppression of viral RNA below 50 copies/μL of plasma. Such suppression minimizes selection of resistant mutants, causes immune reconstitution and avoidance of morbidity and mortality.
10. *Studies.* Antiretroviral treatment continues to evolve toward greater simplicity and efficacy. Patients should be encouraged to participate in clinical studies that aim to optimize therapy.

INDICATIONS FOR STARTING TREATMENT
(SEE TABLES 17-11 AND 17-12)

- The course of HIV infection can be compared to a train speeding toward a fallen bridge.
  - The CD4 count represents the distance from the locomotive to the site of the fallen bridge and potential train wreck.
  - The viral load represents the speed.
- The CD4 count indicates the degree of immune deficiency, and predicts short-term risk of opportunistic disease. Without treatment the risk is:
  - $< 1\%$/year when the CD4 count > 500/mm^3
  - 30%/year when the CD4 count < 100/mm^3
- In the long term, prognosis is also determined by the viral load because HIV destroys CD4 cells and the lymph node architecture.
  - In population studies, elevated viral load predicts more rapid progression toward AIDS.
  - However, variations from individual to individual are enormous.
- Antiretroviral treatment
  - Suppresses viral replication
  - Prevents further destruction of the immune system
  - Allows for considerable repair in patients who are already immunosuppressed
- Recommendations of Table 17-11 are only approximations.
- Possible advantages and disadvantages of early start of treatment are outlined in Table 17-12.
- At present, four different classes of drugs are available (see Table 17-13):
  1. Nucleoside reverse transcriptase inhibitors (NRTI), such as abacavir (ABC), didanosine (ddI), lamivudine (3TC), stavudine (d4T), zalcitabine (ddC), and zidovudine (AZT)
  2. Nonnucleoside reverse transcriptase inhibitors (NNRTI), such as efavirenz (EFV) and nevirapine (NVP)
  3. Protease inhibitors (PI), such as amprenavir (APV), atazanavir (ATZ), indinavir (IDV), lopinavir/ ritonavir (LPV/r), nelfinavir (NFV), ritonavir (RTV), and saquinavir (SQV)
  4. Fusion inhibitors (FI): T-20 or enfuvirtide blocks fusion of HIV-1 with CD4+ cells
- Optimal suppression of viral replication requires the use of at least three drugs:
  - 1 or 2 NRTIs with 1 or 2 PIs, or with an NNRTI, or possibly 3 NRTIs
  - Factors considered in the decision:
    - Drug interactions
    - Dosage intervals (e.g., by the need to accommodate professional activity)
    - Future therapeutic options, or possible pregnancy
  - A double-blind controlled trial has shown initial treatment with 2 NRTIs (AZT, 3TC) and 1 NRRTI (EFV) to have a lower rate of development of resistance and lower incidence of side effects than 2 NRTIs and 1 PI.
- In other circumstances there are no clear criteria to choose between protease inhibitors and NNRTIs. Advantages and disadvantages of the two classes of drugs are shown in Table 17-14.
- The following treatment options are not recommended:
  - Therapy with only 1 or 2 drugs
  - Combinations of ddI plus ddC, or ddC plus d4T (added toxicity), zidovudine plus d4T (antagonism), or ddC plus 3-TC (no data)
  - Use of saquinavir, particularly the hard-gel capsule (Invirase®) without concomitant ritonavir (insufficient drug levels)
  - Use of agenerase or saquinavir, without concomitant ritonavir, in combination with efavirenz (insufficient drug levels)

TABLE 17-11
INDICATIONS FOR STARTING ANTIRETROVIRAL TREATMENT

Clinical stage	Laboratory values	Recommendations		
Acute HIV infection	Irrelevant	Consider HAART, obtain specialized consultation		
	CD4 count	*Viral load*		
		<50000	<50000	>50000
Chronic asymptomatic HIV infection (stage A)	>500	Wait	Wait	Wait
	350–500	Wait	Wait	Consider HAART
	<350	Treat	Treat	Treat
Symptomatic chronic HIV infection (CDC stage B or C)	Irrelevant	Treat		

TABLE 17-12
POTENTIAL ADVANTAGES AND DISADVANTAGES OF EARLY ANTIRETROVIRAL TREATMENT

Possible advantages of starting treatment early	Possible disadvantages of starting treatment early
Maximal suppression of viral replication; as a consequence, lesser risk of selection of resistant mutants	Risk of resistance as a consequence of suboptimal compliance
Prevention of immune deficiency and more complete immune reconstitution	Duration of efficacy of treatment may be limited
Less risk of side effects in patients whose general state of health is excellent	Loss of quality of life through short-term side effects, and possible long-term toxicity
	Cost
Healthy carriers are less contagious when treated; lesser number of new infections?	Transmission of new infections with drug-resistant viruses

TABLE 17-13
ANTI-HIV DRUGS AVAILABLE IN 2002

Generic name (Abbreviation)	Trade name	Usual dosage in the absence of renal failure	Class
Abacavir (ABC)	Ziagen	300 mg bid	NRTI
Didanosine (ddI)	Videx	300–400 mg qd*	NRTI
Lamivudine (3-TC)	3-TC	150 mg bid	NRTI
Stavudine (d4T)	Zerit	40 mg bid**	NRTI
Tenofovir (TFV)	Viread	300 mg qd	NRTI
Zalcitabine (ddC)	Hivid	0,75 mg tid	NRTI
Zidovudine (AZT)	Retrovir	250 mg bid	NRTI
AZT + 3-TC	Combivir	1 tab bid	NRTI
AZT + 3-TC + ABC	Trizivir	1 tab bid	NRTI
Efavirenz (EFV)	Stocrin	600 mg once daily	NNRTI
Nevirapine (NVP)	Viramune	200 mg bid	NNRTI
Amprenavir (APV)	Agenerase	900 mg bid***	PI
Atazanavir (ATZ)	Reyataz	400mg qd	PI
Indinavir (IDV)	Crixivan	800 mg bid***	PI
Lopinavir/ritonavir (LPV/r)	Kaletra	400/100 mg bid****	PI
Nelfinavir (NFV)	Viracept	1250 mg bid	PI
Ritonavir (RTV)	Norvir	100 mg bid*****	PI
Saquinavir hard gel (SQVh)	Invirase	400 mg bid***	PI
Saquinavir soft gel (SQVs)	Fortovase	1600 mg bid	PI
Enfuviritide (T-20)	Fuzeon	90 mg subQ bid	FI

NRTI = nucleoside reverse-transcriptase inhibitors; NNRTI = nonnucleoside reverse-transcriptase inhibitors; PI = protease inhibitors; FI = fusion inhibitors.

* 250–300 mg qd if weight < 60 kg; adjust dose in case of renal failure.

** 30 mg bid if weight < 60 kg; adjust dose in case of renal failure.

*** When coadministered with RTV.

**** 533/133 mg bid (4 pills bid) when coadministered with efavirenz.

***** 100 mg bid when coadministered with APV, IDV, or SQVs; 400 mg bid when coadministered with SQVh.

TABLE 17-14
PIs COMPARED TO NNRTIS IN INITIAL TREATMENT,
WHEN COMBINED WITH NRTIs

	Advantages	Disadvantages
Protease inhibitors	• Well-documented clinical efficacy • Relatively slow selection for resistance when treatment is suboptimal • Partial cross-resistance only; possible efficacy of a second PI in case of failure	• Heavy pill burden • GI side effects • Elevation of serum cholesterol and triglycerides • Glucose intolerance • Lipodystrophy • Osteopenia?
Nonnucleosides	• Only a few pills to swallow • Better compliance • Possibly less lipodystrophy	• Rapid development of resistance when treatment is suboptimal • Cross-resistance among currently used NNRTIs • Cutaneous side effects, including rare cases of Stevens-Johnson syndrome

TOLERANCE AND SIDE EFFECT MONITORING (SEE TABLE 17-15)

- NRTIs can be toxic to mitochondria, producing:
  - Liver damage
  - Lactic acidosis more strongly associated with d4T than with other NRTIs
  - Lipoatrophy more strongly associated with d4T than with other NRTIs
  - Polyneuropathy
- PIs cause:
  - Nausea, vomiting, and diarrhea
  - Elevated plasma cholesterol and triglycerides
    - Treatment with statins can result in toxic drug interactions.
  - Insulin resistance and glucose intolerance
  - Contribute, together with NRTIs, to the redistribution of fatty tissue; more frequent with the combination of saquinavir and ritonavir
  - Atrophy in the face and extremities and fat accumulation in breasts and abdomen

TABLE 17-15
FREQUENT SIDE EFFECTS OF ANTI-HIV DRUGS

Clinical symptom	Reverse Transcriptase Inhibitors NRTIs						NNRTIs		Protease Inhibitors						
	ABC	AZT	DdC	ddI	d4T	3TC	EFV	NVP	APV	ATZ	IDV	LPV	NFV	RTV	SQV
Abdominal pain															
Alterations of taste															
CNS symptoms															
Diarrhea															
Drug rash															
Fat accumulation							?	?							
Fat loss							?	?							
Fatigue															
Fever															
Headaches															
Hypersensitivity syndrome															
Kidney stones															
Myalgia															
Nausea															
Pancreatitis															
Paresthesias															
Polyneuropathy															

Key: Black = principal side effect, gray = side effect in >5% of patients

Row labels:
- Sleep disturbances
- Stomatitis
- Vertigo
- Vomiting
- **Laboratory tests**
- Amylase ↑
- Bilirubin ↑
- Cholesterol ↑
- Creatinine ↑
- Cytopenias
- Glucose ↑
- GOT/GPT ↑
- Lactate ↑
- Macrocytosis
- Triglycerides ↑

- T-20 (enfuvirtide) often causes inflammatory reactions at the injection site, causing some discomfort.
  - Forces discontinuation in 3% of patients
- All drugs produce various specific side effects; an overview is presented in Table 17-15.
  - Light shading means that the corresponding side effect has been reported in > 5% of patients.
  - Black shading designates the drug's principal side effect.
  - Because the drugs have usually been tested in combination, assignment of a particular side effect to a particular drug is often uncertain.
- The potential side effects necessitate regular patient visits.
  - When drugs are first begun, visits after 1, 2, and 4 weeks of treatment are recommended to monitor toxicity.
  - If no toxicity, the intervals may then lengthen to every 2–3 months.
  - Should monitor complete blood count, liver enzymes, lactate, and serum cholesterol and triglycerides.

DRUG INTERACTIONS

- Protease inhibitors and NNRTIs are preferably metabolized by cytochrome P3A.
  - Rifamycins or hypericum (St. John's wort) induces cytochrome P3A and may lower PI and NNRTI concentrations.
  - Ergotamines and benzodiazepines are also metabolized by cytochrome P3A and their levels may increase.
- Drug-drug interactions are constantly being updated, and should be periodically checked on the Internet.
  - (www.hiv-druginteractions.org) (and)
  - (http://medscape.com/home/topics/aids/aids.html)
- Ritonavir is the most powerful inhibitor of cytochrome P3A known in medical therapeutics.
  - Inhibits metabolism of other PIs, increasing indinavir, lopinavir, saquinavir, and amprenavir serum levels.
  - Other PIs can be combined with small doses of ritonavir (100 mg twice daily) to boost plasma drug levels and to lengthen intervals between doses.

COMPLIANCE

- Largely determines the long-time success or failure of HAART.
- More than 95% of dosages need to be taken correctly in order to guarantee optimal results.
- Patients must be educated in:
  - The pathogenesis of HIV
  - The goals of HIV treatment
  - Pharmacokinetics
  - Recognition of the most frequent side effects and know how to manage them

EFFICACY

- Above 20–50 copies/mm^3, the nadir of the viral load achieved by treatment predicts duration of viral suppression.
- Combination treatment should reduce viral load to:
  - <400 copies/mm^3 after 12 weeks
  - <50 copies/mm^3 after 24 weeks
- Viral load measurements and CD4 counts are recommended every 3 months.

RESISTANCE TESTS

- Low drug concentrations allow continued viral replication and selection of resistant mutants and is caused by:
  - Suboptimal treatment
  - Lack of compliance
  - Insufficient bioavailability
  - Drug interactions
- Resistance testing is mainly useful for excluding drugs to which the virus is resistant.
  - Less helpful for finding drugs to which the virus is sensitive
- Resistance tests are recommended in patients:
  - Infected in 1997 or later when first initiating therapy
  - After early treatment failure

MEASUREMENT OF PLASMA DRUG CONCENTRATIONS

- Drug levels are not routinely recommended. Should be ordered when there are:
  - Unexpected toxicities
  - Suspected problems with compliance that cannot be investigated otherwise
  - Multiple medications producing unforeseeable pharmacokinetic interactions

TREATMENT MODIFICATION AND SIMPLIFICATION

- Once viremia is suppressed, simplification of treatment can be considered.
  - Risky to replace triple therapy (with a PI and 2 NRTIs) with just 2 drugs
  - PI can be replaced by an NNRTI, and viral suppression usually persists for at least 2 years.
  - In formerly drug-naïve patient may replace the PI/2NRTI combination with the three NRTIs ABC/AZT/3-TC
    - Insulin resistance, serum cholesterol, and triglycerides tend to normalize.
    - Fat redistribution is usually irreversible.
  - Strategic treatment interruptions are not recommended in routine practice.

PROCEDURES IN CASE OF FAILURE

- Changes are often required for intolerance, drug interactions, or side effects.
  - If viremia is below 50 copies/mm^3, a single offending drug can be replaced.
- In cases of virologic failure (viral load is not <50 copies/mm^3 after 6 months or after 9 months in patients with an initial viral load > 1,000,000 copies/mm^3):
  - A new combination should be chosen, containing, if possible, a drug from a class that had not been used previously. T-20 may be useful in these patients.
  - At least 1 additional drug should also be replaced by 1 to which the patient is unlikely to be resistant on the basis of his/her drug history and resistance tests.
  - A virologically failing regimen should be maintained, if there is no alternative. Often preserves the CD4 count

START AND END OF PROPHYLAXIS FOR OPPORTUNISTIC INFECTIONS

- Prophylaxis of opportunistic infections can be discontinued after the CD4 count has risen above specific levels for at least 3 months.
  - 100 CD4 cells/mm^3 for stopping prophylaxis of cytomegalovirus and nontuberculous mycobacteria
  - 200 CD4 cells/mm^3 for stopping prophylaxis of *P. carinii* pneumonia and Toxoplasma encephalitis

CONCLUSIONS CONCERNING THERAPY

- A durable antiviral effect requires complete abolishment of viral production.
  - Emergence of resistance becomes much less likely.
  - Patients may be treated for many years without viral breakthrough.
  - Despite optimal therapy, the virus persists in reservoirs that are not accessible to current treatment, making eradication by continuous treatment unrealistic.

REFERENCES

Some of the best (certainly the most up-to-date!) resources can be accessed via the Internet, for instance:

1. http://hivinsite.ucsf.edu/InSite or http://medscape.com/home/topics/aids/aids.html for general information
2. www.hiv-druginteractions.org is particularly useful for information about drug interactions
3. www.unaids.org for the latest statistics on epidemiology
4. www.hivatis.org/trtgdlns.html#Adult for the latest treatment guidelines

Shafer RW, Smeaton LM, Robbins GK, De Gruttola V, Snyder SW, et al: Comparison of four-drug regimens and pairs of sequential three-drug regimens as initial therapy for HIV-1 infection. *N Engl J Med* 2003; 349:2304–15.

INDEX

Note: Page numbers followed by *f* indicate figures; those followed by *t* indicate tables.

A

Abscesses, 82
  brain, 162–165
  epidural, 166
  hepatic, 205
  intra-abdominal, 94
  lung, 102
  pancreatic, 205
  peritonsillar, 141
  skin, 240*t*, 244
  spinal epidural, 166–167
  subdural, 166
Acanthamoeba, 138
Acidosis, metabolic, 74
Actinomycosis, 118
Acute pneumonias, 97–125
Acyclovir, 61–62, 160
Acylostoma duodenale, 276
Adjunctive therapies for sepsis syndrome, 78
Adult respiratory distress syndrome (ARDS), 74
AIDS. *See also* HIV infection
  indicator conditions in the case definition of, 341*t*
Air sinus infections, 95
Alkalosis, respiratory, 74
Allergic conjunctivitis, 137
Amantadine, 69–70
Amebiasis, 197–199
Amikacin, 28, 29, 53
Aminoglycosides, 3, 25–29
Aminopenicllins, 13–14
Amoxacillin, 13, 14

Amoxacillin-clavulanate (Augmentin), 13, 14
Amphotericin B, 55–56, 133, 134
Ampicillin, 13, 14
Ampicillin-sulbactam (Unasyn), 14
Anal carcinoma, 358
Anaphylaxis, 12
Anemia, hemolytic, 46
Angiomatosis, bacillary, 298, 299, 369, 372
Animal bites, 245–246
Anogenital warts, 235
Anthrax, 303–307
  cutaneous, 304–305, 305*f*, 307
  gastrointestinal, 306–307
  inhalation, 305–306, 306*f*, 307
  treatment of, 308*t*
Antibiotic-associated diarrhea, 201–202
Antibiotics
  for bacterial meningitis, 156*t*
  basic strategies for, 5, 6*f*, 7
  β-lactam, 11, 177
  for bioterrorist bacterial agents, 308–309*t*
  cidal, 177
  classification of, by spectrum of activity, 8*t*
  classification of oral, by cost, 10*t*
  cost ranges for intravenous and oral, 8*t*
  for ear infections, 142–143*t*
  for gastrointestinal infections, 195–196*t*
  glycopeptide, 29–31
  for hematogenous osteomyelitis, 252*t*
  for infective endocarditis, 178–179*t*
  mechanisms of resistance, 1–3, 2*f*
  for nose infections, 142–143*t*
  for sepsis syndrome, 76*t*, 77

for skin and soft tissue infections, 240t
specific, 11
for throat infections, 142–143t
for zoonotic infections, 290–291t
Antifungal agents, 54–60
Anti-HIV therapy, 372–374, 378, 380–382
drugs available in 2002, 376t
Anti-infective therapy, 1–70
algorithm for initial use, 6t
classification of parenteral, by cost, 9t
factors determining dosing, 3–5, 4f
Anti-influenza viral agents, 69–70
Antimicrobial resistance
biochemical mechanisms for, 2–3
genetic modifications leading to, 1–2, 2f
Antimycobacterial agents, 48–54
first-line medications, 49–53
second-line medications, 53–54
Antipyretics, 92
Antiretroviral treatment, potential advantages and disadvantages of early, 375t
Antiviral drugs, 61–70
Anus, infections of, 358
Aphthous stomatitis, 356
Arbovirus, encephalitis caused by, 161t
Arthritis, septic, 257–261
Ascaris, 275
Aseptic meningitis, 362
Aspergillus, 138
Aspiration pneumonia, 116–117
Astroviruses, 197
Atrial myxoma, 84
Atypical mycobacteria (MOTT), 132, 357
Atypical pneumonia, 121–122
Autoimmune diseases, 84–85
Azithromycin, 31, 33–34, 109, 119
Azoles, 56
Aztreonam, 22

B
Babesiosis, 268–269
Bacillary angiomatosis, 298, 299, 369, 372
Bacteremia, 72
causes of, leading to potential endo-carditis, 171t
Bacterial aspiration pneumonia, 117

Bacterial conjunctivitis, 137
Bacterial diarrhea, 189–194
Bacterial endocarditis, subacute, 82
Bacterial infections, 337
Bacterial meningitis, 151–157
antibiotic treatment for, 156t
CSF profiles, 154t
etiologies, 151–152, 152t
pathogenesis, 153–154
Bacterial pharyngitis, 141
Bacterial pneumonias, 346, 350
Bacterial sinusitis, 13, 14, 148
Bacteriophages, 1
Bannworth's syndrome, 288
Bartonella infections, 298–300
treatment of, 291
Benzathine penicillin G, 13
β-lactam antibiotics, 11, 177
β-lactamases, 2
Biliary system infections, 82
Biochemical mechanisms for anti-microbial resistance, 2–3
Bioterrorism, 303–315
antibiotic treatment of agents, 308–309t
Bites
animal, 245–246
human, 245–246
Bithionol, 281
Blood helminths, 276–281
Blood protozoa, 261–269
Bone infections, 247–260
Bone marrow transplantation, infec-tions associated with mixed deficits found in, 333
Borrelia burgdorferi, 287–290, 292
Boutonneuse fever, 295
Bradycardia, 74
Brain abscess, 162–165
neurologic manifestations of, 164t
Brill-Zinsser disease, 295
Bronchial obstruction, 117
Bronchitis, 94
Bronchopneumonia, 102, 106f
Brucellosis, 36, 83, 300–301
treatment of, 291
Brugia malayi, 282–283
Burn infections, 243

C
Campylobacter, 357
Campylobacter fetus, 191
Campylobacter jejuni, 191, 194

Candida albicans, 183, 368
Candida endophthalmitis, 140
Candidiasis, 356
Capreomycin, 53
Carbapenems, 23–25
Carboxypenicillins, 15–16
Carbuncles, 244
Cardiovascular infections, 169–187
    clinical manifestations, 172–173,
        174f
    complications, 175–177
    diagnosis, 175, 176t
    etiologies, 170–171, 172t
    prevention, 180–181
    prognosis, 180
    treatment, 177, 178–179t, 180
Caspofungin, 60
Cat scratch disease, 298–300
Cavernous sinus thrombosis, 146
Cefazolin, 17, 18
Cefepime, 22
Cefipirome, 22
Cefixime, 21, 119
Cefotaxime, 20
Cefotetan, 18, 19
Cefoxitin, 18
Cefpodoxime proxetil, 21, 119
Cefriaxone, 20
Ceftazidime, 20–21
Ceftizoxime, 20
Cefuroxime, 18, 19
Cellulitis, 15, 146, 237, 239
    treatment of, 240t
Central nervous system
    HIV and, 359, 360–361t, 362–366
    infections, 151–168
Cephalexin, 17
Cephalosporins, 16–22
    basic structure, 16f
    chemistry and mechanisms of action,
        16, 16f
    first-generation, 17–18
    fourth-generation, 21–22
    second-generation, 18–19
    third-generation, 19–21
    toxicity, 17
Cephradine, 17
Cerebrovascular diseases, 365
Cervical necrotizing fasciitis, 241
Chagas' disease, 183
Charcot's triad, 206
Chemical burn pneumonitis, 116
Chest x-ray, 348t
Chinese liver fluke, 281

Chlamydia, 36, 83, 141
Chlamydia pneumoniae, 122
Cholangiocarcinoma, 281
Cholangitis, 206, 281
Cholecystitis, 206
Choramphenicol, 36–38
Chronic herpes simplex, 368–369
Chronic pneumonia, 126–135
Cidal antibiotics, 177
Cidofovir, 65–66
Ciprofloxacin, 39–40, 46
Clarithromycin, 32–33, 109, 119
Clindamycin, 34–35
Clinorchis sinensis, 281
Clostridia myonecrosis, 237
Clostridium difficile, 201, 202
Cloxacillin, 15
Coccidioidomycosis, 353
Coccidiomycosis, 134–135
Colitis, cytomegalovirus, 358
Colonization, differentiating from
    infection, 10
Community-acquired pneumonia, 20
    clinical characteristics of acute, clas-
        sified by etiology, 101t
    port assessment of risk factors in,
        104t
    specific causes of acute, 113–122
Concentration-dependent killing, 4
Congyloma acuminata, 235
Conjugation, 1, 2f
Conjunctivitis, 137–138
    allergic, 137
    bacterial, 137
Contact lens abrasions, 138
Corneal infections, 138–139
Coryneacterium diphtheriae, 141
Coxiella burnetti, 297–298
Cryptococcal meningitis, 364–365, 368
Cryptococcal meningoencephalitis, 159
Cryptococcoma, 364
Cryptococcosis, 83
Cryptosporidium, 200
Cryptosporidium parvum, 198f
Cutaneous anthrax, 304–305, 305f
Cyclic neutropenia, 81
Cycloserine, 54
Cysticercosis, 278–279
Cystic fibrosis, 98
Cystitis, 219
    treatment, 221
Cytomegalovirus, 83, 158, 328, 337,
    356, 358
Cytomegalovirus colitis, 358

Cytomegalovirus encephalitis, 362
Cytomegalovirus retinitis, 366–367

D
Dalfopristin, 42
Daptomycin (Cubicin®), 43–44
Depressed cell-mediated immunity, infections associated with, 332–333
Dermatitis, seborrheic, 372
Diabetes mellitus, 241
Diabetic foot infection, osteomyeltis secondary to vascular insufficiency, 253–254
Diarrhea, 357
    antibiotic-associated, 201–202
    bacterial, 189–194
    immunocompromised hosts and, 200–201
    infectious, 189–197
    traveler's, 194
    viral, 197
Dicloxacillin, 15
Digestive system, tumors of, 358
Dirofilariasis, 283
Disseminated gonococcal infection, 259–260
    treatment of, 225t
Disseminated toxoplasmosis, 353
Dog heartworm, 283
Donovanosis, treatment of, 228–229t
Doxycycline, 36
Drotrecogin alpha, 78
Drug fever, 85, 95
Drug reactions, 372

E
Ear infections, 144–145
    antibiotic therapy for, 142–143t
Echinococcosis, 277–278
Echinococcus, 277–278
Efflux pumps, 3
Ehrlichia, 296–297
Elephantiasis, 282
Empiric treatment, 109, 110–111t, 112–113
Empyema, 124–125
Encephalitis, 151, 318
    arboviruses as cause of, 161t
    cytomegalovirus, 392
    herpes, 327
    toxoplasma, 363
    viral, 160–162

Encephalopathy, HIV, 392
Endocarditis
    causes of bacteria leading to potential, 171t
    infective, 169–181, 178–179t
    subacute bacterial, 82
    tricuspid, 177
Endophthalmitis, 139–140
    candida, 140
    fungal, 139
    hematogenous, 140
Entamoeba histolytica, 197, 198f
Entamoeba spp., 198
Enteric adenovirus, 197
Enteric fever, 193–194
Enteritis, regional, 85
Enterobius, 275
Epidural abscess, 166
Epiglottitis, 141
Epithelial hyperplasia, 356
Epstein-Barr virus, 83, 158, 319–320, 356
Erlichia, treatment of, 291
Erythema migrans, 288, 288f
Erythema multiforme, 12, 46
Erythromycin, 31, 32, 109
Escherichia coli, 191–192, 194
Esophagitis, 354, 356
    differential diagnosis, 357
Esophagus, infections in, 356–357
Ethambutol, 52–53
Ethionamide, 54
Ethmoid sinusitis, 146, 148
Extended-spectrum β-lactamases (ESBLs), 2
Eye infections, 137–140
    HIV and, 366–368

F
Factitious fever, 86
Famciclovir, 63
Familial Mediterranean fever (FMF), 85
Fasciola hepatica, 281
Febrile nonneutropenic compromised host, diagnosis and management of the, 336–337
Febrile patient, 79–96
Fever
    benefits of, 80
    factitious, 86
    harmful effects of, 80
    in sepsis syndrome, 74

in surgical intensive-care and medical intensive-care patients, 94–95
treatment of, 80
Fever of undetermined origin (FUO), 81–96
  causes, 82–84, 86f
  diagnosis, 81, 87–92, 88ft
  drugs causing, 85t
  history in, 86
  in the HIV-infected patient, 93
  prognosis, 93
  tests recommended for, 88t
  treatment of, 92
Filariasis, 282–283
Flea-borne typhus, 296
Fluconazole, 56, 57, 58, 135, 356
Flucytosine (5-FC), 59–60
Fluoroquinalones, 115, 119
Focal CNS lesions, 362–364
Folliculitis, 244
Foscarnet, 66–67
Fournier's gangrene, 241
Francisella tularensis, 311–312
Frontal sinusitis, 147, 148
Fungal endophthalmitis, 139
Fungal infections, 337
Fungi, 83
Furunculosis, 244

G
Ganciclovir, 64–65
Gangrene, Fournier's, 241
Gastroenteritis, 193
Gastrointestinal anthrax, 306–307
Gastrointestinal infections, 189–216, 355t
  antibiotic therapy for, 195–196t
  HIV infection and, 354, 356–359
Gastrointestinal M. tuberculosis, 357
Gatifloxacin, 41, 109, 115
Genital ulcers, 230–231
  clinical characteristics of, 232t
  treatment of, 227–228t
Gentamicin, 13, 27, 28, 29
Giardia lamblia, 198f, 199
Glucocorticoids, 92
Glycopeptide antibiotics, 29–31
Gonococcal proctitis, 358
Gonococcal urethritis, treatment of, 225t
Grand mal seizures, 12
Granulomatous diseases, 85

H
Haemophilus influenzae, 119, 152, 157
Hantavirus, 321
Heartworm, 283
Helicobacter pylori-associated peptic ulcer disease, 206–207
Helminths
  intestinal, 272, 273f, 274, 274f, 275–276
  tissue and blood, 276–281
Hematogenous endophthalmitis, 140
Hematogenous osteomyelitis
  antibiotic treatment of, 252t
  of long bones and vertebral bodies, 248–253
Hemolytic anemia, 46
Hepatic abscess, 205
Hepatitis, viral, 207–214, 358–359
Hepatitis A, 207, 208–209, 210t
Hepatitis B, 207, 209, 210t, 211–213, 354
  clinical course of, 212f
Hepatitis C, 207, 210t, 214, 354
Hepatitis D, 210t, 213
Hepatitis E, 209, 210t
Hepatobiliary infections, 189–216
Hepatoma, 84
Herpes encephalitis, 327
Herpes keratitis, 327
Herpes simplex, 138, 326–327, 337, 358
  chronic, 368–369
  type II primary disease, 158
Herpes zoster, 318, 369
Herpetic whitlow, 327
Highly active antiretroviral therapies (HAART), 373, 373t
Histiocytic necrotizing lympadenitis, 85
Histoplasmosis, 83, 132–133, 353
HIV encephalopathy, 362
HIV infection, 339–382
  central nervous system and, 359, 360–361t, 362–366
  fever of undetermined origin in, 93
  gastrointestinal system and, 354, 356–359
  laboratory evaluation of, 341–343
  lung diseases linked to, 347t
  ophthalmology and, 366–368
  pulmonary infections and, 346–354
  stages of, 343t
HIV retinopathy, 366
Hodgkin's disease, 81

Hookworm, 276
Human bites, 245–246
Hyperinfection syndrome, 275
Hypernephroma, 84
Hypersensitivity angiitis, 85
Hypersensitivity reactions, 12
Hypoprothrombinemia, 17
Hypotension, 74

I

Imipenem, 23, 25
Immunocompromised hosts
  diarrheal illnesses primarily associ-
    ated with, 200–201
  infections in, 331–337
Immunodepression, forms of, 331–332
Impetigo, 244
  treatment of, 240*t*
Infections
  bacterial, 337
  bartonella, 298–300
  biliary system, 82
  bone and joint, 247–260
  burn, 243
  cardiovascular, 169–187
  corneal, 138–139
  diabetic foot, 253–254
  differentiating colonization from, 10
  disseminated gonococcal, 259–260
  ear, 142–143*t*, 144–145
  fungal, 337
  heptobiliary, 189–216
  HIV, 339–382
  in the immunocompromised host,
    331–337
  intra-abdominal, 202–207
  intravascular catheter-related,
    181–183
  intravascular device, 94–95
  nose, 142–143*t*
  opportunistic, 343–344, 345*t*,
    368–369, 372, 382
  parasitic, 197–199, 198*t*, 261–284
  in prosthetic joints, 256–257
  pulmonary, 97–136, 346–354
  rickettsial, 83, 293–300
  sinus, 145–148
  skin and soft tissue, 237–246
  throat, 140–143, 142–143*t*
  zoonotic, 287–301, 290–291*t*
Infectious diarrhea, 189–197
Infective endocarditis, 169–181
  antibiotic therapy for, 178–179*t*

Inflammatory demyelinating polyneu-
  ropathy, 365
Influenza, 324–326
Ingestion, nematodes acquired by,
  274–275
Inhalation anthrax, 305–306, 306*f*
Interferons, 68–69
Interstitial lymphoid pneumonia, 352
Interstitial pneumonia, 102
Intestinal helminths, 272–273, 274,
  274*f*, 275–276
Intestinal nematodes, 274, 274*f*
Intra-abdominal abscess, 94
Intra-abdominal infections, 202–207
Intravascular catheter-related infections,
  181–183
Intravascular device infection, 94–95
Invasive aspergillosis, 354
Isoniazid (INH), 49–50
Isospora belli, 198*f*, 200, 201
Itraconazole, 57–58, 133, 135

J

Joint infections, 247–260

K

Kanamycin, 53
Kaposi's sarcoma, 354, 357, 358, 369
  pulmonary, 352
Kartagener's syndrome, 98
Katayama fever, 280
Keratitis
  herpes, 327
  viral, 139
Ketoconazole, 56
Kikuchi's disease, 85

L

Large intestine, infections in, 357–358
Legionella pneumophila, 120–121, 332
Leishmaniasis, 269–271
  cutaneous, 270–271
  mucosal, 270–271
  visceral, 270
Leptospirosis, 292–293
  treatment of, 290*t*
Leukemia, 84
Levofloxacin, 40–41, 109, 115
Linezolid, 41–42
Listeria monocytogenes, 152, 332
Liver, diseases of, 358–359

Loa Loa, 283–284
Lobar pneumonia, 102, 105*f*
Löffler's syndrome, 276
Loiasis, 283–284
Louse-borne typhus, 295
Lung abscess, 102
Lung diseases linked to HIV, 347*t*
Lung fluke, 281
Lyme disease, 36, 83, 287–290, 292
  treatment of, 290*t*
Lymphocytic choriomeningitis, 158
Lymphogranuloma venereum, treatment
  of, 228*t*
Lymphoma, 83, 358
  primary brain, 363–364

M
Macrolides, 31–34
Macular pruritic rash, 12
Malaria, 81, 83, 261–268
  differences in strains, 265*t*
Mastoiditis, 145
Mean bactericidal concentration
  (MBC), 3–4, 4*f*
Medical intensive-care patients, fever
  in, 94–95
Meningitis, 135, 364–365
  aseptic, 362
  bacterial, 151–157, 154*t*, 155*f*, 156*t*
  cryptococcal, 364–365, 368
  nosocomial, 152
  tuberculous, 158–159
  viral, 151, 158
Meningoencephalitis, cryptococcal, 159
Meropenem, 23, 24, 25
Metabolic acidosis, 74
Methicillin, 15
Metronidazole, 44–45, 199
Microsporidia, 198*f*, 200–201
Miliary tuberculosis, 83, 126, 128–129
Minimum inhibitor concentration
  (MIC), 3, 4*f*
Mixed connective tissue disease, 85
Monobactams, 22–23
Mononeuritis multiplex, 365
Mouth ulcers, 356
Moxifloxacin, 41, 109, 115
Mucositis, pathogens associated with,
  332
Mumps, 158
Mycobacteria, atypical, 132
Mycobacteria other than tuberculosis
  (MOTT), 352

Mycobacteria spp., 332
Mycobacterium kansasii, 352
Mycoplasma, 141
Mycoplasma pneumoniae, 121–122
Myelopathy, 366
Myocarditis, 183–184
Myonecrosis, 237, 242–243
  treatment of, 240*t*

N
Nafcillin, 15
Natural penicillins, 12–13
Necator americanus, 276
Necroses, retinal, 367–368
Necrotizing fasciitis, 237, 239,
  241–242
  due to *Steptococcus pyogenes*, 75
  treatment of, 240*t*
Neisseria gonorrhoeae, 141
Neisseria meningitidis, 151, 157
Nematodes
  acquired by ingestion, 274–275
  acquired by skin penetration,
    275–276
  intestinal, 274, 274*f*
Nephrotoxicity, 25–26
Netilmicin, 28
Neuramidase inhibitors, 70
Neuromuscular blockade, 26–27
Neuropathy, peripheral, 365–366
Neutropenia, 5, 331
  diagnosis and treatment of, 333–336,
    334*f*
  pathogens associated with, 332
Nocardia, 118–119, 332
Nocardia asteroides, 353
Nodular lesions, 102
Nongonococcal urethritis, treatment of,
  226*t*
Noninfectious causes of fever, 95
Nonnucleosides, 377
  tolerance and side effect monitoring,
    377, 378–379*t*
Norwalk virus, 197
Nose infections, antibiotic therapy for,
  142–143*t*
Nosocomial meningitis, 152
Nosocomial pneumonia, 122–124

O
Onchocerca volvulus, 283
Onchocerciasis, 283

Opportunistic infections, 343–344
  prophylaxis of, 345*t*
  with skin or mucosal involvement,
    368–369, 372
  start and end of prophylaxis for, 382
Optic neuritis, 52
Oral candidiasis, 354
Oral cavity, infections in, 356–357
Oral hairy leukoplakia, 354, 356
Oral thrush, 356
Orbital cellulitis, 146
Oroya fever, 298
Oseltamivir, 70
Osteomyelitis, 82, 247–256
  diagnosis, 249–251, 250*f*, 251*f*
  general principles for the manage-
    ment of, 255–256
  microbiology of, 248*t*
  secondary to a contiguous infection,
    253
  treatment, 251, 252*t*, 253
Otitis externa, 144
Otitis media, 13, 144–145
Ototoxicity, 26
Oxacillin, 15
Oxazolidones, 41–42

P
Pancreatic abscess, 205
Pansinusitis, 147*f*
Papular gu lesions, 235
Para-aminosalicylic acid (PAS), 54
Paragonimus westermani, 281
Parasites, 83
Parasitic infections, 197–199, 198*t*,
    261–284
Pel-Ebstein fever, 81, 83
Pelvic inflammatory disease (PID), 36,
    224, 230
  treatment of, 226–227*t*
Penciclovir, 63
Penicillinase-resistant pencillins, 15
Penicillin G, 13
Penicillin-resistant *S. pneumoniae*, 155
Penicillins, 11–16
  basic structure of, 11*f*
  natural, 12–13
  penicillinase-resistant, 15
Penicillin V-K, 13
Pericardiocentesis, 186
Pericarditis, 185–186
  purulent, 185, 186
  tuberculous, 185, 186

Peripheral neuropathy, 365–366
Peritonitis, primary or spontaneous,
    202–203
Peritonsillar abscess, 141
Pharyngitis, 140–141
  bacterial, 141
Phlebitis, 29
Pinworm, 275
Piperacillin, 15
Plague (*yersinia pestis*), 308–309*t*,
    310–311
Plasmid, 1
Plasmodium falciparum, life cycle of,
    263*f*
Pneumocystis carinii, 337, 346,
    349–350, 368
Pneumocystis carinii pneumonia, treat-
    ment of, 348*t*
Pneumonia, 74, 94, 318, 349–350
  acute, 97–125
  aspiration, 116–117
  atypical, 121–122
  bacterial, 350
  chronic, 126–135
  community-acquired, 20, 113–122
  empiric treatment, 109, 110–111*t*,
    112–113
  interstitial, 102
  interstitial lymphoid, 352
  lobar, 102, 105*f*
  nosocomial, 122–124
  pneumocystis carinii, 349–350
  viral, 325
Pneumonic plaque, 310–311
Point mutations, 1
Polyarteritis nodosa, 84
Polymyalgia rheumatica, 84
Postantibiotic effect, 4
Praziquantel, 281
Primary brain lymphoma, 363–364
Primary peritonitis, 202–203
Primary tuberculosis, 127
Procaine penicillin G, 13
Progressive multifocal leukoen-
    cephalopathy, 364
Prostatitis, 221, 223
Prosthetic joints, infections in, 256–257
Protease inhibitors, 377
  tolerance and side effect monitoring,
    377, 378–379*t*
Protozoa, 358
  blood, 261–269
  tissue, 269–272
Prozone phenomenon, 234

Pulmonary infections, 97–136
HIV infection and, 346–354
Pulmonary Kaposi's sarcoma, 352
Purulent pericarditis, 185, 186
Pyelonephritis, 219, 221
subacute, 82
Pyrazinamide, 51–52

Q
Q fever, 36
treatment of, 291
Quinolones, 38–41, 39f, 53
Quinupristin, 42

R
Rabies, 160
Rectal carcinoma, 358
Rectum, infections of, 358
Red man syndrome, 29
Regional enteritis, 85
Relapsing fever, 83
Respiratory alkalosis, 74
Respiratory viruses, 122
Retinal necroses, 367–368
Retinitis, cytomegalovirus, 366–367
Retinopathy, HIV, 366
Reye's syndrome, 325
Rhodococcus equii, 354
Ribavirin, 67–68
Rickettsial infections, 36, 83, 293–300
Rickettsialpox, 295
Rifabutin, 368
Rifamycins, 50–51
Rimantadine, 69–70
Rocky Mountain spotted fever, 36, 293, 294–295
treatment of, 290–291t
Rotavirus, 197
Roundworms, 274, 274f

S
Salivary glands, infections in, 357
Salmonella, 190, 357
Schistosomiasis, 280–281
Scrub typhus, 296
Seborrheic dermatitis, 372
Secondary peritonitis, 203–205
Secondary tuberculosis, 129–132
Sepsis, 72
severe, 77
Sepsis syndrome, 71–78

clinical manifestations, 74–75
diagnosis, 75
pathophysiology, 73f
treatment, 76t, 77–78
Septic arthritis, 257–261
Septic cavernous sinus thrombosis, 146
Septic shock, 72
Serum sickness, 12
Severe acute respiratory syndrome (SARS), 321–324
Severe sepsis, 72, 77
Sexually transmitted diseases (STDS), 223–235, 358, 372
treatment regimens for, 225–229t
Shigella, 190–191, 194, 357
Sickle cell disease, 265
Sinus infection, 145–148
air, 95
Sinusitis
bacterial, 13, 14, 148
ethmoid, 146, 148
frontal, 147, 148
sphenoid, 147, 148
Skin abscesses, 244
treatment of, 240t
Skin and soft tissue infections, 237–246
antibiotic treatment of, 240t
classification of, 237, 238f
HIV infections and, 368–369, 370–371t, 372
less severe, more common, and localized skin infections, 244–246
severe, 239, 241–243
Skin penetration, nematodes acquired by, 275–276
Small intestine, infections in, 357–358
Smallpox, 313–315, 314f
Soft tissue infections. See Skin and soft tissue infections
Specific antibiotics, 11
Sphenoid sinusitis, 147, 148
Spinal epidural abscess, 166–167
Spirochetes, 83, 287–293
Spontaneous peritonitis, 202–203
Staphylococcus aureus, 119–120, 183, 237
Sterile hematoma, 95
Stevens-Johnson syndrome, 12, 46
Still's disease, 84
Streptococcus pneumoniae, 113–116, 151
Streptococcus pyogenes, 237
Streptogramins, 42–43

Streptomycin, 27, 28, 29
Strongyloides, 275–276
Subacute bacterial endocarditis, 82
Subacute pyelonephritis, 82
Subacute thyroiditis, 85
Subdural abscess, 166
Sulfonamides and trimethoprim, 45–48, 45f
Surgical intensive-care patients, fever in, 94–95
Swimmers' itch, 280
Syndercid, 42
Syphilis, 231, 233–234, 358, 372
    treatment of, 229t
Systemic inflammatory response syndrome (SIRS), 72
Systemic lupus erythematosis, 84

T
Tachycardia, 74
Tachypnea, 74
Taenia solium, 278–279
Teicoplanin, 30, 31
Temporal arteritis, 84
Tetanus, 244–245
Tetracyclines, 35–36
3-day rule, 7
Throat infections, 140–143
    antibiotic therapy for, 142–143t
Ticarcillin, 15
Tissue helminths, 276–281
Tissue protozoa, 269–272
Tobramycin, 28, 29
Toxic shock syndrome, 75
Toxoplasma encephalitis, 363
Toxoplasmosis, 83
Transduction, 1, 2f
Transformation, 1, 2f
Traveler's diarrhea, 194
Treponema pallidum, 141, 231, 233–234
Trichinella, 183, 276–277
Tricuspid endocarditis, 177
Trimethoprim, 47–48
Trimethoprim-sulfamethozazole, 119
Trypanosoma cruzi, 183, 271–272
Trypanosomiasis, 83, 271–272
Tuberculosis, 126–132, 346, 351–352
    gastrointestinal *M.*, 357
    miliary, 83, 126, 128–129
    primary, 127
    secondary, 129–132
Tuberculous meningitis, 158–159

Tuberculous pericarditis, 185, 186
Tularemia, 27, 309t, 311–312
Tumors of the digestive system, 358
Typhus, 295–296
    flea-borne, 295
    louse-borne, 295
    scrub, 296
    treatment of, 291

U
Ulcers
    genital, 227–228t, 230–231, 232t
    mouth, 356
    peptic, 206–207
Ureidopenicillins, 15–16
Urethritis, 219, 223–224
Urinary tract infection (UTI), 95, 217–223
    common urinary pathogens, 218t
    diagnosis, 219–220, 220f
    treatment, 221, 222t, 223
Urticaria, 12

V
Vaginitis, 219
Valacyclavir, 61–62
Valganciclovir, 64–65
Vancomycin, 3, 13, 29, 30, 31, 115
Varicella zoster virus (VZV), 317–319
Vascular insufficiency, osteomyeltis secondary to, 253–254
Venereal warts, 358
Verruga peruana, 298
Vibrio cholerae, 192, 194
Vibrio parahaemolyticus, 192
Vincent's angina, 140
Viomycin, 53
Viral diarrhea, 197
Viral encephalitis, 160–162
Viral hepatitis, 207–214, 358–359
    clinical characteristics of, 210t
Viral keratitis, 139
Viral meningitis, 151, 158
Viral pneumonia, 325
Voriconazole, 57, 58
VZV, 337

W
Warts
    anogenital, 235
    venereal, 358

Weil's disease, 293
White blood cell count (WBC), 5
Woolsorters' disease, 305–306, 306f
Wuchereria bancrofti, 282–283

Y
Yersinia enterocolitica, 192, 194
Yersinia pestis, 310–311

Z
Zalcitabine, 356
Zanamivir, 70
Zoonotic infections, 287–301
    antibiotic treatment of, 290–291t